Medicine from the Black Death to the French Disease

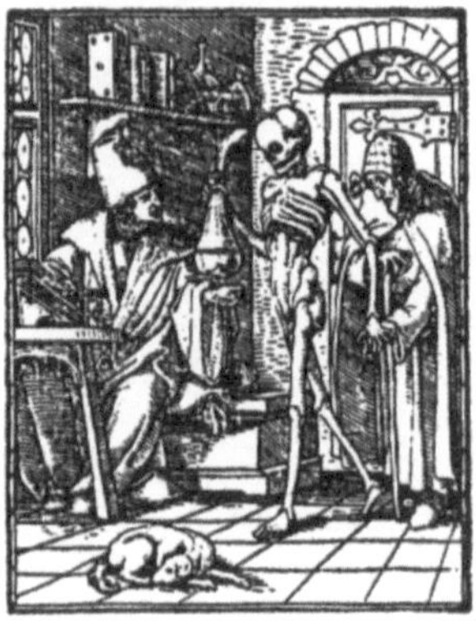

The History of Medicine in Context

Series Editors: Andrew Cunningham and Ole Peter Grell,
Wellcome Unit for the History of Medicine,
Department of History and Philosophy of Science,
University of Cambridge

Titles in this series will include:

Faith, Medical Alchemy and Natural Philosophy:
Johan Moriaen, Reformed Intelligencer and the Hartlib Circle
J. T. Young

The Making of the Dentiste, *c. 1650–1760*
Roger King

'The Battle for Health': A Political History
of the Socialist Medical Association, 1930–51
John Stewart

Medicine from the Black Death to the French Disease

Edited by

ROGER FRENCH, JON ARRIZABALAGA,
ANDREW CUNNINGHAM and
LUIS GARCÍA-BALLESTER

Routledge
Taylor & Francis Group
LONDON AND NEW YORK

First published 1998 by Ashgate Publishing

Reissued 2019 by Routledge
2 Park Square, Milton Park, Abingdon, Oxon, OX14 4RN
52 Vanderbilt Avenue, New York, NY 10017

Routledge is an imprint of the Taylor & Francis Group, an informa business

A Library of Congress record exists under LC control number:

Typeset in Sabon by Manton Typesetters, 5–7 Eastfield Road, Louth, Lincolnshire, LN11 7AJ

ISBN 13: 978-0-367-19504-5 (hbk)
ISBN 13: 978-0-429-20299-5 (ebk)

Contents

Contributors

Jon Arrizabalaga
Consejo Superior de Investigaciones Científicas, Barcelona, Spain

Ron Barkai
Tel Aviv University, Israel

Monsterrat Cabré
Universitat Autònoma de Barcelona, Barcelona, Spain

Ann G. Carmichael
Indiana University, USA

Andrew Cunningham
Wellcome Unit for the History of Medicine, Cambridge University, UK

Roger French
Department of History and Philosophy of Science, Cambridge University, UK

Luis García-Ballester
Universidad de Cantabria, Santander, Spain

Peter Murray Jones
King's College, Cambridge, UK

Michael R. McVaugh
The University of North Carolina at Chapel Hill, USA

Katherine Park
Wellesley College, Massachusetts, USA

Michela Pereira
University of Siena, Italy

Vivian Nutton
Wellcome Institute for the History of Medicine, London, UK

Fernando Salmón
Universidad de Cantabria, Santander, Spain

CHAPTER ONE

Introduction: The 'Long Fifteenth Century' of Medical History

Roger French

The Black Death of 1348–49 was a watershed in Western history. Since it killed perhaps a third of the population it perhaps could hardly have been otherwise. Its economic and demographic effects were great. In medical terms it marks the end of a period when the medical faculties were instituted and developed in the universities. The university physicians had established themselves on the narrow rung at the top of the medical ladder. It marked the height of scholastic medicine. The form of the commentary reached a degree of elaboration that was never exceeded.

The 'long fifteenth century' of European medicine (i.e. *c.*1348–*c.*1500) saw a slow recovery from the major effects of the Black Death, despite recurrent outbreaks. It saw the spread of universities, often modelled on that of Paris, across Europe. Scholastic medicine retained its form but was increasingly challenged from outside by new intellectual movements like Italian civic humanism and eventually by Hellenism. The long century was ended by the introduction of new ideals within medicine and the collapse of some features of the scholastic mode of instruction, events symbolized by the appearance of the *editio princeps* of the printed Greek Galen and the disappearance of the medieval textbook. The long century ended, as it had begun, with the arrival of a dreadful new disease; both had their effects on European medicine.

One of these effects was to put pressure on the medical hierarchy. The university-trained doctors claimed a monopoly of the practice of internal medicine on the grounds of the superior effectiveness of their medicine. But their claim could only be enforced under certain circumstances, normally where there was an important faculty. The university physicians were few in number and competed for custom with a range of other practitioners, from travelling purveyors of nostrums to surgeons and medical specialists who had legitimate but partial licences from corporations other than the faculty, mostly guilds and civil examination boards. Minorities like Jews and women could practise legitimately, or at least without harassment, in niches of the medical market.

But the market could be disturbed at moments of medical crisis, as by the two epidemics we consider here. Scholarly medicine before the Black

Death was not designed to cope with general catastrophes. University physicians believed that disease was a personal imbalance of humours: they studied their patients' particular constitutions and managed their regime over a long period of time. Indeed, an ideal career was to become attached to a court or a household of a great man as a medical retainer with constant advice on his lips. The great epidemics did not fit this pattern. The Black Death killed its victims in a few days. The French Disease stubbornly resisted attempts to achieve a balance of the humours. Both were entities, diseases that happened to people, rather than individuals submitting to their own innate or acquired weaknesses and hence coming to have 'unbalanced' humours. And both were widespread, happening much more, in absolute terms, to the mass of people who could not afford the physician's fees than to those who could.

The physicians were uncertain about what to do. Some took their own advice and fled quickly, stayed away a long time, and came back slowly. Those who stayed could not easily identify either of the new diseases and accordingly could not agree on a treatment. Other kinds of practitioners took advantage of the absence or uncertainty of the physicians. Empirics often had their favoured remedies, and in the absence of elaborate and impressive theory they now had what was marketable: specific medicines for a specific disease, at a price well below the level of the physician's fees.

In the long medical fifteenth century the physicians' strategy ultimately worked, and they maintained their position. They sold their medicine in the market on the grounds of its rationality and learning. It was ultimately an Aristotelian rationality, recognized by all who had been to a university as the proper way to argue. Deep learning in the accepted Greek and Arabic authorities persuaded the patient that the doctor knew about his case. This medicine was scholastic in a good sense, before a pejorative meaning had been attached to that term and before the term 'middle ages' had been introduced. The physicians' image was attractive. When towns began to hire medical men, they wanted ones trained in the universities. If they gave a contract to a bachelor of medicine, sometimes they paid him also to go back to university and become a doctor. Successful surgeons who had been trained as apprentices, often indentured to their fathers, not infrequently sent their sons for a medical training at a university. Women who practised illegally aped the learned language of the doctors to impress their patients. Jews, excluded from the schools, often learned scholastic medicine in their own way, obtained civil licences by examination and rose to eminence.

One of the reasons that communes engaged medical men was to treat the poor, generally free of charge. The commune was buying the constant attention of a resident doctor, which meant that he could practise his preferred long-term, regimen-based medicine. But he also had to face sudden epidemics among the poor and had to think in terms of public health – what could be done to avert an epidemic, whether to segregate the sick, and related questions. The poverty of the sick poor was met not only by the town's doctor but by charitable actions of the townsfolk. Hospitals, once refuges for the deserving needy, increasingly became medical institutions, some specializing in acute cases (where the charitable 'turnover' was rapid) and others acting as charitable medical establishments for the chronically ill. The doctors and surgeons who attended hospitals, like those hospitals set up for victims of the French Disease, or who were under contract to towns that faced repeated epidemics of plague, necessarily had a notion of medicine that differed from that of the medical men who were concerned with confirming a place for their subject in the new universities, and who thus preferred the largely literary revival of Greek medicine.

The history of medieval medicine is not yet at a point where these changes can be explored in detail. What must come first is putting the various kinds of practitioner into their contexts and seeing how they interacted with society at large, both in normal times and at moments of crisis. Some of these contexts are met with in the chapters that follow, and here we can only suggest some of their diversity.

One common thread is the medical marketplace, concerned with supply and demand, and the structures that allowed exchange to take place. It is notorious that in the ancient world there was no control over the practice of medicine: there was a free market and no licensing. It is also well known that the twelfth and thirteenth centuries were a period of the corporation: guilds, voluntary associations, fraternities; the legal person in general. The members of such bodies had some interest in common and collectively controlled entry into the body. They also gained authority by being recognized at some superior level in society. The universities were bodies of this kind, and in the North, where they were closely connected with the Church, the bishop or his chancellor claimed the right of granting the licence. This extended to medicine, and a common procedure for medical licensing was examination of the candidate by an agent of the bishop advised by a panel of medical men.

The consortium of medical men licensed in this way was the faculty of medicine. The power of their monopoly was maintained by the small number of full licences given, a number controlled by the length and expense of a full medical education (which was used in turn to justify the monopoly). The university physician claimed that his knowledge encompassed that of the surgeon and apothecary and that *their* ignorance of *his* high theory not only justified his monopoly but explained why surgeons and apothecaries were often dangerous to their patients. In practice surgeons and other specialists often got their licences on the grounds of competent practice, and before a panel of established surgeons, set up by a guild, or other civic authority, or chaired by the king's physician.

The medical marketplace centred in towns. Here there were those who could pay fees and the concentration of people in a small area provided even specialists (who often combined their specialism with another trade) with a steady, if small, niche. In the countryside the market was much more diffuse. There could be such a thing as a 'general practitioner', a man who prescribed, made up and administered internal medicines and at the same time undertook surgical cases. If he was a full-time practitioner he probably had to travel from place to place to make a living. Probably few university-trained physicians found such a practice attractive or saw such practitioners as competitors; the country doctor without a full licence did not suffer the persecution of the urban empiric by the learned physicians.

Despite the physicians' claim that their medical knowledge was all-inclusive, in practice medical knowledge was exercised in a compartmentalized way. Surgical knowledge was partly that gained by practical training and experience, and this is what the licence rewarded. Morphological anatomy was important to the surgeon and was often learned formally alongside the physicians. But in practice the surgeon's anatomy was a business limited to comparatively superficial structures and the bodily orifices; when he placed too much credence on what he was told by anatomists he could be misled.

Anatomy indeed was a specialism that did more than serve surgery and medicine. Anatomical knowledge was a compartment of medical knowledge that served anatomists, just as medical knowledge of the rational and learned practitioner served to identify the kind of doctor he was. In an age of guilds and strict separation of the arts, knowledge of the arts was technical know-how that was the protected stock-in-trade of the knower, the artisan. It mattered in the marketplace: not only to make the art effective, but to persuade the customers it was so. Anatomists, surgeons, empirics, specialists and learned doctors all used knowledge in these ways. The learned doctor was seen as having the best corner of the market, both by those below, who emulated him, and by those lawmakers above, to whom he had been convincing about the superiority of scholastic medicine. When the first successful attacks on school medicine were made, at the end of the long fifteenth century, they came at the top, with powerful figures being persuaded by groups of activists that the Latin, disputatious and commentatorial medicine of the schools was in fact not the most effective. The new Greek Galen and the Hellenists were only partly successful in their attack, and school medicine, with its disputations and Arab authors, lasted for well over another century. But the Hellenists and classicists, in identifying their own time and preferences with the ancient world, had begun to see the period between in a new and unattractive light. The 'middle' ages had been invented.

The invention was not noticed by the men of the schools. They were proud to call themselves scholastic because in medicine it meant mastery of a technically difficult discipline. They recognized the linguistic skill of the Hellenists outside the universities but suspected that they could not handle the finer points of philosophy or medicine. The medical establishment continued in its admiration of the systematic and vastly detailed Arabic textbooks. The demand for scholastic writings of the high Middle Ages continued undiminished until well after the French Disease had arrived. Works of Taddeo Alderotti, Gentile da Foligno, Dino del Garbo, Jacobus de Partibus and others were printed in quantity by men who knew the state of the medical market. These works sold because of the very subtlety and comprehensiveness of their discussions. Scholars of the thirteenth and fourteenth centuries who could 'conciliate' differences between philosophers and physicians, or 'speculate' further into theory than others or simply out-comment the others remained valuable assets for Renaissance printing-houses. Indeed, there is a strong sense in which the height of medical reasoning reached by scholasticism before the plague was never reached again afterwards.

CHAPTER TWO

Jewish Treatises on the Black Death (1350–1500): A Preliminary Study*

Ron Barkai

> In 1347 there was such a great pestilence and mortality throughout almost the whole world that in the opinion of well-informed men scarcely a tenth of mankind survived. The victims did not linger long, but died on the second or third day. The plague raged so fiercely that many cities and towns were entirely emptied of people ... Some say it was brought about by the corruption of the air; others that the Jews planned to wipe out all the Christians with poison and had poisoned wells and springs everywhere. And many Jews confessed as much under torture: that they had bred spiders and toads in pots and pans, and had obtained poison from overseas ... God, the lord of vengeance, has not suffered the malice of the Jews to go unpunished. Throughout Germany, in all but a few places, they were burnt.[1]

In these words, the Franconian Franciscan friar, Herman Gigas, describes in his chronicle (1349) the plight of the Jews of Europe while the plague was raging at its worst. Not only did they – along with the rest of the population – fall victims to the fatal disease; they were also accused of having brought it on, and many thousand of Jews were slaughtered by the ignorant, horrified mob. The double distress of Europe's Jews, plague on the one hand, and persecution on the other, is reflected in various genres of Jewish literature.[2] However, the medical literature on the Black Death written by medieval Jewish physicians was almost completely neglected by modern historians, a fact which gave birth to the idea that 'After 1348, when Jews were accused of initiating the plague, some Jewish writers composed original works, like Abraham Caslari's *Pestilential Fevers* ... These were isolated efforts, however, and did not amount to a genuine medical tradition'.[3] However, a careful examination of the available Jewish medical manuscripts demonstrates that the Jews of Christian lands, especially of Spain and southern France, showed a great deal of interest in the medical aspects of the plague: relatively to their number in the population, they possessed a considerable quantity of treatises, translated from Latin and Arabic or originally written by Jewish physicians. My intention in the following pages is to survey these treatises, most of them never published or studied, and to underline their peculiarities.[4]

Translated works on the plague

Most popular of the translated treatises on the Black Death was that of John of Burgundy, written in 1365.[5] It was, in fact, translated twice: first by Benjamin ben Rabbi Isaac Karkashoni (of Carcassonne), in 1399;[6] and later by Joshua of Bologna in the fifteenth century.[7] The first translation is titled *'Ezer elohī, ma'mar be-'ipush ha-avir ve-ha-dever* (Divine Help: A Treatise on the Corruption of the Air and the Plague), to which the Jewish translator added an introduction. This preface indicates that the original treatise was written 'in the year 1349, and that along with the medical treatise, its author wrote an astrological chapter explaining the forces of Nature which had brought the plague'. Referring to the motivation of the translation, Benjamin of Carcassonne states that having observed that this work was kept locked away by the Christians, and that it had been 'examined and verified by noteworthy physicians', he had made the effort 'to take it out of their hands and to translate it from their language into the Holy Tongue, so that it might be of help and benefit to us and to our successors as well'.[8]

At least two of the treatises available to the Jewish physicians of the time were originally written in Spain. The first was not translated into Hebrew, like most translations made by Jewish physicians: only the opening lines and the summary appear in Hebrew, and the treatise *per se* is written in Judeo-Spanish – that is, in Castilian dialect transcribed in Hebrew letters. The opening attests to the author's identity: 'A treatise on the plague, written by Maestri *Goan de Tornamira*, on the advice of the townspeople ... at the request of the King, *Don Enrique, King of Castilla*.'[9] The reference is apparently to Enrique II, called Enrique de Trastámara, who began to rule Castile in 1369. The author, Jean de Tournemire, a French physician who taught at the Montpellier school of medicine, wrote his treatise *Preservatio contra pestilenciam*, in 1370.[10] This work had a considerable effect on the practice of medicine in Castile and Aragon. Regrettably, we do not know the identity of the Jewish author who translated it into Judeo-Spanish; the two Hebrew lines concluding the translation consist solely of an appeal to God, and cite neither the translator's name nor the date of his work.

The second treatise of Spanish origin is a Hebrew translation of a work on *Regimen sanitatis* in the plague time (*Ha-hanhaga ha-divrit*), that is, how to stay healthy during the epidemic.[11] In the title, the translator attributed the work to 'Maestri Pablo de Sipaya'. More details on the author appear in his own statement within the work:

> I, Pablo of Sipaya, although unworthy of composing this treatise which I had begun, was moved by the strength of passion to compose it for two reasons. The first is the work of God, may he

> be blessed; the second, for the general good, and especially that of this illustrious town of Jaca, in which I dwell.[12]

We do not have any information about a Spanish author of a medical text on the plague called Pablo, and this Hebrew translation is the unique trace of that work. Unfortunately, also the identity of the Jewish translator remains unknown. Appearing as a motto to the treatise are quotations from Aristotle ('The Philosopher') on the good to which all aspire, and by Arnaldo de Villanova ('The Sage Arnav de Villanova') on the conservation of physical health. The author explains:

> And I shall state that the health of the body will give rise to the health of the soul; and, as this is a good thing, it is definitely worthwhile for us to devote great study to conserving the health of the body ... and I shall also state that, as health is one reason for the peace of soul ... [13]

It should be noted that almost all the *materia medica* are listed by their Spanish names, in Hebrew transcription. This may be because the translator was not familiar with the Hebrew terms, which had already been used in Hebrew medical writings since the thirteenth century, or simply he found it more convenient to employ the Spanish terms, which were well known to the Jewish physicians of this country.[14]

This problem of using foreign terms transcribed in Hebrew letters is discussed in detail by Solomon the Physician (*Shelomoh ha-Rofé*), son of Moses Shalom of Spain, who translated into Hebrew a treatise on the plague written by Antonio Guaineri of Pavia. The Italian author composed in the fifteenth century two works: *Summarium de febribus* and *Tractatus de peste*,[15] of which only the first one was translated, under the title *Ha-klal me-ha-kadaḥot* (The Whole [Knowledge] on Fevers).[16] Solomon the Physician gives two motives for his translation: the first is its quality, the translator states that he had read the treatise several times and had been quite impressed by its content; this is the well-known theme appearing in the prefaces of many translations into Hebrew in the Middle Ages – the competition with their learned Christian colleagues:

> And I have seen also many of the Christian sages boasting and bragging of it, and condemning us by saying that we cannot reach perfection in the curing of fevers, as Ibn Sina, Galen, Hippocrates and the other sages ... Therefore, I was seized with internal torment and great envy, and I undertook to translate it, to the best of my ability, into our Holy Language ... [17]

As to the linguistic problem involving the frequent use of foreign terms, the translator apologizes to the reader for this practice, giving two reasons for its necessity. First, is the lack of terms in 'our Holy

Language': in a clearly apologetic manner, Solomon the Physician explains that all these terms originally did exist in Hebrew, but were lost over the many generations in which that language remained in disuse.[18] Secondly, even if such terms were to be found in Hebrew, they would be 'utterly strange', dating from the Hebrew of the Talmudic sages. Therefore, their use would not be justified, even assuming the work would be read by a Jewish physician familiar with biblical and Talmudic literature. Certainly, should the treatise come into the hands of a physician ignorant of that old language, 'of which kind there are uncountably many', the reader would never understand it, but would be like one speaking with a Greek or a German, without knowing their languages.[19]

An anonymous translator produced a Hebrew version of the Latin *Concilium contra pestilenciam*, written in 1348 by Gentile da Foligno in Perugia, Italy.[20] The unique manuscript conserved of this translation is made from the fifteenth century, and it bears the Hebrew title *'Eṣah 'al ha-dever* (Advice on the Plague).[21] According to the translator, he was moved to compose the Hebrew version by the horrors of the Black Death, the physicians' fear of approaching its victims, and the nature of the work itself:

> As this illness, the plague, is the most frightening and the most dangerous of illnesses, and the most frequently to come newly to the world, none of the physicians will come near to it, out of their fear. Anyone who approaches its dwelling shall die, as it is among the contagious illnesses, as it is apparent from both supposition and experience ... Therefore, my heart moved me to seek and inquire which is the right way ... And I found a treatise, whose author is called Foligno, a Christian and a great sage in the science of medicine ... renowned for his importance, and the said sage has done a marvelous thing ... as he compiled and selected all the ancient dicta ... that which was saved from experience comprises twelve chapters ... in the proper order, concise and illustrative ... [22]

Two other Latin treatises on the plague were translated into Hebrew without any comment or explanation by the translators. One is Velescus de Taranto's text *Compendium utilissimum contra pestilentia*, which in the manuscript which has come down to us, bears the Hebrew title *Hanhagt ha-dever* (Regimen for the Plague).[23] The second was originally written by Francisco de Cenellis of Bologna, and translated by Samuel ben Jacob, under the title *'Eṣah 'al ha-dever*, of which two manuscripts have been conserved.[24]

The translations from Arabic and Latin into Hebrew were an important component in the medical library of medieval Jewish physicians from the twelfth to the fifteenth centuries. The translators examined carefully the medical literature to be found in their milieu, written by Christians and Muslims, in order to supply Jews interested in studying medicine with the best, most up-to-date theoretical and practical texts. This tendency is clearly expressed by the anonymous translator from Provence, who translated between 1197 and 1199 seven books on medical theory and seventeen practical books.[25] The examination of the Latin treatises on the plague translated into Hebrew demonstrates that the same attitude prevailed in Jewish society from the middle of the fourteenth to the end of the fifteenth centuries. One may notice that the first 'Christian' text on the plague, Jacme d'Agramont's *Regiment de preservació de pestilencia* (Spain, Lerida, 24 April 1348),[26] was not translated into Hebrew. The reason seems to be quite obvious and indicates another tendency of Jewish medical literature in this period: a short time after Jacme d'Agramont completed his treatise, a prestigious Jewish physician, Abraham ben David Caslari, wrote in the same geographical area a Hebrew text on the Black Death. The public using this literature preferred, of course, the 'Jewish-Hebrew' work.

Original Hebrew treatises

The most important Jewish author in the field of epidemiology during the Black Death years was undoubtedly Abraham ben David Casalri. His father, David ben Abraham Casalri, had been active as a physician and translator in the Kingdom of Aragon and in southern France (Narbonne).[27] The surname indicates that the family originated in the town Caslar, in the province of Tarragona; Abraham himself lived principally in the town of Besalu in the Kingdom of Aragon. In consideration of his valued services as a physician, King Jaime II granted him an exemption from taxes for the years 1320–36.

Abraham Caslari wrote at least two medical works. One of these, a brief and concise text, was written before the Black Death (1326), bearing the title *'Ale ra'anan; ma'mar qaṭan ba-qadaḥot* (A Fresh Leaf: A Little Treatise on Fevers).[28] The second, a long and detailed treatise called *Ma'mar be-qadaḥot divriot u-minei qadaḥot* (A Treatise on Pestilential Fevers and Other Kinds of Fevers).[29] Abraham's own words in the introduction to the treatise indicate that he wrote it soon after the outbreak of the Black Death:

> My heart awakened me to write this treatise because of what happened in the summer and the late spring. Fevers overcame the entire province and all of Catalunia and Aragon, and there was no city which was safe from the fevers ... And those fevers were lethal; they would not pass away for ten days, and many would die of them; and the fevers were incessant, with much fainting and distress.[30]

In other words, only a few months elapsed between the outbreak of the plague and the writing of the treatise.

An anonymous author wrote the Hebrew text entitled *Ha-ma'mar be-qadaḥat ha-dever* (The Treatise on Plague Fever). The unique known manuscript of this work bears no explicit clue as to the identity of its author.[31] Nevertheless, the context of the manuscript, the handwriting, and the foreign terms appearing provide some useful information. The manuscript is written by a Jewish-Spanish scribe, most of the foreign terms mentioned in it are Arabic; moreover, the medical authorities cited therein refer exclusively to Arab authors. All this brings us closer to the source, which should reasonably be Spanish-Arabic. Indeed, the general structure of the treatise is quite similar to that of Aḥmad ibn 'Ali ibn Khātimah (1323/4–69?), a theologian, historian and physician from Almería, who wrote the *Kitāb Taḥsīl al-ġaraḍ al-qāṣid fī tafṣīl al-marāḍ al-wafīd* in February 1349.[32]

The Arabic treatise, written as a dialogue between the author and a friend, opens with an explanation that his friend had approached him and asked him to explain the sources, development and treatment of the disease. The author of the Hebrew text also begins with the story of his friend, who asked him to write a book on the Black Death:

> You have asked me, dear brother, to write to you an overall regime for use in plague time; and – though I am very busy and my heart is not with me; I have almost succumbed to old age, and my forces have become weakened, and I am tired and weary – for the great urging which you have urged me, and for my pity on you and the beloved members of your household, here is your regime, written in great haste and with great diligence, a brief and concise way that, should you wish to study it once daily, will facilitate the matter for you and you shall be able to save yourself and others ...[33]

This sort of opening, presenting the treatise as having been written at the request of a friend, is a frequent topos in medieval Hebrew medical literature.[34] Nevertheless, the fact that a preface of this type also appears in the Arabic treatise is significant. And, in fact, comparison of the two texts shows that the Hebrew one is essentially a concise summary of ibn Khātima's work. The Hebrew author 'sifted out' of the Arabic treatise the theoretical chapters and the passages referring to Muslim tradition and left only six practical chapters: 'And these necessary things without which no person of the human species can survive are as follows: the surrounding air, sleeping and waking, food and drink, movement and rest, voiding and continence, and movement of the soul.'[35] The treatise was given a Jewish character by citing passages from the Bible and by traditional Jewish appeals to God:

> with the help of God, from whom I shall ask help, in Him I put my trust, and I shall say: Know my brother, that God shall keep you from all evil and shall keep your soul, and He in His mercy shall save you from '*the pestilence that walketh in darkness, or [from] destruction that wasteth at noonday*' [Psalms 91:6].[36]

It should be noted that the citation taken from Psalms was employed in medieval Jewish tradition as an opening to a magical incantation to avoid plague and other calamities.[37]

Especially important among the Hebrew medical treatises on the Black Death is *Be'er la-ḥay* (A Well for Life), written by Isaac ben Todros.[38] We do not have much data on the author himself. He lived in the second half of the fourteenth century in Avignon in southern France; there in his youth, he studied Bible and Talmud, and later devoted himself to the study of French and Latin, philosophy and medicine. His philosophical training is reflected in the first, theoretical part of his work; his great knowledge of medical literature, both ancient and that written after the outbreak of the plague in 1348, led him to a rather severe criticism of the positions held by contemporary doctors, although his personal feelings towards some of them were those of honour and appreciation. Isaac ben Todros was familiar with Arabic medical literature in Latin and Hebrew translation, and frequently quoted it while arguing with his contemporaries.[39] To these we may add ibn Khātima's treatise, transmitted to him directly or indirectly, as the six chapters constituting the general framework of the anonymous Hebrew text *The Treatise on Plague Fever* and parallel to those in the original Arabic, are also included, with small changes, in Isaac ben Todros's work.

Indeed, one of the most interesting aspects of the treatise *A Well for Life* is its author's critical attitude toward the epidemology of his time, this criticism in fact being what had impelled him to write the work. In his opinion, contemporary physicians do not take into consideration the various circumstances and manifold causes of the plague; yet precisely these, he feels, should dictate the nature of treatment:

> The custom of the physicians who practise today, and of those who were before us, according to what our ears have heard, is to behave in the same manner in all times of plague, equally for all natures, one constitution and one law for all, without examining the differences of natures and the inherent changes of the times, and without seeking the reasons for the loss ... [40]

Isaac ben Todros's criticism is directed primarily against three Latin treatises. The first of these criticisms refers to the work compiled by the physicians of the University of Paris: *Compendium de epidemia per collegium medicorum parisius ordinatum*,[41] which claimed that the plague resulted from a loss of balance of dryness, and that the excessive dryness had given rise to red fever.[42] The second 'was written by a doctor from Italy, whose name is Maestro Fiorenzo, to several of the great men of this country',[43] in which he claimed that the conjunction of Saturn and Mars in Scorpio had brought about an excess of sanguine humour. The third is the work 'which was written a year ago by the great doctor, the physician of our Master the Pope (*sic*), whose name is *Maestro Jan Turna Mira*, who has ascended to the throne at the head of the doctors of our present day ... '.[44] These and other contemporary physicians, claims Isaac ben Todros, 'all walk one path and tend to creating cold and dry and continuous blood-letting and abstention from meats and wines and things which heat, all of them being health-giving in nature, as if the air which had become unbalanced by a single cause requires constant loss'.[45] His criticism is directed especially at Jean of Tournemire, 'who writes on the treatment of the plague occurring today and commands continuous blood-letting and things which subtract from the blood ... ', and at the French physicians for 'having given advice from afar', without becoming acquainted with local circumstances.[46]

Isaac ben Todros demonstrated a relatively optimistic attitude concerning the possibility of overcoming the Black Death, and in his preface he emphasizes the practical motives for writing the work:

> I decided in my heart to seek and to enquire into the wisdom of medicine, and to compose a brief treatise, devoid of commentary, which provides, in a proper and generally complete form, an abridgement of the compiled sayings of the early sages. My intention is to recall those matters easily conceived and implemented, which have been verified by experience, according to the ideas of the ancient doctors. And I have called it by the name *A Well for Life*, as everyone who follows its advice and omits nothing of that which is written therein is guaranteed to be saved from the pestilential affliction and to remain alive and well.[47]

The treatise is concluded with a prayer, not only for healing from the plague, but for the redemption of the People of Israel and the end of its suffering in the diaspora.[48]

The terrors of the plague and human futility in the face of it are reflected in the opening lines of a brief and practical treatise on the Black Death by Abraham ben Rabbi Salomon Ḥen: 'A sudden scourge shall befall the inhabitants of this world from time to time, and shall strike at the roots of the human species, and its face is that of a flying seraph in a wheel, whose turning from afar nullifies us ... '.[49] Although the manuscript gives no information as to the date on which this text was written, the preface appears to indicate that the author had already experienced several waves of pestilence; he may, in fact, have written it in the late fourteenth century. Rather pessimistically, he explains the need for his work:

> I saw the need to write down how God has made it possible to survive, and especially in taking precautions in advance, which will make it easier to remove the illness if the advice is taken before the plague than during the plague, and which should be practised permanently by almost everyone.[50]

The text is simple in nature and explains the symptoms of plague and their stages of development, the various types of illness and their causes; yet, most of the work is devoted to preservation of health and prevention of the disease. It was apparently written in southern France or Christian Spain, as its author demonstrates a good knowledge of both Arabic and Latin terms, which he uses alternatively. For the word 'plague', for example, he employs both the Arabic term *ta'ūn* and the Latin *epidemia*.[51] The word 'preservation' is explained by the Latin *preservatio*; similarly, 'northern' and 'southern' are *septemtrional* and *meridional* respectively; all foreign terms are, of course, transcribed in Hebrew letters.[52] Undoubtedly, the author made use of both original Arabic and Latin sources in the treatise.

The study of science among medieval Jews and of medieval Hebrew, traditionally emphasized the revolution wrought in both those areas by the shift to Hebrew as the language of science among the Jews from the twelfth to the fifteenth centuries. Recent historical research, however, has demonstrated that the picture is more complex. Admittedly, the Jews of France, Italy and Christian Spain wrote their scientific works chiefly in Hebrew. But the facts indicate that Arabic continued as a language in which scientific texts – primarily in the field of medicine – were read and written by Jews in Christian Spain until the end of the fifteenth century. In his pioneering research on Arabic manuscripts in Christian Spain, Peter Sj. van Koningsveld comes to the conclusion, after examining 128 manuscripts, that Arabic medical and scientific manuscripts of Christian Spain almost exclusively circulated in Jewish circles.[53]

No less important is the fact that eminent Jewish physicians of Christian Spain preferred to write their important medical works in the Arabic language. The most remarkable of these medical treatise is the *Kitāb al-ṭibb al-qaštālī al-malūkī*, written in the beginning of the fourteenth century, probably by a member of the famous family of Jewish physicians, the Banū Shushan of Toledo.[54] This tradition of writing medical treatises in Arabic among Spanish Jews was continued by Joshua ha-Lorqi, who served Pope Benedict XIII as his personal physician. In 1412, ha-Lorqi was baptized under the name of Hieronymus de Sancta Fide.[55] While still a respectable member of the Jewish community, he was asked by its dignitaries to write an up-to-date book on medicine for the benefit of Jewish physicians.[56] Significantly, he wrote the treatise in

Arabic, rather than in Hebrew. Unfortunately, the original Arabic was lost, but its Hebrew translation entitled *Guerem ha-ma'qlot* (The Staircase), has been preserved in 18 manuscripts. The author included in this work a detailed chapter on the Black Death, its causes, symptoms and therapy.[57]

The last medieval Jewish medical treatise on the plague was also written in Arabic: *Kitāb majannat al-ṭa'ūn wa-l-wbā'*.[58] It was composed by a Spanish Jew, Elijah ben Abraham, as attested by his Arabic appellation – Ilyās ibn Ibrāhīm al-Yahūdī al-Išbānī (*sic*) – and dedicated to the Ottomon Sultan Selim I.[59] The author gives a detailed account of his medical training. From the information about his theoretical studies (*al-mumārasa al-'ilmiya*), it is possible to reconstruct the library to which 'qualified doctors' of his time were expected to refer. It contained the basic literature of the ancients (*al-mutaqaddimūn*) and of later writers (*al-muta'akhkhirūn*), that is to say, Muslim, Christian and Jewish writers of the Middle Ages.[60] By contrast, it is interesting to note that he seems not to have been familiar with the three important treatises on the plague written in Arabic in al-Andalus: that of ibn Khātima, mentioned above; Muḥammad ibn al-Khaṭīb of Granada's work *Muqni'at al-sā'il 'an al-maraḍ al-hā'il* (1359–62?);[61] and, finally, that written by Muḥammad ibn 'Alī al-Shaqūrī, a student of al-Khaṭīb, who served as a physician in Granada: *Taḥqīq al-naba' 'an amr al-waba'*.[62] He studied the complementary course of practical medicine (*al-mumārasa al-'amalīya*) in various Spanish cities under the tutelage of Christian masters.[63] After his expulsion from Spain in 1492, Ilyās ibn Ibrāhīm practised medicine in Naples,[64] and finally, at the beginning of the fifteenth century, he settled in the Ottoman Court in Constantinopole, where he wrote a philosophical treatise and a work on the plague. This last one is divided into four sections (*abwāb*):

1. The definition and causes of the plague.
2. The symptoms of the disease.
3. Preservation of health in plague-time.
4. A [scholastic] study of ten questions regarding the plague.

One of the things that makes Ilyās ibn Ibrāhīm's treatise unique is that, apart from the chapters generally found in every medical book dealing with the bubonic plague (aetiology, identification and classification of the plague and its causes, public health during outbreaks, treatments for plague victims), he included the following ten rationalistic–scholastic discussions. These discussions in fact deal with the plague, but they have extensive philosophical and medical aspects as well:

1. Does pestilent fever belong to the category of diurnal and putrid fevers?
2. Are thunder, lightning and columns of fire seen in the air portents of the plague or not?
3. Is putridity naturally air-borne or not?
4. Does the living soul spring from within the heart or not?
5. If someone is exhausted and takes long baths, is he more susceptible to the disease?
6. Is there a significant change in pulse rate or urine as result of being ill with the plague?
7. At which time of the year does the plague appear more often?
8. Is blood-letting efficacious in the cure of the plague?
9. Are vinegar and other acid [materials] beneficial for the plague fevers or not?
10. Is it efficacious or not to treat plague victims with the *theriaka* called *al-farūq*.[65]

Paradoxically, the treatise of Ilyās ibn Ibrāhīm is an excellent expression of medieval scientific–rationalistic views of the plague, on the one hand; but one the other hand, he completely accepts the religious idea that this epidemic is no less than a divine punishment, in the face of which medicine is hopeless. Thus, after the presentation of accepted scientific causes of the plague, the author stresses his own position:

> The fourth cause is not allied to the conjuction of the stars, nor the terrestrial causes, nor to the fire of the stars nor the colour [of the sky], rather, God sent the disease to weary sinners so that they might return to Allah (may he be exalted), and *that is the real reason* [my italics] as the noble Isidorus recounted in *The Book on the Form of the Earth:* and know that the plague is a special, unknown disease, sent unto the world by God. And we found this in the Law of Moses and in the Psalms of David (may he rest in peace), because whenever God wants to punish sinners, He deliberately sends the sickness called the Plague. And the eyes of all mortals are bleared and they do not understand the causes of the plague nor its remedies ... *And all the doctors are lost and helpless to cure a person sick with the plague, because even if his heart beat is constant and his urine normal, even so he dies* [my italics] ... [66]

The Jewish author was aware of the difficulty of such a position for the reader when presented in a medical treatise whose function was to give an immediate therapeutic solution. At the end of the chapter on the cure of the plague he repeats almost word for word the impossibility of curing the disease; however, there are two reasons why he viewed the treatment of the plague victims as important, one ‘psychological’ and the other practical:

I was taught [when studying medical treatment] to value and appreciate two things: one is that if the disease is acute and the physician does not try to find a cure for it, the patient no longer has the will to live, and many die because of hallucinations and heart failure. For it is the role of the expert physician to strengthen the heart [of the patient] by giving him medicines, as Galen the wise said: encouraging the heart is superior to stronger treatments ... The other ... is that a person sick with an epidemic is like a person fighting in a battle. Those who are wounded in battle are not necessarily mortally wounded. Thus people sick with the epidemic do not [necessarily] suffer from putridity, and if it does not invade the heart, the person can possibly be cured.[67]

Magical treatment of the plague

Theoretical and practical magic, throughout the Middle Ages, was a constant companion to scientific medicine. I do not intend to discuss the manifold and complex relationship between the two methods of healing, one based on the 'natural' and the other on the 'supernatural'. Michael Dols's statement in this regard is correct: 'In general, the magical beliefs and practices indicate a common need to supplement or replace inadequate medical knowledge with supernatural devices for protection and relief from plague.'[68] The fatal nature of the plague, the unprecedentedly ubiquitous death, and the obvious helplessness of contemporary medicine made magic a precious commodity in all three monotheistic cultures.[69]

The Jews, naturally enough, made use of two main sources: biblical methods of controlling plague, and the Book of Psalms. The use of these materials is reflected both in adjurations and prayers specially composed for the purpose of fighting the Black Death. The basic premise of all the manuscripts of this type is that God was the one who brought down the plague on humanity, as punishment for its sins. Accordingly, the aim of these magical texts was to mollify God by means of prayer, repentance, and especially by the mention of 'historical' precedents appearing in the Holy Scriptures.

An anonymous adjuration *To Remove the Plague*,[70] apparently dating from the second half of the fourteenth century, is especially interesting in light of its universal nature. Its author asks for salvation and healing, not only for his own people, but for the Gentiles as well:

Please, God, banish from our homes and from the homes of all who dwell within this city, and from the homes of all its borders and all its surroundings, and from the homes of your People ... wherever they may be, plague and the sword and famine and evil and commotion and looting and ruin and epidemic and Satan and the Evil Impulse and evil disease ... [71]

This kind of appeal to God to save the non-Jewish population is exceptional in medieval Hebrew literature, and it might be explained by the persecution of the Jews during the plague: They probably believed that with the abolition of the plague the persecution would cease.

The plague, admittedly, was viewed as divine punishment; but at the same time, it was linked with the forces of Hell: Satan, demons and evil spirits. Whether because the latter were said to tempt humanity to sin, or because they were thought to bring the plague – the formulas of appeal to God often included sections such as the following passage, specially written by Solomon ben Isaac in the fifteenth century, in order to combat the epidemic:

> And save me from all great misfortune, and from epidemic and plague ... from demons and devils and spirits of evil and from the Evil Eye and from fear and horror ... and save my soul from all that is evil, and from Evil Impulse, and from an evil woman, and from Satan the Destroyer.[72]

Special importance was attributed to the Book of Psalms in the entire procedure of invocations, adjurations and magical operations, as practised in Jewish and Christian cultures. The Middle Ages saw the compilation of the most important book of Jewish magic, based entirely on the Book of Psalms, *Sefer shimush Tehillim* (The Book of Use of Psalms), which also gained popularity in its Latin–Christian version: *De usu Psalmorum*.[73] The versions of this treatise dating from the fourteenth and the fifteenth centuries added magical formulas against the plague. Thus, for example, in the fifteenth century Spanish–Jewish version, Psalm 96 was devoted exclusively to combatting the plague which attacked the city:

> To relieve the city from a plague which has come to afflict them in their many sins in our days, he will say that Psalm, and after it, he will say: Ḥasdiel, Yasriel, Ḥayayel [names of angels], relieve the men of this city of the plague which has come to afflict them, and reprove Satan who plagues them, in the name of the Brave and Powerful King ... [74]

The 'historic' example often referred to by Jewish magical texts and quoted as a way to stop the plague is the story appearing in Numbers 17:3–15. The biblical passage tells how Moses and Aaron halted the plague which had afflicted the People of Israel by using incense taken from the altar. This passage, together with various Psalms which were considered useful to fight the plague, were also frequently woven into scientific medical texts.

Hebrew terminology of the plague

The terms and concepts used to define and describe the Black Death in Hebrew texts are somewhat vague. The two most common terms are taken from the Bible: *magefa* and *dever*. Both these words appear indiscriminately in medieval Hebrew treatises, especially in those written after 1348. The word *magefa* (from the root *N-G-F*, meaning 'to strike' or 'to strike down') is more general, relating to any type of disease afflicting many persons within the same geographical area at the same time. *Dever* is even less clear, as, despite its many occurrences in the Bible, we do not know the precise illness(es) to which the term refers. In the medieval texts this term is often used to describe the Black Death of 1348. Obviously, then, the word *magefa* is a generic term for epidemic diseases, whereas *dever* referred primarily to the bubonic plague.[75]

This matter of confusion in definition and diagnosis was adopted by Abraham Caslari as one of the central topics for his work on the plague. It should be noted that this author, and many subsequent Jewish physicians in his footsteps, linked the plague (*magefa* or *dever*) with fever (*qadaḥat*, sing. *qadaḥot*, plur.). The disease is referred to as 'plague fever' (*qadaḥat divrit*); to be more exact, these authors distinguished between several different types of *qadaḥot divrit*, according to their symptoms: trembling of the body and protracted sweat, disordered capacity of judgement, nosebleed, vomiting, diarrhoea, great thirst and dryness of the tongue, watery or white urine, severe headaches, and fevers developing so rapidly that the physician is unable to treat the patient.[76] Given this confusion, he seeks to define the 'plague fever': 'some have used the word *dever* for any suddenly fatal illness, which spreads throughout city or province or provinces'.[77] However, says Caslari, a distinction should be made between diseases propagated as a result of 'loss of air to corruption' and those caused by bad foods or medically improper behaviour.

The Jewish guilt

Strangely, none of the Jewish authors of medical treatises attempted to refute directly the accusation that the Jews were responsible for the outbreak of the Black Death. No less surprising is the complete silence of the Jewish religious authorities regarding the plague: contrary to the abounding literature on the plague written by both Muslim 'ulama and Christian clergy, the epidemic has left no traces in rabbinical writings.[78] It is, indeed, difficult to explain this phenomenon. Undoubtedly, the

Black Death was largely treated in rabbinical preaching (*derashot*) in the synagogues and in the *Responsa* of the Jewish religious authorities, since both are dealing with daily life. But in none of the conserved *derashot* and the *Responsa* is there any treatment of the plague. It is possible, therefore, the general atmosphere of accusation and suspicion against the Jews deterred them from keeping this kind of literature.

Only one Jewish physician, Isaac ben Todros, refers indirectly to the fate of his co-religionists during the Black Death. In a way of apology he states that not only did the epidemic make no distinction between Jews and Christians, but it afflicted the Jews first, and even more severely than the Gentiles:

> And indeed, ... we have seen the impression that this fever flares up in all our dwelling places, and actually among our people first. Marvellously, it is within our camp and strikes us a vast, severe and overwhelming blow, and He [God] has not stretched out his saving hand to the most noble of the Children of Israel, and calamity began with them, and after them the Christians ... [79]

This difficulty, claims the author, may be regarded from two different directions. The first is a religious one: the plague is a divine decree, and therefore its outbreak among the Jews is no more than 'a trick from which it will arise to give us a remnant of the land, as some times an evil thing will be arranged which will draw good after it ... And all this is of the wisdom of God'.[80] The second is the scientific one: if we accept the view that astrology is the determining factor, the twelve zodiacs and the seven planets control not only individual lives, but the lives of countries and nations. The fate of the Jews in the plague, then, is determined 'from the conjunction of Saturn and Mars, which will be in the House of Capricorn'. After all, astrologers, Jews and non-Jews alike, agree that the planet affecting the Jewish people is Saturn, which is also the planet of 'the poor and miserable and of all contemptible and valueless things', whereas the planet in conjunction with Saturn 'is the sign of the world in general, and the sign of Israel ... '. This astrological constellation explains why Jews were more severely afflicted than others, as well as why they were struck down first.[81]

The quantity of Hebrew treatises on the plague, both translated and original, and their quality, as well as other Hebrew writings on all branches of medicine, demonstrate unmistakably that 'rational-scientific' medicine continued to have a central place in Jewish culture from the outbreak of the Black Death to the end of fifteenth century. In fact, most Hebrew medical manuscripts known to us were occupied or composed in this area. A first reading of these manuscripts reveals that their authors were quite familiar with the theories circulating in Latin Europe and the Muslim world concerning the causes of this mortal disease, its aetiology, therapy and prevention. However, we may underline already at this stage of our study two interrelated characteristics of the Jewish writings on the Black Death:

1. *None* of them mentioned the contagious nature of the plague, while this idea was accepted by some of the Christian and Muslim physicians.[82]
2. Most of the Jewish physicians who describe the causes of the plague, ultimately attribute it to God.

Thus, for example, Isaac ben Todros, after a long discussion on the astrological causes of the plague, concludes that 'the heavenly hosts do not themselves have strength, but are as an axe in the hands of the Hewer, and they have no ability to harm or to benefit except what is given them by the Creator ... '.[83] We have seen that the same position was held by Ilyās ibn Ibrāhīm, who, in consequence described the physician who treated the people afflicted by plague as 'a blind man, trying to find his way in the darkness'.[84] In any case, only a thorough analysis of the Hebrew treatises on the plague, and their comparison with Muslim and Christian writings would give us more accurate answers regarding some essential questions, such as: which were the medical sources used by the Jewish authors? Did they have a monolithic position concerning fundamental problems such as the individual and communal conduct during the plague time?

Notes

* In memory of Michael W. Dols, a colleague and a friend.

1. *The Black Death*, translated and edited by R. Horrox, Manchester University Press, Manchester and New York, 1994, p. 205.
2. On the fate of the European Jewish communities in the times of the plague, see: P. Ziegler, *The Black Death*, London, 1969, pp. 84–100; A. Rubio, *Peste negra, crisis y comportamiento sociales en la España del siglo XIV. La ciudad de Valencia (1348–1401)*, Collins, Granada, 1979, pp. 97–100; J. Shatzmiller, 'Les juifs de Provence pendant la peste noire', *Revue des Etudes juives*, **133** (1974), pp. 457–80; S. Guerchberg, 'La controverse sur les prétendus semeurs de la "Peste Noire" d'après les traités de peste de l'époque', *Revue des études juives*, **108** (1948), pp. 3–40; English translation: 'The Controversy Over the Alleged Sowers of the Black Death in Contemporary Treatises on the Plague', in S. Thrupp, *Changes in Medieval Society. Europe North of the Alps, 1050–1500*, London, 1965, pp. 208–24. Of special interest is E. Wickersheimer, 'Les accusations d'empoisonnement portées pendant la première moitié du XIVe siècle contre les lépreux et les juifs; leur relation avec les épidémies de peste', *Compte-Rendus du quatrième congrès international d'histoire de la médecine*, 1927, pp. 76–83.

3. J. Shatzmiller, *Jews, Medicine, and Medieval Society*, California, 1994, p. 54.
4. Actually, I am working on a book analysing the content of the original Jewish writings on the plague and comparing them to the treatises which were written by Muslims and Christians.
5. K. Sudhoff, 'Pestschriften aus den ersten 150 Jahren nach der Epidemie des "schwarzen Todes" 1348: III', *Archiv für Geschichte der medizin*, 5 (1911–12), pp. 62–9. For an English translation of the treatise see Horrox, *The Black Death*, pp. 184–93.
6. Bibliothèque Nationale, Paris, MS héb. 1191/10, ff. 141r–146r; MS héb. 1124/7.
7. Vienna, MS 175/7.
8. Bibliothèque Nationale, Paris, MS héb. 1191/10, f. 142r.
9. The Institute of Hebrew Manuscripts, Jerusalem, mic. 3479, f. 1r.
10. On his career, see L. Dulieu, *La médecine à Montpellier, vol. I: Le Moyen-Age*, Montpellier, 1975, pp. 97–100, 294.
11. The Institute of Hebrew Manuscripts, Jerusalem, mic. 3479, f. 1r.
12. Ibid.
13. Ibid.
14. In fact, Spanish Jewish physicians employed in medical treatises both Arabic, Spanish dialects and Hebrew. See R. Barkai, *A History of Jewish Gynaecological Texts in the Middle Ages*, Leiden, 1998, pp. 13–37.
15. See J.-N. Biraben, *Les hommes et la peste en France et dans les pays européens et méditerranéens, vol. II: Les hommes face à la peste*, Paris, La Haye, 1976, p. 189.
16. Parma, MS 1365/7, ff. 104r–123r. Cf. M. Steinschneider, *Die hebraeischen Ubersetungen des Mittelalters*, Berlin, 1893, repr. 1956, p. 799.
17. Parma MS 1365/7, f. 104v. On this theme see also J.-P. Rothschild, 'Motivations et méthodes des traductions en hébreu du milieu du XIIe à la fin du XVe siècle' in *Traductions et traducteurs au Moyen Age*, Actes du colloque international du CNRS, Paris, 1986. Textes rèunis par G. Contamine, Paris, 1989, pp. 279–302.
18. According to the Medieval Jewish tradition, Hebrew, the Holy Language, was the language used by God to create the universe, therefore, it contains the whole existing knowledge. See especially M. Idel, *Language, Torah and Hermeneutics in Abraham Abulafia*, Tel Aviv, 1994 (Hebrew).
19. Parma MS 1365/7, f. 104v. On the formation of the Hebrew medical language in the Middle Ages see Barkai, *A History of Jewish Gynaecological Texts*, pp. 6–37.
20. See Sudhoff, 'Pestschriften', pp. 83–7, 332–5; P. Lugano, 'Gentile Fulginas Speculator e le sue ultime volunà', *Bolletino della Regia Deputatione di Storia Patria per l'Umbria*, **14** (1908), pp. 195–260; L. Thorndike, *History of Magic and Experimental Science*, New York, 1922–23, vol. III, pp. 233–52.
21. Vienna, MS 175/7a.
22. Ibid., f. 1v.
23. New York, Jewish Theological Seminary of America, MS 2669/1, ff. 1r–17v.
24. Paris, Bibliothèque Nationale, MS héb. 1124/8, ff. 135r–139v; Vienna, MS 175, 7c, ff. 220v–232r.
25. Paris, Bibliothèque Nationale, MS héb. 1190/10, ff. 44r–46r. For an

English translation and analysis of the document see Barkai, *A History of Jewish Gynaecological Texts*, pp. 20–34.

26. *Regiment de preservació de pestilència de Jacme d'Agramont (S. XIV)*, Introducció, transcripció i estudi lingüístic, by J. Veny i Clar, Tarragona, 1971.
27. A. Cardoner i Planas, *Historia de la medicina a la Corona d'Arago (1162–1479)*, Barcelona, 1973, p. 40.
28. The text has not yet been pubished; it seems to have had a great popularity in the Middle Ages, since we know of at least eight manuscripts.
29. Paris, Bibliothèque Nationale, MS héb. 1191/9, ff. 134v–141r; Leiden, Warn. 40/7 (Cod. or. 4778), ff. 115r–123v. The treatise was edited by H. Pinkhof (*Abraham Kashlari over pestachtige Koortsen*, Amsterdam, 1891), basing himself solely on the Leiden manuscript. Cf. J. O. Leibowitz, 'A. Caslari's Hebrew Manuscript of His Acolyte's "Pestilential Fevers" edited by H. Pinkhot', *Koroth*, 4 (8–10), 1968, pp. 517–20 (Hebrew).
30. Paris, Bibliothèque Nationale, MS héb. 1191/9, ff. 135v.
31. Berlin, MS 232/10 (Qu. 836), ff. 123r–129v.
32. T. Dinānah, 'Die Schrift von Abī Ja'far Ahmed ibn 'Alī ibn Moḥammed ibn 'Alī ibn Ḫatimah aus Almeriah über die Pest', *Archiv für Gschichte der Medizin*, 19 (1927), pp. 27–81. Cf. M. W. Dols, *The Black Death in the Middle East*, Princeton, 1977, pp. 321–2.
33. Berlin, MS 232/10 (Qu. 836), ff. 123r.
34. On the use of this topos see R. Barkai, 'La obra científica del granadino Šelomoh ben Yosef ibn Ayyub', in *La ciencia en la España medieval: Musulmanes, judío y cristianos*, edited by L. Ferre, J. R. Ayaso and M. J. Cano, Granada, 1992, pp. 93–101.
35. Berlin, MS 232/10 (Qu. 836), ff. 123r.
36. Ibid., f. 124r.
37. See R. Barkai, *Medieval Magic: The Uses of Psalms*, forthcoming (Hebrew).
38. Moscow, Ginzbourg MS 165/15, ff. 375r–400r; Oxford, Bodleian Library, MS or. 2585/3. The Moscow manuscript was published by D. Ginzbourg in *Tif'ert seivah, Studies in the Honour of Yom Tov Lipman Zunz*, Berlin, 1844, pp. 91–126.
39. A part of his medical library was indentified by Ginzbourg, see *Be'er la-ḥay*, p. 101–2.
40. Ibid., p. 104.
41. Edited by H. E. Rebouis in *Etude historique et critique sur la peste*, Paris, 1888, pp. 70–145. Cf. Horrox, *The Black Death*, pp. 158–63.
42. For the position of Paris' doctors see Ziegler, *The Black Death*, pp. 70–74.
43. Nicolas de Florence(?), see Biraben, *Les hommes et la peste*, p. 188.
44. Be'er la-ḥay, p. 105. Cf. note 38.
45. Ibid.
46. Ibid.
47. Ibid., p. 104.
48. Ibid., p. 126.
49. Leiden, MS Warn. 40/8, f. 124v.
50. Ibid.
51. Ibid., f. 125r.
52. Ibid., ff. 125r, 125v, 126r.

53. P. Sj. van Koningsveld, 'Andalusian-Arabic Manuscripts from Christian Spain: A Comparative Intercultural Approach', *Israel Oriental Studies*, 12 (1992), pp. 75–110.
54. This work is evaluated as 'a highly elaborated intellectual product, an expression of mature Galenism, based on direct knowledge of Galen's medical corpus ... it is indeed a singular piece of medical literature of the Late Middle Ages, whether Latin, Arabic or Jewish', L. García-Ballester and C. Vázquez de Benito, 'Los médicos judíos castellanos del siglo XIV y el galenismo árabe: El kitab al-tibb al-qastali al-maluki (Libro de medicina castellana regia) (*c.*1312)', *Asclepio*, 1 (1990), p. 120.
55. Y. F. Baer, *The History of the Jews in Christian Spain*, trans. L. Schoffman, Philadelphia, 1961, vol. II, pp. 139–50.
56. Paris, Bibliothèque Nationale, MS héb. 1143, f. 86r.
57. Ibid., ff. 51v–54r.
58. Dublin, Chester Beaty, MS 3676/6, ff. 185r–216r. Cf. Dols, *The Black Death*, pp. 332–3. I am currently preparing a critical edition and translation of this text.
59. R. Barkai, 'Between East and West: A Jewish Doctor from Spain', in B. Arbel (ed.), *Intercultural Contacts in the Medieval Mediterranean*, 1996, pp. 49–63.
60. For his book list see ibid., pp. 54–5.
61. Dols, *The Black Death*, pp. 322–3.
62. Ibid., pp. 323–4.
63. Dublin, Chester Beaty, MS 3676/6, ff. 185r.
64. Ibid., f. 190v.
65. Ibid., ff. 194v–199r.
66. Ibid., ff. 186v–188r. As to the position of the Muslim physicians, Michael Dols writes: 'When confronted by the Black Death, Muslims generally ascribed its ultimate cause to God. The manner by which God caused it to occur among men, however, was the subject of innumerable and often contradictory explanations' (*The Black Death*, p. 84).
67. Dublin, Chester Beaty, MS 3676/6, f. 195r.
68. Dols, *The Black Death*, p. 121.
69. For a representative text on the religious and magical responses to the Black Death in Latin Christianism, see Horrox, *The Black Death*, pp. 111–57; cf. Biraben, *Les hommes et la peste*, pp. 56–84. For the magical treatments of the plague in Islam, see Dols, *The Black Death*, pp. 121–42.
70. New York, Jewish Theological Seminary of America, MS 4634, ff. 1r–4v.
71. Ibid., ff. 3r–3v.
72. Florence, Lorenziana, MS Plut. A42/7, f. 43v–44r.
73. On the history of the various versions of this text and the magical procedures employed in it see R. Barkai, *Medieval and Early Modern Magic: The Book on [Magical] Uses of Psalms*, forthcoming.
74. London, The Wellcome Institute for the History of Medicine, MS Well. Heb. A. 34, f. 32r.
75. The same phenomenon appears in Arabic medical texts: 'The common designation of *plague* in Arabic is *ṭā'ūn* (pl. *ṭawā'īn*). It is derived from the verb *ṭa'ana*, which has the general meaning of 'to strike' or 'to pierce'. Although *ṭā'ūn* may have the generic sense of epidemic, it is used consistently in the late medieval Arabic texts in the sense of 'a plague' ... The general term for 'epidemic' or 'pestilence' is *wabā'* or *waba'*. The follow-

ing statement, which is found in these treatises, makes the distinction clear: 'Every *ṭā'ūn* is *wabā'*, but not every *wabā'* is a *ṭā'ūn*' (Dols, *The Black Death*, p. 315).

76. Paris, Bibliothèque Nationale, MS héb. 1191/11, f. 135v.
77. Ibid., ff. 135(i)r–135(i)v.
78. On the Muslim religious reaction, see, Dols, *The Black Death*, pp. 109–21. For a selection of Christian texts, see Horrox, *The Black Death*, pp. 111–57; cf. P. Ziegler, *The Black Death*, London, 1969 (1972), pp. 259–65.
79. *Be'er la-ḥay*, p. 111.
80. Ibid., pp. 111–12.
81. Ibid., p. 112.
82. Biraben, *Les hommes et la peste*, pp. 18–26; Dols, *The Black Death*, pp. 92–4.
83. *Be'er la-ḥay*, p. 112.
84. Dublin, Chester Beaty, MS 3676/6, f. 195r.

CHAPTER THREE

Mater Medicinarum: English Physicians and the Alchemical Elixir in the Fifteenth Century

Michela Pereira

At the beginning of the fifteenth century the English King Henry IV (1399–1413) had forbidden the practice of alchemy, which had been permitted, and even fostered, by his predecessors since the time of Edward III (1327–77).[1] Yet after the end of the Hundred Years War an increasing number of alchemists filed petitions to the king to obtain licence to make artificial gold and silver, perhaps with the hope that King Henry VI (1422–61) would be interested in an activity that promised an easy increase of wealth. Several petitions of this kind may be found in the Patent Rolls from 1444 on.[2] All of them are written according to the same formula: the alchemists promise to transmute base metals into silver and gold.[3]

One of these petitions, however, dating from 1456, develops in a quite unexpected manner: though its authors were also referring to the artificial gold-making, their interest was clearly focused on the medical use of the *lapis philosophorum* (the 'philosophers' stone', that was grounded in a development of alchemy tracing back to the late thirteenth and early fourteenth centuries:

> Know ye, that the sages and most famous philosophers of ancient times have taught, and recorded in their writings and books under signs and symbols, that many glorious and noteworthy medicines can be made from wine, precious stones, oils, vegetables, animals, metals, and certain minerals; and especially a most precious medicine, which some of the philosophers have called the mother and Empress of medicines; others have named it the inestimable glory; others, indeed, have named it the quintessence, the philosophers' stone, and the elixir of life.

A patent letter, granting the solicited permission was eventually signed by Henry VI (31 May 1456): the text of the letter, largely modelled on that of the petition,[4] granted the king's protection to 'some talented men, sufficiently learned in natural sciences, and willing and disposed to practise the said medicines; men who fear God, seek truth, and hate deceitful work and false tincturing of metals'.[5]

Though twelve petitioners were mentioned in the patent letter,[6] only three of them, John Faceby, John Kirkeby and John Rayny, are recorded in the parchment as bearers of the licence.[7] Six out of the twelve petitioners were physicians, and three of them were appointed to the king or to his family: John Faceby, physician to the king in 1443 and 1460; William Hathclyff, licensed in Padua in 1447, was required 'to minister about the king's person in his sickness' together with John Faceby and others on 6 April 1453 and appointed physician to the queen in 1457; and the famous Gilbert Kymer, who wrote a regimen of health for Humphrey, Duke of Gloucester.[8] Among the three holders of the king's patent letter, two were physicians (Faceby and Rayny), while the third, John Kirkeby, was chaplain to the king.[9]

The episode I am referring to is well known in the history of medicine in fifteenth-century England; my first approach to it was due to the necessity of outlining the history of a manuscript Oxford, Corpus Christi College 244, that is a very important document within the pseudo-Lullian alchemical tradition.[10] Alchemy and medicine have been closely linked in the western scientific tradition since the time of Roger Bacon, and their link is the main concern of alchemical writings focusing on the theme of the elixir, like those attributed to Arnald of Villanova and Raimond Lull. Therefore this chapter is intended to be a contribution to the understanding of one of the 'intellectual factors' that characterize the English medical history of the fifteenth century – i.e., the period immediately preceding the 'medical Renaissance' fostered in England by humanist physicians like Caius and Linacre.[11]

I shall illustrate the meaning of the elixir in the western alchemical tradition; the place of the pseudo-Lullian *Testamentum* in this tradition; its bearing on the 1456 episode; and I shall give some other examples of the link between medicine and alchemy from the thirteenth to the fifteenth century.

The alchemical elixir in the western tradition[12]

The name 'elixir' already appeared in the first treatises on alchemy that were translated from Arabic into Latin (such is the case for the well-known *Morienus*)[13] or arranged from Arabic sources (like the pseudo-Avicenna, *De anima in arte alchemiae*, written in Spain during the twelfth century).[14] In the Hellenistic tradition, *iksìr* was the name of the 'immortality powder' that Zosimus was looking for: yet, as it seems, Zosimus' immortality is to be understood as concerning the spiritual salvation of mankind. When the term used by Zosimus reappeared in the Latin West, it had undergone a change in its form, modified by the prefix al- of clearly Arabic origin (*alexir* in pseudo-Avicenna,[15] 'arabice nominatur acir' in the *Morienus*,[16] *elixir*, *iccir*, *yaccir* in the thirteenth century *Liber secretorum alchimiae*).[17] It was the most important product of the alchemical *opus*, also called *lapis philosophorum* (philosophers' stone), the real agent of transmutation. 'Alexir est res quam iactamus super corpus maius, ut mittat rem de sua natura in aliam',[18] says pseudo-Avicenna, who refers to the Greek origin of the word: 'Alexir verbum Graecum, et dividitur in ic xir, et vult dicere magnus thesaurus.'[19]

The word 'elixir' is used by Albert the Great in his *De mineralibus*, meaning the 'medicine of metals';[20] its preparation is detailed in the pages of the *Summa perfectionis*, by the Latin Geber (the Franciscan friar Paul of Taranto, according to William Newman).[21] In the encyclopedia written by Vincent of Beauvais in the middle of the thirteenth century, the *Speculum Naturale*, we find a thorough, although random exposition of knowledge concerning the elixir. It is defined as the means through which alchemy imitates nature and abbreviates its process.[22] None of these authors, however, speaks of the elixir other than as an agent of metal transmutation.

Islamic alchemists, whose translated writings re-established in the Latin West the written tradition of alchemy (interrupted after the Hellenistic flourishing), had probably been influenced by the Far Eastern ideas concerning the *soma*, a drink conferring immortality on the human body.[23] The obscurity of their language and the novelty that alchemy represented during the twelfth and early thirteenth centuries for the Latins, prevented them from perceiving this side of the alchemical research. In the West, then, alchemy was first considered almost exclusively as the art of transmutation of base metals into silver and gold.[24] Yet the idea of a medicine of long life and rejuvenation came to the surface in the western culture during the first half of the thirteenth century, when at the papal court a treatise *De retardatione accidentium senectutis* appeared, that would later be considered a writing by Roger Bacon.[25] In fact, Bacon was not the author, but he extensively used this work, as well as the pseudo-Aristotelian *Secretum secretorum*, considering both 'experimental' *auctoritates*: he referred to them especially in his search for a 'medicine' capable of conferring the perfect balance of humours (*perfectum temperamentum*), and of restoring mankind to the state of Adamite perfection. This search was also rooted in ancient western beliefs, like that of the fountain of life or the herb of immortality,[26] that were the mythical grounds on which a man like Bacon might accept the 'scientific' proofs for the existence of a substance conferring long life and perfect health.

As has been shown elsewhere,[27] Roger Bacon considered alchemical doctrine as a parallel to natural philosophy and medicine; according to him, the alchemical language hides the general truth about elementary generation and corruption, being the veritable root (*radix*) of every natural and medical knowledge. This consideration is parallel to those expressed by Agostino Paravicini Bagliani in his research on Bacon and the tradition of prolongevity (*prolongatio vitae*);[28] and by Faye M. Getz, who has shown Bacon's contribution to the English learned pharmacology, describing him as the first supporter of a 'speculative pharmacology' that, opposing the multiplicity of procedures used by apothecaries, developed 'a rational enquiry into how to quantify pharmaceutical practice'.[29]

Speculative alchemy, which Bacon for the first time distinguished from its practical side, teaches the unitary character of the generation of all natural beings, that depends on the elements and humours: thus the generation of living beings is linked to that of all others.[30] In the *Opus Tertium* he affirms that he is revealing the common roots of the great sciences, i.e. natural philosophy, medicine and alchemy, urging people to teach these roots as if they were only natural and medical.[31]

Accordingly, Bacon's theory of alchemy was broader than his contemporaries': while Albert the Great, Vincent of Beauvais and the Latin Geber tried to sanction the scientific validity of alchemy as a part of the physical science (subordinated to the theory of the origin of metals outlined by Aristotle, *Meteor IV*), and limited the use of the alchemical elixir to the making of precious metals, gold and silver, Bacon developed a more general doctrine of material change. It was based on the idea that it was possible to go back from elementary bodies to their unitary root, first matter (*prima materia*), to separate the four elements and then refine and unite them again, producing a more balanced mixture.[32] The material thing so obtained was not only perfect in itself, but also capable of giving perfection to bodies of every kind, i.e., not only were base metals transmuted into gold or silver, but human bodies were given health and longevity: therefore it was called 'the greatest of the secrets'.[33]

After Bacon, this idea of alchemy reappeared in some writings of the early fourteenth century, such as the *Rosarium* attributed to Arnald of Villanova, the pseudo-Lullian *Testamentum* and the works of the English alchemist John Dastin. All of them assume as the aim of the alchemical *opus* the production of an agent of material perfection, the *elixir* or *lapis philosophorum*, that can purge metals of their impurities as well as restore the perfect balance of elementary qualities (*perfectum temperamentum*) to human bodies and precious stones. In the Arnaldian *Rosarium* (a text dating back to the early fourteenth century, whoever may have been its author)[34] the alchemical medicine is extolled as a thing that has a more active virtue than every other remedy, because of its occult and subtle nature.[35] The pseudo-Lull describes the virtues of this 'medicine' in a long passage of the *Practica Testamenti*, where he stresses the character of the alchemical remedy that is most opposed to traditional pharmacology: its simplicity. It is unique, yet it can treat all diseases and more quickly than any traditional remedy.

> This is the greatest stone kept hidden from the unlearned people by all the ancient philosophers, yet revealed to you, my son. It transmutes every base and imperfect metal into an agent that can produce an infinite quantity of gold and silver. Moreover we say that it has more efficacious virtue than all other remedies, and that it is capable of healing all illnesses that affect the human body - illnesses of hot as well as of cold nature. And this is the reason: it is of the subtlest and noblest nature ... It treats in one day an illness dating from one month, in twelve days a one-year one; should the illness be more ancient, it would be treated in one month. Therefore don't wonder if this remedy was sought for more eagerly than any other, because in it all other remedies are encompassed. My son, if you can get it, you will own an everlasting treasure.[36]

The simplicity of the elixir or *lapis philosophorum* is obtained through the extraction of the pure, essential virtue that constitutes the core of material elements (defined as *elementum virgo* and fifth essence):[37] this is the ultimate meaning of the alchemical *opus*.[38] The alchemical medicine is called, as it was by pseudo-Avicenna, a treasure – moreover, an everlasting treasure (there seems even to be an echo here of the evangelical treasure that thieves cannot plunder); its value is stressed by similar definitions in Arnaldo's and Dastin's *Rosaries*: the most precious secret, the philosophers' treasure,[39] the most valuable jewel.[40]

The same virtues were attributed to the fifth essence described in the *Liber de consideratione quintae essentiae*, written by John of Rupescissa about 1351–52.[41] Although John of Rupescissa uses only the name 'fifth essence', his views fit exactly the idea of elixir: the goal of his research is to produce a material thing that fits the needs of men, so that it can preserve their mortal bodies from corruption, confer on them incorruptibility and health, cure their diseases and restore their strength, until the day of their death ordained by God.[42] Compared to our bodies, that are composed of four elements, this thing is 'essentia quinta ... sicut caelum incorruptibile';[43] and, like heavens towards elementary bodies, its simplicity makes it efficacious towards every kind of elementary alteration.[44]

The elixir, then, may be defined in very general terms as a material thing that, unlike things produced by nature, is not a compound of material elements (*elementatum*), but results from the extraction and mixture of their inner virtues, and therefore it is something superior, capable of developing each elementary action, according to the necessity of the body to which it is applied.[45]

Arnald of Villanova, John Dastin and John of Rupescissa have been indicated by Joseph Needham as the first western supporters, after Roger Bacon of course, of the theory of the *elixir*, later developed in the Paracelsian pharmacological research:

> By the +13 century, especially with Roger Bacon, the elixir idea was clearly implanted in Europe even though necessarily restricted by Western cosmology and theology to the attainment of longevity rather than material immortality ... After this time the theme of elixirs goes continuously on. In the following century the Villanovan *corpus* has a *Liber de Conservatione Juventutis et Retardatione Senectutis*. About +1320 John Dastin wrote a letter on alchemy to John XXII ... By this time alcohol had become widely known and used. John of Rupescissa (*fl.* +1345) was perhaps the first to identify it with the quintessence or missing fifth element, and though gold leaf suspended in alcohol was more impressive as an elixir symbolically than effectually, the new solvent did give access to higher concentrations of many active substances from the plant and animal world. Henceforward the elixir idea becomes a universal commonplace.[46]

Then Needham continued with quotations from the *Ordinal of alchemy*, by Thomas Norton (who, as we have seen,[47] cited Gilbert Kymer as a follower of Lull). Norton, together with George Ripley, were celebrated English alchemists of the second half of the fifteenth century: both of them declare themselves followers of Lull, and their alchemical writings extol the virtues of the elixir.

The *Testamentum* attributed to Raimond Lull

Oddly enough, Raimond Lull (i.e., pseudo-Lullian alchemy) was not mentioned by Needham as one of the authors belonging to the elixir tradition, yet the alchemical writings attributed to him are surely among the most important witnesses to the birth of this tradition in the western world. The earliest of them, the *Testamentum*, that purports to have been written in 1332 and cites Arnald of Villanova as an alchemical authority, seems indeed, in many respects, the most relevant text fully developing the idea of elixir: it brings forth Bacon's ideas, conceiving a true 'alchemical philosophy', that explains the fame of Lull in all the following Hermetical tradition, even till the eighteenth century; it gives a detailed set of practical processes and recipes, whose attempt at clarity gave them a wide diffusion, as its manuscript tradition clearly shows.[48]

Alchemy as developed in the *Testamentum* shares with that in Bacon's works the broad theory of the reduction of substances to the first matter and its separation into the four elements; an important difference from Bacon, however, concerns the substances that are to be taken as the point of departure of the *opus*. Roger Bacon, influenced by pseudo-Avicenna and by the treatise *De retardatione*, considered organic substances as the best point of departure.[49] The author of the *Testamentum*, by contrast, clearly rejects the use of such substances as blood, hair, urine, and states that the alchemist must begin his *opus* from things that nature has endowed with perfection (i.e. incorruptibility): henceforth he will take silver and gold, that like seeds of perfection can, by means of a defined set of manual operations, give birth to the elixir – the dynamically perfect body capable of multiplying its perfection and of conferring it on all natural bodies. This is explained according to the general rule, that everything generates something similar to itself.[50]

Standing in the background of this affirmation there is an idea of the relationship between the alchemist and nature, that cannot be reduced to the imitation theory, nor to a pure external intervention; rather the alchemist accomplishes nature's work, acting from inside nature itself and according to its rules.[51] When this ability of the alchemist is applied to human bodies, he reveals himself to be a perfect physician.

There are in the text many hints that the author of the *Testamentum* might have been a physician, or at least that he was endowed with medical knowledge; but there is also a vein of polemicism towards *mundani medici*, clerks and lawyers, made from the point of view of someone who has become, as he defines himself, *filius Hermetis*. Defining alchemy at the beginning of the second part of his work (*Practica*), he affirms that alchemy is a hidden part of natural philosophy, that teaches how to confer perfection to gems, how to heal human bodies and to transmute base metals, by means of a universal remedy that encompasses all other remedies.[52] In the third part, *Liber mercuriorum*, where he teaches how to proceed in the *opus*, he goes so far as to affirm that the good physician does not need to make a diagnosis, because nature has given the philosophers' stone the capability of healing any disease.[53]

So we have in the *Testamentum* a full theory of alchemy, based on mineral substances and applied to the preparation of a medicine for human bodies that in the same *Liber mercuriorum* is defined as 'matrem et imperatricem omnium medicinarum'[54] – the first of the names used by English petitioners to define the elixir.

The *Testamentum* and John Kirkeby's manuscript

The *Testamentum* is the work of an alchemist probably of Catalan origin, who wrote during the second or third decade of the fourteenth century; the colophon, appearing in all the fifteenth-century manuscripts, gives the date 1332, which could as well refer to its composition as to the date of a dedicatory copy to the English king, Edward III.[55] In some writings of the pseudo-Lullian alchemical *corpus*, that can be dated approximately to the second half of the fourteenth century, some passages from the *Testamentum* are quoted in Catalan.[56] Although the first known Latin manuscript is dated 1435, Latin seems to be the original language of the text, which as early as the fourteenth century was translated into Catalan and into French.[57] The earliest copy of the Catalan text known at present is preserved in the already cited manuscript Oxford, Corpus Christi College 244, written in 1455: a very important document in the pseudo-Lullian tradition, not only for the text of the *Testamentum*, but for that of several early pseudo-Lullian alchemical works. It includes, among other items, a very carefully arranged text of the *Liber de secretis naturae seu de quinta essentia*, whose author put together the alchemical theory and practice developed in the *Testamentum* with John of Rupescissa's treatise on distillation, and tried to arrange all this material by means of trees, combinatory figures and tables in a truly Lullian style. This text, together with the *Testamentum*, may be considered a pivot of the pseudo-Lullian *corpus*.[58] Figures of true Lullian mien had also been used by the author of the *Testamentum*, and several of the fifteenth-century manuscripts are enriched by them:[59] the Oxford manuscript is one of them.

The story of the manuscripts is closely linked to the 1456 petition of physicians and alchemists to Henry VI: in fact, this manuscript was owned and at least partially written by one of them, John Kirkeby, the year before.[60] Almost half of the volume is occupied by a double version of the *Testamentum*, with the Catalan text preceding chapter by chapter a Latin version slightly different from that preserved in other manuscripts; the first part of the work (*Theorica*) is finely written, yet it contains some faults typical of a copy – so that it seems to be the work of a scribe. The second and third parts (*Practica* and *Liber mercuriorum*) are more correct, albeit quickly written by a hand that has also recorded many marginal notes: that of John Kirkeby, who signed his name at the end of this section in a long colophon which will be considered below.

The entire text is carefully annotated not only by Kirkeby (who, unlike all subsequent readers, added some notes to the Catalan chapters too), but by at least three other hands. Two of them may be identified:

one of the readers of the manuscript was the alchemist Robert Green de Welbe, who signed his name at fol. 37r;[61] the other was John Dee, who owned the manuscript at the end of the sixteenth century (fol. 81r).[62] Both of them made a few annotations to the text; a large number of marginal additions is on the contrary due to an unknown reader, who stresses the relevant points of the Latin text, interprets difficult passages and adds recipes, showing a deep concern for and a broad knowledge of alchemy. This reader is not, at present, identifiable; his handwriting is a tiny cursive, easily readable. It would be interesting to compare this handwriting with autographs – if they exist at all – of Kirkeby's partners in the petition to Henry VI.[63]

In the colophon at the end of the *Testamentum*, John Kirkeby explained the reason why he had also copied the Catalan text: he wrote that the 'original' text had first been translated into Latin by an otherwise unknown Lambertus 'at the priory of St Bartholomew' in 1443.[64] Unfortunately the archival documents of St Bartholomew (Smithfield) cannot help to identify this translator,[65] and we are left to mere hypotheses and questions concerning his work: did Lambert own the Catalan version, while not being aware of the existence of a Latin text circulating in continental Europe?[66] Why did he turn back to an alchemical text supposedly written in a foreign language? How was it possible that a Catalan copy of the *Testament* had reached the Hospital of Saint Catherine at the Tower, remaining unheard of for more than a century after it was written, according to the author's colophon?[67] Or rather was there a Latin text, dedicated to the king, and had the Catalan supposed original been recovered somehow by Lambert's time?[68] Or was the entire story conceived by John Kirkeby, and, if so, why?

The dedication of the *Testamentum* to King Edward III raises no problems, as has been shown elsewhere.[69] It is not unlikely that a Catalan alchemist, fleeing away from his land at the beginning of the fourteenth century, when alchemy was increasingly suspected, found a shelter in the *hospitium* of Saint Catherine at the Tower, that was under the custody of the queen (in 1332 it was still under the influence of the queen mother, Isabel). According to the statutes rewritten by Queen Eleonor in 1273, Saint Catherine should have given hospitality to twenty four 'poor people', six of whom should be *pauperes scholares*.[70] At the court of Edward III the interest in alchemy is shown by such episodes as the king's order to bring before him two alchemists, Jean le Rous and William de Dalby, willingly or unwillingly.[71] Foreigners were often employed as apothecaries at the English court in that period;[72] the queen mother, Isabel, as well as Henry of Lancaster, were interested in cosmetics and pharmacology.[73] Yet, even if the author of the *Testamentum* found hospitality in England, the events of the following years, with the outbreak of the Hundred Years War, might have quickly shrouded his text in oblivion. How, then, did it reappear a hundred years later?

Kirkeby gives no account of the reason why Lambert translated the text; neither does he give any account of the reason why he himself was so interested in it, as to revise its translation and copy it in both languages. As we have seen,[74] he only wrote that Lambert's 'translation' was disappointing to him in many respects, but nowhere does he say why they both turned back to this text. Kirkeby was chaplain to the king in the years 1455–57, after having been prior at St Frideswide's Hall at Oxford (1436–37);[75] he is the only member who certainly was not a physician, in the group who submitted to Henry VI the petition to make the elixir. We can suppose that, stimulated by the growing interest in the artificial gold-making (possibly due to the monetary difficulties subsequent to the war), Kirkeby planned to collect for the king the most important works by 'Raimond Lull', whose fame as an alchemist was spreading. The Oxford manuscript is a deluxe volume, very likely as a dedication copy. Moreover it shows a considerable research effort, perhaps aimed at impressing the king: a double text is given both for the third part of the *Liber secretorum naturae* and for the *Compendium animae transmutationis metallorum*; long notes are added to both texts, where Kirkeby explains how he got *exemplaria* different from each other, respectively in England and in the Iberian peninsula, 'de regno Portugaliae'.[76] On the other side Lull, to whom the *Testamentum* was by now attributed (the first clear statement is in the *Liber de secretis naturae seu de quinta essentia*), was a Catalan like Arnald of Villanova, who had already gained fame as an alchemist in England,[77] and the *Testamentum* clearly refers to Arnald's teaching.[78]

Can we then suppose that:

1. after a century of oblivion the discovery of the marvelous alchemical elixir was made accidentally by Kirkeby who, like the people who submitted other alchemical petitions, was initially searching for a recipe to make gold?
2. he shared his findings with some of the physicians who attended the royal household?
3. the idea of the petition came from this discovery?

I think that the answer to these questions may be affirmative, because these conjectures might well explain the difference between the 1456 petition and those concerning metallurgical alchemy as well as the fact that the same Kirkeby was one of the people who eventually obtained the royal grant to make the elixir. His notes to the text of the *Testamentum* do not show a special medical interest, but he was the editor of the bilingual *Testamentum* and the owner of the precious manuscript; moreover, his rather central position in the 'Sloane Group' shows that he was highly reputed for his knowledge of alchemy and natural philosophy.[79]

Alchemy and pharmacological research

Whatever the reason, Kirkeby's involvement with alchemy is surely borne witness to by his manuscript. It is clearly a fruit of the enthusiasm that led him to search for older manuscripts even abroad; to put himself to work to copy them; to spend his money to get the help of an illuminator for the coloured figures that improve the understanding of the texts. At first sight it is more difficult to understand how a number of distinguished physicians could become so enthusiastic for the elixir praised in the *Testamentum*. Gilbert Kymer, John Faceby, John Rayny, William Hathclyff, Wolfard Cook and John Morer were graduated doctors, and alchemy was not taught at the faculty of medicine, nor at the faculty of arts: what did these physicians search for in alchemy, that they had not found in the academic teaching? I propose that the answer to this question is to be found in the character of the alchemical medicine, or elixir, compared to traditional pharmacology.[80]

Alchemy – especially its metallurgical side – was indeed a suspicious knowledge in the fifteenth century. Its inclusion in the scholastic curriculum had been prevented, although an initial interest had been shown in it even in some university environments. As the recent edition of Constantine of Pisa's *Liber secretorum alchimiae* has shown, the notebook of a student of medicine, probably of the Italian university of Bologna around the middle of the thirteenth century, might include much alchemical material;[81] and the whole development of the *Quaestio de alchimia* had attracted the interest of philosophers and physicians, like Pietro Bono de Ferrara, who in his *Pretiosa Margarita Novella* tried to make a kind of alchemical *Conciliator*.[82] Despite so many efforts, alchemy had eventually been rejected, perhaps on a theological basis – i.e., because of the problems implicit in the idea of man's capacity to act upon the inner processes of nature.[83] The negative attitude of the Church towards this possibility is well shown in the Bull 'Spondent', by Pope John XXII, that in 1319 rebuked the alchemists as forgers, and in subsequent documents, like the short treatise against alchemists written by the Inquisitor in the Kingdom of Aragon, Nicholas Eymerich.[84] However, this disapproval was not directed towards the search for the medicine of human bodies, that we have seen becoming the leading feature of the alchemical elixir.

Moreover it seems that, contemporary with the scholastic debate on gold-making, the promises of alchemy in the field of pharmacological research began to be explored: Danielle Jacquart has stressed, in her *Supplement* to Ernest Wickhersheimer's *Dictionnaire*, the names of several fourteenth-century physicians who were interested in alchemy.[85] This interest was not only of a bookish kind, as is now witnessed by the archaeological findings described by Isabelle Rouaze. On the site of the Louvre, in Paris, the vestige of a distiller's laboratory destroyed about 1360 has been found, whose vessels still contain traces of chemical substances: Rouaze declares herself unable to decide whether it was the laboratory of an alchemist or of an apothecary, but perhaps this is not the point.[86]

In fact, about this period alchemical research was joined by John of Rupescissa to an already extant tradition of *aquae medicinales*, using a primitive technique of distillation. Of this tradition we shall recall here the recipes for twelve medicinal waters in Peter of Spain (1215–77; Pope John XXI in 1276–77), *Liber de oculo*; those of Vitalis de Furno, in his *Pro conservanda sanitate*;[87] and those of Teodorico Borgognoni[88] and Taddeo Alderotti.[89] The fiery water of ancient origin, produced through distillation of wine, was considered a remedy for cold diseases; according to C. Ann Wilson, it was included in medical practice as a counterpart to the distilled rosewater of Arabic origin, that was used for treatment of hot diseases.[90] Three kinds of *aqua vitae* appear to be used to prepare the healing waters, and sometimes they were compared to silver, gold and balsam: this graduation in perfection (of alchemical flavour) may be referred to the increasing refinement of the alcohol of wine via fractioned distillation, or to the addition of precious substances to the distilled wine: so that 'silver' should mean distillation of pure wine, 'gold' wine distilled with medicinal herbs, 'balsam' wine distilled with Eastern spices.[91] We may add two examples to those that Wilson has taken from the medical literature: that of an *aqua* for healing fevers, eyes and skin diseases in the pseudo-Avicenna *De Anima*,[92] dating back to the twelfth century; and the treatise on waters by Bonaventura de Iseo, *Liber Compostellae*, written in the thirteenth century and still unedited,[93] that is usually ascribed to the alchemical tradition.

In his treatise on medical waters, Alderotti calls the alcohol of wine *medicinarum mater*: the same words we have seen used in the *Testamentum* and in the 1456 petition to define the wondrous elixir made through alchemical processes. Yet distilled waters are not the same as the alchemical elixir, because they have elementary qualities: as Wilson reports, 'the principle underlying the treatment is that of medieval Galenic medicine, whereby imbalance in one of the four humours was cured by remedies of the opposite quality'.[94] Only in John of Rupescissa's treatise on the fifth essence do we find the fusion of both traditions.

Arnold of Villanova, with his authentic writings on wines and his pharmacological texts, might provide the most interesting link between the tradition of distilled medical waters and that of the alchemical elixir; he is in fact also the supposed author of writings on alchemy, which some scholars are inclined to attribute to him at least in part. Yet the possible relation between his authentic medical writings and the oldest alchemical texts attributed to him has not been explored since Paul Diepgen's studies.[95] Also, a text on medicinal waters attributed to Lull, the *Ars operativa medica*, refers to Arnald's teaching; though it is included in the range of Lull's alchemical works, it really does not say anything about transmutation or elixir.[96] This short book is formed of two parts, a prologue describing the virtues of *aqua vitae*, and a text giving the twelve traditional recipes of healing waters. The prologue seems a later addition; its author introduces himself as Raimond Lull, disciple of Arnald of Villanova, and writes of a vision in which Saint Gilles showed him medical secrets.

This *Ars operativa medica* is extant in the oldest dated English manuscript including pseudo-Lullian alchemical texts that we know; this manuscript was written about 1440.[97] Although this manuscript bears no visible signs of being linked to Lambert or to Kirkeby, it needs to be closely examined, being almost contemporary with the period that we are studying. It is a miscellaneous manuscript, written in Latin and in English by a fine English hand. Beyond the pseudo-Lullian text, it contains recipes of pure medicinal character, written in both languages; a short text *De retardanda senectute et iuventute conservanda secundum Arnaldum Catellanum*; a medical text *Regimen speciale et conservacio oculorum secundum magistrem* [*sic*] *Johannem Sandryve, doctorem in theologia et medicina*; and a recipe for preparing a remedy against the plague.[98] In the Summary of the description of the manuscript it is stated that 'both the fifteenth century English writers of [this manuscript] were primarily interested in medicinal cures, both wrote fluently in Latin and English, and both may well have been physicians ... After the Lull text was copied, the volume was used as a medical commonplace book'.[99]

The recipe of a remedy against the plague in this manuscript introduces another question: what, if any, link had the search for alchemical remedies with the problems posed by the plague to traditional pharmacology? In the *Liber de consideratione quintae essentiae*, John of Rupescissa included an important chapter on the remedy against the plague:[100] in a period when 'medicine seemed largely inefficient against plague'[101] it was possible indeed that research on alchemical medicines might attract the interest of the physicians, even if – or just because – it was definitely separate from Galenic pharmacology.[102]

Physicians and alchemy in France and Italy

The interest of fifteenth-century physicians in alchemy is not at all limited to England: as has been recently shown by Danielle Jacquart, alchemy was regarded by outstanding physicians in Italy and in France as a means to help medicine to produce new, perhaps more efficacious remedies.[103] Antonio Guainieri tells of some recipes he had learnt from a hermit who, practising alchemy, had become a physician and healed paralyses by means of alchemical remedies. Michele Savonarola, who explicitly refused to believe in the transmutation of metals, was notwithstanding interested in alchemical procedures applied to the production of remedies, and he himself wrote a treatise on distillation. The French physician Jacques Despars used alchemical metaphors, beyond showing interest in the distillation of remedies and in other alchemical processes.

To these examples we can add William Fabri de Die, physician to the Antipope Felix V (1439–49), who wrote a *Liber de lapide philosophorum et de auro potabili*, where he opposed the more efficacious alchemical remedies to the traditional Galenic ones.[104] The prelate questions Fabri about a paralysis that affects his own hand.[105] Felix goes on, comparing traditional physicians to others, who possess a secret method for healing:[106] the distinction between traditional physicians and the others is thus presented as a distinction according to their native land – Italian vs French physicians, traditional vs alchemical medicine. It should be noted that the disease referred to by Fabri is a paralysis, like that treated by the hermit's ointment reported by Guainieri. Fabri's long answer to his patron is a true example of *quaestio de alchimia*, but his ultimate aim is to explain terms such as elixir and *aurum potabile*, answering another clear request of Felix, who wished to know Fabri's opinion about 'that philosophers' medicine called elixir'.[107] In his answer, Fabri refers more than once to 'Arnaldum, Raymondum and Johannem de Testym (Dastin)',[108] and seems to identify the elixir definitely with the potable gold,[109] that gold which is to the human body like the sun to the body of the world.[110]

Another episode, the sudden fame gained in Florence during the 1520s by Lorenzo da Bisticci, from a silversmith become a physician, shows that alchemy might even be the main path leading someone to become a healer, and a reputed one; once again we find a tract similar to that of Guainieri's hermit, though the Florentine healer, unlike the unnamed hermit, met his town physicians' opposition rather than their favour.[111] Lorenzo da Bisticci distilled a remedy that his fans called *Christus medicinarum*, probably a compound of wine distillate and gold. This story is told by the scribe of a Venetian manuscript, Bartholomeus Marcellus, who wrote that

> this Bistichius was still working as a goldsmith, when he began to use these medicines. He succeeded in preparing all the remedies described in the *Ars operativa*; then, experimenting sublimations with great commitment, he strenuously searched for the great Christ according to the rules of the work *De philosophiae famulatu* – a remedy almost divine and completely unknown today – and, with God's consent and the help of fortune, he found the Christ of medicines that heals even the helpless sick. Therefore he is reputed the king of today's physicians.[112]

The preparation of this remedy, whose action against incurable diseases recalls the virtues of the elixir, was discovered by Lorenzo perusing the pseudo-Lullian *Ars operativa medica* and Rupescissa's *Liber de consideratione quintae essentiae*.

As Richard Palmer has shown, in sixteenth-century Venice 'the tradition of medicine borrowing from alchemy, which owed so much to Ramon Lull, Arnoldus of Villanova and John of Rupescissa was also well established'.[113] According to him, the tradition of the alchemical distillation of remedies was one of the factors underlying the diffusion of Paracelsian medicine. Moreover Charles Webster, noting 'the importance of medicine in achieving official sanction for practical alchemy', has stressed the narrow link between the practical and esoteric features of alchemy and 'the unity of metallurgical and medical aspects of alchemy' – both themes that are central to the alchemy focused on the elixir.[114] We may then conclude that the physicians' interest in alchemy and alchemically prepared remedies, starting in the fourteenth century and reaching a climax in the fifteenth, was probably a factor that fostered the survival of the alchemical tradition, while contributing to modify deeply this same tradition in the transition from the Middle Ages to the Renaissance.

Notes

1. Some records concerning alchemy in fourteenth- and fifteenth-century England can be found in D. Waley Singer, *Catalogue of Latin and Vernacular Alchemical Manuscripts in Great Britain and Ireland, Dating from before the Sixteenth Century*, 3 vols, Brussels, 1928–31: vol. 3, appendix II. Lynn Thorndike gives several additional notices in his *History of Magic and Experimental Science*, 8 vols (New York, 1923–58), especially vol. III, chaps 1, 3, 5–7.
2. *Calendar of Patent Rolls* (hereafter CPR), Henry VI, vol. 5 (7 April 1444; 6 July 1444; 4 July 1446); vol. 6 (30 April 1452; 9 March 1457; 2 November 1457; 3 September 1460). On 18 August 1452, on the contrary, the same Henry VI gave an order to prosecute people who pretended to be capable of transmuting base metals. Some of the petitions are recorded also in Thomas Rymer, *Foedera, conventiones, litterae et*

cuiuscumque generis acta publica inter Reges Angliae et alios quosvis Imperatores, Reges, Pontifices, Principes vel Communitates, ab ineunte saeculo duodecimo viz. ab anno 1001 ad nostra usque tempora habita aut tractata (several editions).

3. Cf. CPR cited in the previous note: 'Metalla imperfecta de suo proprio genere transferre, et tunc ea, per dictam artem, in aurum vel argentum perfectum transmutare, ad omnimodas probationes et examinationes, sicut aliquod aurum vel argentum, in aliqua minera crescens'. See also Thomas Rymer, *Foedera ... editio tertia* (The Hague, 1741), vol. 5, part I, p. 136.
4. 'Cum antiqui sapientes et famosissimi philosophi, in suis scriptis et libris, sub figuris et integumentis docuerint et reliquerint ex vino, ex lapidibus prectiosis, ex oleis, ex vegetabilibus, ex animalibus, ex metallis et ex mediis mineralibus multas medicinas gloriosas et notabiles confici posse. Et praesertim quandam pretiosissimam medicinam, quam aliqui philosophorum matrem et imperatricem medicinarum dixerunt, alii gloriam inaestimabilem eandem nominarunt, alii vero quintam essentiam, alii lapidem philosophorum et elixir vitae nuncupaverunt eandem'. CPR Henry VI, 31 May 1456; cf. Rymer, *Foedera*, vol. 5, part II. p. 68; the text from the original vellum manuscript, Oxford, Museum of the History of Science, 84, has been published and translated into English by D. Geoghegan, 'A Licence of Henry VII to Practise Alchemy', *Ambix*, 6 (1957), pp. 10–17; the passage is quoted from Geoghegan, p. 15 (slightly modified).
5. Geoghegan, 'A Licence', p. 16.
6. Cf. Geoghegan, 'A Licence', pp. 13–14. Some biographical data on most of them can be obtaind from A. B. Emden, *A Biographical Register of the University of Cambridge to A.D. 1500*, 2 vols (Cambridge, 1963) (hereafter BRUC); A. B. Emden, *A Biographical Register of the University of Oxford to A.D. 1500*, 3 vols (Oxford, 1957–59) (hereafter BRUO); *Dictionary of National Biography* (hereafter DNB); C. H. Talbot and E. A. Hammond, *The Medical Practitioners of Medieval England*, Wellcome History of Medicine Library (London, 1965) (hereafter TH); F. M. Getz, 'Medical Practitioners in Medieval England', *Social History of Medicine*, 3 (1990), pp. 245–83 (hereafter Getz). The petitioners seem to be subdivided into two groups, nine of them being defined as 'viri in scienciis naturalibus eruditissimi', the other three as trustworthy and discreet men. The first nine are: **Gylbert Kymer** (BRUO. DNB s.v. Rymer, *Foedera*, 12 June 1455: required as physician at Windsor [not in CPR?]. TH, pp. 60–63: M.D., principal of Hart Hall, Oxford in 1411, dead 1463; many books and manuscripts owned by him are now at the Bodleian Library, Getz, pp. 259–60; Geoghegan, 'A Licence', pp. 11–12: 'not only Duke Humphrey's personal friend and physician, but a man of eminent scholastical and clerical influence'); **John Faceby** (BRUO: physician to the king 1443, 1460. CPR Hen. VI, vol. 6, pp. 147, 291, 398. TH, p. 143: 'one of the most trusted of the medical advisers to Henry VI'. The identification with J. Fauceby, signatory of the petition, is dismissed by TH because of the different spelling of the name, vs BRUO, Getz, p. 265 and Geoghegan, 'A Licence', p. 11); **William Hatclyff** (BRUC, 292. CPR Hen. VI, vol. 6, pp. 147, 339: required 'to minister about the king's person in his sickness' together with John Faceby and

others, 6 April 1453; appointed physician to the queen in 1457. TH, pp. 398–9: licensed in Padua, 1447; recipes by him in British Museum, MS Harley 168, ff. 155–6; Getz, p. 281. Cfr. Geoghegan, 'A Licence', p. 12); **John Kirkeby** (BRUO, p. 1078: chaplain to the king in 1455, d. 1459. Getz, p. 266: natural scientist. Cfr. Geoghegan, p. 11); **Wolfard Cook** (TH, p. 421: Wolforde Cooke [Coke], Master, Doctor of Medicine, London, about 1465. Getz, p. 283); **Henry Welles** (CPR Hen. VI, vol. 6, p. 524: 23 June 1460, 'H. W. late of Canterbury, co. Kent, fisician'. TH, pp. 85–6); **John Fouler** (or Fowler) (Unknown); **John Rayny** (Cfr. TH, p. 178: physician in the Isle of Wight, about 1451; Getz, p. 267: John Ragny, natural scientist); **John Morer** (CPR Hen. VI, vol. 6, p. 280. TH, p. 173: 1429–72, M.A., M.D.; inception: 6 Feb. 1455, New College, Oxford). The following three are **Henry Bourgchier** (DNB: H. B., count of Essex, d. 1483. CPR Hen. VI, vol. 6, p. 378: H. B., knight, 18 Nov. 1457. Geoghegan, 'A Licence', p. 13: 'It is possible that this H. B. may have been related to the Lord Chancellor, Archbishop Thomas Bourgchier ... but no evidence can be advanced in support of this conjecture'); **John Solers** (Perhaps J. S. from Racheford, imprisoned with others, 11 Aug. 1455: CPR Hen. VI, vol. 6, p. 259); **William Lynde** (Unknown).

7. Geoghegan, 'A Licence', p. 10.
8. Kymer was mentioned by Thomas Norton in his *Ordinal of alchemy*: cf. Charles Webster, 'Alchemical and Paracelsian Medicine', in Charles Webster, ed., *Health, Medicine, and Mortality in the Sixteenth Century* (Cambridge, 1979), p. 302; and F. M. Getz, 'To Prolong Life and Promote Health: Baconian Alchemy and Pharmacy in the English Learned Tradition', in *Health, Disease and Healing in Medieval Culture* (New York, 1991), p. 141. Both Webster and Getz briefly refer to the 1456 petition as an outstanding episode in the medical history of fifteenth-century England.
9. On the identification of John Kirkeby, see the thorough discussion (eventually agreeing with my conclusion) by L. E. Voigts, 'The "Sloane Group": Related Scientific and Medical Manuscripts from the Fifteenth Century in the Sloane Collection', *The British Library Journal*, **16** (1990), pp. 26–57; esp. pp. 33–7 (p. 36 on the 1456 episode).
10. Cf. M. Pereira, *The Alchemical Corpus Attributed to Raimond Lull* (London, 1989), p. 3n; *Eadem*, 'Lullian alchemy: aspects and problems of the corpus of alchemical works attributed to Ramon Lull (XIV–XVII century)', *Catalan Review*, **4** (1990), pp. 41–54.
11. Cf. *The Medical Renaissance of the Sixteenth Century*, ed. by A. Wear, R. K. French, I. M. Lonie (Cambridge, 1985); *The History of the University of Oxford, vol. III, 'The Collegiate University'* (Oxford, 1986): 4.2, G. Lewis, 'The Faculty of Medicine'. On English medieval medicine see V. L. Bullough, 'Medical Study at Mediaeval Oxford', *Speculum*, **36** (1961), pp. 600–612; and F. M. Getz, 'Medicine at Medieval Oxford', in *History of the University of Oxford, vol. II: 'Late Medieval Oxford'*, edited by J. I. Catto and T. A. R. Evans (Oxford, 1993).
12. On the Western tradition of the elixir see now: M. Pereira, 'Teorie dell'elixir nell'alchimia latina medievale', *Micrologus. Natura, scienze e società medievali*, **3** (1995), pp. 103–48.
13. *A Testament of Alchemy, Being the Revelation of Morienus, Ancient Adept and Hermit of Jerusalem to Khalid ibn Yazid Mu'Awiyya, King of*

the Arabs, of the Divine Secrets of the Magisterium and Accomplishment of the Alchemical Art, ed., trans. and comm. by L. Stavenhagen (Hanover, New Hampshire, 1974).

14. *Liber Abuali Abincine De Anima in Arte Alchimiae, in Artis Chemicae principes Avicenna atque Geber* ... (Basel, Petrus Perna, 1572). On Avicenna and alchemy see J. Ruska, 'Die Alchemie des Avicenna', *Isis*, 21 (1934), pp. 14–51; G. Anawati, 'Avicenne et l'alchimie', in *Oriente e Occidente nel Medio Evo*, (Rome, 1971), pp. 251–83; P. Carusi, 'Animalis Herbalis Naturalis. Considerazioni parallele sul 'De anima in arte alchimiae attribuito ad Avicenna e sul "Miftah al-Hikma" (opera di un allievo di Apollonio di Tiana)', *Micrologus. Natura, scienze e società medievali*, 3 (1995), pp. 45–74.
15. *De Anima*, p. 108.
16. *A Testament*, p. 34.
17. Constantine of Pisa, *The Book of the Secrets of Alchemy*, Intr., critical ed., trans. and comm. by B. Obrist (Leiden, 1990), pp. 86, 111, 112; cfr. p. 212n.
18. *De Anima*, p. 108.
19. Ibid.
20. Albertus Magnus, *De mineralibus et Rebus Metallicis*, in *Opera Omnia*, ed. Borgnet, (Paris, 1899) vol. 5, III. i, ch. 7: 'propter quod dicunt aegra esse metalla quae in materia non habent formam auri et studuerunt ad medicinam quam elixir vocant per quam egritudines metallorum ... removent'; ch. 9: 'Sed tunc oportet nos dicere quod alchimicorum periti operantur sicut periti medicorum.' (English translation by D. Wyckhoff, *Albertus Magnus Book of Minerals* [Oxford, 1967], pp. 171, 178).
21. *The Summa Perfectionis of Pseudo-Geber*, critical ed., trans. and study by W. R. Newman (Leiden, 1992): the problems concerning the identity of 'Geber' are reported in the Introduction; on the preparation of the elixir see book 3, chs 71–81.
22. Vincentii Bellovacensis, *Speculum Doctrinale, Historiale, Morale, Naturale* (Douai, 1624), col. 476. 'In corporibus itaque mineralibus, ut supra dictum est, ad instar operationis naturae, conati sunt alchymistae facere brevi tempore, quod natura facit in annis mille: unde et docuerunt rem quandam, quae corpora super quibus proicitur transmutet. Haec vocatur ab eis elixir'.
23. J. Needham, *Science and Civilisation in China* (Cambridge, 1974), vol. 5, p. 74. The importance of medicine for Arabic alchemy is also affirmed by A. Debus, *The Chemical Philosophy. Paracelsian Science and Medicine in the Sixteenth and Seventeenth Centuries* (New York, 1977), ch. 1.
24. Cf. R. P. Multhauf, *The Origins of Chemistry* (London, 1966), chs 8, 9. Cfr. also C. Crisciani and M. Pereira, *L' arte del sole e della luna. Alchimia e filosofia nel Medioevo*, (Spoleto, 1996).
25. Cf. A. Paravicini Bagliani, *Medicina e scienze della natura alla corte dei Papi del Duecento* (Spoleto, 1991), esp. the essays nos VI, VII, IX, X; by the same author, 'Ruggero Bacone autore del "De retardatione accidentium senectutis?"', *Studi Medievali Serie Terza*, 28 (1987), pp. 707–28.
26. Cr. A Paravicini Bagliani, 'Ruggero Bacone, Bonifacio VIII e la teoria della "prolongatio vitae"', in *Medicina e scienze*, pp. 327–61; G. J. Gruman,

'A History of Ideas about the Prolongation of Life. The Evolution of Prolongevity to 1800', *Transactions of the American Philosophical Society* 56, part IX (1966), pp. 1–97; J. Needham, *Science and Civilisation*, 5, pp. 491–509 ('Comparative Macrobiotics, 3: Macrobiotics in the Western World'). For the Western mythical background of the search for an agent of immortality see F. Cardini, 'Faust e il Santo Graal. Nota storico-antropologica al mito dell' Elixir'; M. Ariani, 'Il "fons vitae" nell' immaginario medievale'; M. Centanni, 'Da Achille ad Alessandro. Storie di morte e di immortalità', all in *Exaltatio essentiae. Essentia exaltata*, edited by F. Cardini and M. Gabriele (Pisa, 1992).

27. M. Pereira, *L' oro dei filosofi. Saggio sulle idee di un alchimista del Trecento* (Spoleto, 1992), ch. 2; *Eadem*, 'Un tesoro inestimabile. Elixir e "prolongatio vitae" nell' alchimia del "300"', *Micrologus. Scienze, natura e società medievali*, 1 (1993), pp. 161–87.
28. See above, n. 25.
29. Getz, *To Prolong Life*, p. 137.
30. R. Bacon, *Opus Tertium*, in *Opera quaedam hactenus inedita*, ed. J. S. Brewer (London, 1859), p. 39: 'Generatio enim hominum, et brutorum, et vegetabilium est ex elementis et humoribus, et communicat cum generatione rerum inanimatarum.'
31. R. Bacon, *Un fragment inédit de l' Opus tertium précédé d'un étude sur ce fragment*, ed. P. Duhem (Quaracchi, 1909), pp. 180–83: 'hic aperiuntur magnarum scientiarum radices, scilicet naturalis Philosophie, Medicine et Alkimie ... Nam quia communicant in radicibus naturalis Philosophia, Medicina et Alkimia, ideo simulavi me tradere radices has tanquam essent solum naturalia et medicinalia, cum tamen sint alkimistica.'
32. Ibid., p. 182: 'Accipe igitur lapidem, qui non est lapis; et est in quolibet homine, et in quolibet loco, et in quolibet tempore; et vocatur ovum philosophorum, et terminus ovi. Divide igitur ipsum in quatuor, scilicet terram, aquam, aerem, ignem. Et cum hoc diposueris, vivificabis et albificabis, Domino concedente.'
33. R. Bacon, *Opus Maius*, ed. J. H. Bridges (Oxford, 1897–1900; reprint Frankfurt am Main, 1964), p. 215: 'Et vere est secretum maximum, nam non solum procuraret bonum reipublicae et omnibus desideratum propter auri sufficientiam, sed quod plus est in infinitum, daret prolongationem vitae.'
34. Scholarly views concerning the alchemical corpus attributed to Arnald may be grouped into two opposite trends: a) that of accepting a few works, including the *Rosarium*, as authentic (P. Diepgen, 'Studien zu Arnald von Villanova: III. Arnald und die Alchemie', *Archiv für Geschichte der Medizin*, 3 (1910), pp. 369–96; cf. L. Thorndike, *History*, vol. 3, pp. 52–84; J. García Font, *Historia de la alquímia en España*, (Madrid, 1976) pp. 103–22; R. Halleux, *Les Textes alchimiques* (Turnhout, 1979), pp. 105–6); and, b) that of denying that Arnald wrote anything alchemical: J. A. Paniagua, 'Notas en torno a los escritos de alquimia, atribuidos a Arnau de Vilanova', *Archivo Iberoamericano de historia de la medicina*, 11 (1959), pp. 404–19; J. J. Payen, '"Flos Florum" et "Semita semite". Deux traités d' alchimie attribués à Arnaud de Villeneuve', *Revue d' histoire des sciences*, 12 (1959), pp. 289–300. See now M. Pereira, 'Arnaldo da Villanova e l'alchimia. Un'indagine preliminare', in *Actes de la I Trobada Internacional d'Estudis sobre*

Arnau de Vilanova (Barcelona, 1995), pp. 95–174. Anyway, whether or not one accepts Arnald as author of the *Rosarium*, the origin of this text dates back to a fourteenth-century tradition: see M. Berthelot, 'Sur quelques écrits alchimiques, en langue provençale, se rattachant à l' école de Raymond Lulle', in *La Chimie au Moyen Age* (Paris, 1893; reprinted Amsterdam, 1967), p. 354; Payen, cited above; G. Camilli, 'Il *Rosarius philosophorum* attribuito ad Arnaldo da Villanova nella tradizione alchemica del Trecento', in *Actes de la I Trobada*, pp. 175–208.

35. Arnaldi de Villanova, *Rosarium Philosophorum*, in J. J. Manget, *Bibliotheca Chemica Curiosa* (Geneva, 1702), vol. 1, p. 676: 'habet virtutem efficacem super omnes alias medicorum medicinas ... eo quod est occultae et subtilis naturae'.
36. R. Lulli, *Testamentaum*, MS Oxford, Corpus Christi College, 244, f. 57rb–va: 'Iste est lapis summus omnium [philosophorum] occultatus ignorantibus et indignis et tibi revelatus, quod transformat quodlibet corpus diminutum in infinitum solificum et lunificum verum, secundum quod elixir fuerit preparatum et subtiliatum. Et consimiliter tibi dicimus, quod habet virtutem et efficaciam super numerum omnium aliarum medicinarum, sanandi realiter omnem infirmitatem corporis humani, sive sit frigide, sive calide nature. Quamobrem, quia est subtilissime et nobilissime nature, omnia reducens ad summam equalitatem, conservat sanitatem et confortat virtutem et eam multiplicat, in tantum quod de sene facit iuvenem; et aliam quamlibet (f. 57va) infirmitatem expellit a corpore; omni veneno resistit; et humectat arterias cordis; et illud, quod stat in pulmone congelatum, dissolvit; et illum volneratum confortat et consolidat; et mundificat sanguinem; et confortat omnes spiritus et eos custodit et servat in sanitate. Et si infirmitas sit unius mensis, ista medicina sanat in uno die; et si sit unius anni, sanat pure in duodecim diebus; et si sit a longo tempore, realiter sanat in uno mense. Quare non est mirum, si ista medicina super omnes medicinas alias ab homine sit merito perquirenda, cum omnes alie universaliter reducantur ad istam. Si igitur, fili, tu habeas istam, thesaurum habes perdurabilem.' Cf. the same passage in the vulgata text edited by Manget, *Bibliotheca*, vol. 1, pp. 776–7.
37. R. Lulli, *Testamentum*, MS cit., f. 25ra.
38. Ibid., f. 68vb: 'Noster lapis, fili, manet in omnibus suis elementis et totus est in quolibet illorum per separacionem eorum ... Si ergo qualitates excellentes omnes insimul debite copulentur in uno mixto, videlicet quod lapis calidus et lapis frigidus et lapis siccus et lapis humidus equaliter omnes insimul in se temperent, erit complexio peculiosa, que portat nascenciam veri temperamenti per actionem actualem qualitatum primarum excellencium, que sunt in elementis.'
39. Arnaldi de Villanova, *Rosarium*, in Manget, *Bibliotheca*, vol. 1, p. 676: 'arcanum pretiosissimum, quod est super omne huiusmodi arcanum impretiabile pretium, et omnium philosophorum thesaurus'.
40. Johannis Dausteni, *Rosarium (Desiderabile desiderium)* in Manget, *Bibliotheca*, vol. 2, p. 324: 'In hoc completum secretum secretorum naturae maximum, quod est super omne huis mundi pretiosum pretiosissimum.'
41. Johannis de Rupescissa, *De consideratione quintae essentiae* (Basel, 1562);

on Rupescissa see R. Halleux, 'Les ouvrages alchimiques de Jean de Rupescissa', in *Histoire Littéraire de la France*, vol. 41 (Paris, 1981), pp. 241–84.

42. Johannis de Rupescissa, *De consideratione*, p. 15: 'Hoc est in quo laboraverunt omnes, quaerere rem creatam ad hominum usum aptam, quae possit corruptibile corpus a putrefactione servare; servatum, sine diminutione conservare; conservatum, si foret possibile, perpetuare in esse ... quae citra terminum vitae nostrae a Deo praefixum, possit corpus nostrum sine corruptione servare, sanare et conservare, infirmum curare, deperditum restaurare, donec veniat ultima dies mortis in termino praefixo a Deo.'
43. Ibid., p. 19.
44. Ibid.: 'quando necesse est, influit qualitatem humidam, aliquando calidam, aliquando frigidam, aliquando sicca. Talis est radix vitae, Essentia quinta.'
45. Cf. the definition of the elixir given by J. Needham, 'Il concetto di elixir e la medicina su base chimica in oriente e in occidente', *Acta Medicae Historiae Patavinae*, 19 (1973–74), pp. 9–41.
46. J. Needham, *Science and Civilisation*, p. 74.
47. Cf. above, n. 8.
48. After the nineteenth century scholarly catalogue by E. Littré and B. Hauréau (in *Histoire Littéraire de la France*, vol. 29, Paris, 1885), the manuscript tradition of the alchemical writings attributed to Lull was studied by L. Thorndike (*History*, vol. 4, ch. 1) and by myself (*The Alchemical Corpus*). For the *Testamentum* see especially Thorndike pp. 28–31 and Pereira, pp. 6–11 and Catalogue, I.61. Cfr. also D. W. Singer, 'The Alchemical "Testamentum" Attributed to Raymond Lull', *Archeion*, 8 (1929–29), pp. 43–52; the 'alchemical philosophy' developed in the *Testamentum* is the main focus of my book, *L'oro dei filosofi*.
49. R. Bacon, *Un fragment*, p. 186: 'Vel maius opus dicitur quando fit operatio super partes animalis ut queratur medicina; minus vero, quando super arsenicum vel suphur, vel aliud inanimatum, vel super plura eorum, quia numquam tam nobilis medicina potest haberi per hec inanimata, sicut per partes animalium.' Cf. Abuali Abincinae *De Anima*, pp. 252–3. According to Multhauf (*The Origins*, p. 192), 'It was possible that Bacon was held by that [fourteenth] century to represent a group which it particularly abhorred, the school which advocated elixirs of organic origin.'; and cf. ibid., pp. 139, 142, 190. See also Pereira, 'Teorie dell'elixir', cit., especially pp. 121–4, 128–30, 147.
50. *Testamentum*, MS Oxford CCC 244, f. 9vb: 'Nulla res convenit ei, nisi illa que ei est propinquior in sua natura. Quia ex homine non potest generari nisi homo; et ab aliis animalibus nisi sua similia. Et sic quelibet res potest generari, que concepit filium simile. Iccirco dicimus, fili, quod opereris cum nobili natura.' (cf. Manget, *Bibliotheca*, vol. 1, p. 719). Cf. John Dastin, 'Epistola boni viri' (in W. R. Theissen, 'John Dastin's letter on the philosophers' stone', *Ambix*, 33 (1986), pp. 76–87), p. 79, 81; *Rosarium* (in Manget, *Bibliotheca*, vol. 2, pp. 309–24), 2, p. 310; Arnald of Villanova, *Perfectum Magisterium* (in Manget, *Bibliotheca*, vol. 1, pp. 679–83), p. 680.
51. *Testamentum*, MS Oxford CCC 244, f. 50ra: 'Quoniam hoc, quod natura facit, nos possumus bene destruere; et hoc post reformare, ponendo infra naturam, sine qua nullus phisicus poterit curam facere.' (cf. Manget, *Bibliotheca*, vol. 1, p. 768).

52. Ibid., f. 46ra: 'Alchimia est una para celata philosophie naturalis magis necessaria, de qua constituitur una ars, que non apparet omnibus, que docet mutare omnes lapides preciosos et ipsos reducere ad verum temperamentum; et omne corpus humanum ponere in multum nobilem sanitatem; et transmutare omnia corpora metallorum in verum solem et in veram lunam per unum corpus medicinale universale, ad quod omnes particulares medicine reducuntur.' (Cf. Manget, *Bibliotheca*, vol. 1, p. 763).
53. Ibid., f. 64rb, 66ra: 'Hic iacet totum regimen sanitatis, ad quod omnis bonus phisicus debet multum suum intellectum applicare ... Et non cures cognoscere infirmitatem, quoniam discreta natura suo instinctu dedit virtutem lapidi dissoluto sanandi omnem infirmitatem.' (The *Liber Mercuriorum* is not published in Manget, *Bibliotheca*).
54. Ibid., f. 64va. Note that in the *Consilia* written by (or attributed to) Taddeo Alderotti the same definition is given to the alcohol of wine or *aqua ardens* (cf. below, n. 89).
55. Ibid., f. 81r: 'Fecimus nostrum Testamentum per voluntatem de A in insula Anglie in Ecclesia Sancte Katerine prope Londonum versus partem castri ante Tamisiam [regnante *add. inter lineas*] iam Rege Eduvardo de [Woodstoc] per graciam Dei. In cuius manus mittimus in custodiam per voluntatem de A presens Testamentum anno post Incarnacionem domini 1332 cum omnibus suis voluminibus, que nominata fuerunt in presenti Testamento, cum Cantilena, que sequitur. Deo gracias.'
56. Cf. M. Berthelot, *La Chimie au Moyen Age* (Paris, 1893; reprint Amsterdam, 1967), vol. 1, pp. 351–6: 'Sur quelques écrits alchimiques, en langue provençale, se rattachant à l' école de Raymond Lulle'; R. Halleux, 'L'Alchimie', in *Grundriss der Romanischen Literaturen des Mittelalters*, vol. 8, part 1, *La Littérature Française aux XIVe et XVe siècles. Partie historique* (Heidelberg, 1988), pp. 336–45.
57. Prague, Universitnì Knihovna, XXIII 132. The debate concerning the original language of the *Testamentum* was opened by P. Bohigas ('El repertori', cit. below n. 60: p. 34), who considered the Catalan version as the original one. Yet more recent analysis by the philologist Barbara Spaggiari, aimed at the edition of the bilingual manuscript Oxford, CCC, 244, shows that the original was Latin (her essay is published as a part of the introduction to the edition prepared in collaboration with myself for 'Società Internazionale per lo Studio del Medioevo Latino', Edizioni del Galuzzo, Florence, 1998).
58. Cf. M. Pereira, 'Filosofia naturale lulliana e alchimia. Con l'inedito epilogo del "Liber de secretis naturae seu de quinta essentia"', *Rivista di storia della filosofia*, 41 (1986), fasc. 4, pp. 747–80; *Eadem*, '"Opus alchemicum" i "Ars combinatoria". El "Liber de secretis naturae seu de quinta essentia" en la tradició lul·liana', in *Del Frau a l' erudició. Aportacions a la història del lul·lisme dels segles XIV al XVIII*, *Randa*, 27 (1990), pp. 45–55.
59. Cf. Pereira, *L' oro dei filosofi*, p. 153–4; *Eadem*, 'Le figure alchemiche pseudolulliane. Un indice oltre il testo?', in *Fabula in tabula. Una storia degli indici dal manoscrito al testo elettronico*, edited by C. Leonardi, M. Morelli and F. Santi (Spoleto, 1995), pp. 111–18.
60. MS Oxford, Corpus Christi College 244 is a vellum and paper manuscript, written in the XVth sec. (1455); it has ix+136 pages (14 booklets)

in folio format; Gothic handwriting by at least two hands (one of which is Kirkeby's), with some later additions (ff. ii r–ix v and 84r–84ter) by John Dee (cf. *John Dee's Library Catalogue*, ed. by R. J. Roberts and A. G. Watson, The Bibliographical Society, London, 1990, p. 181). Many marginal notes, some of which are by the same Kirkeby, others by John Dee, others by Robert Greene de Welbe, others (the great majority) by an unidentified hand. The manuscript is decorated with red and blue titles and capitals, and it includes many figures (some of them are in black ink, others are coloured). There are four signatures by Kirkeby, at folios 81r, 107rb, 124vb, 131rb. Other owners' signatures at fol. 1r: '26° Rober ... ; Raymundi Testamentum. N° 1711.244. W.C.4.3.'; at fol. 37r: 'Sir Robert grene de W.'; 'Jo. royden' [in Greek letters]. The manuscript contains seven pseudo-Lullian treatises (I give only the folios and the numbers from my Catalogue in *The Alchemical Corpus*, pp. 61–96): I. 61 (ff. 1ra–81rb); I. 7 (ff.81rb–82ra); II. 6 (ff. 82rb–82vb); I. 39 (ff. 85ra–124vb); I. 4 (ff. 125ra–126r); I. 12 (ff. 127ra–133va); I. 45 (ff. 133va–136ra). It contains also an alchemical treatise in English (ff. ii r–ix v: Hic incipit Arcium Alkamie, *Inc.*: All the Wisdome in the Worlde comith of our Lorde); an alchemical poem (f. 82v, *Inc.* Duc nutrimento limpinandi septem horarum); a series of Lullian alphabets referring to the attributed alchemical treatises (ff. 82vb–83va); an alchemical note (f. 83va–b: *Inc.*: Fili nota secretum in operando datum a Deo videlicet quod extrahendo oleum); alchemical writings in English (ff. 84r–84ter r: (i) Gemma salutaris, *Inc.*: The firste monde that is workd that the book); (ii) Gemma salutaris qui nascitur orbicularis et Notabilia Philosophorum, *Inc.*: Pictigoras in the take the combuste fugitive; (iii) Septem condiciones huius materiae, *Inc.*: The firste condicon is that yt); an alchemical epistle (f. 126rb–v: *Inc.*: Admetus fortunato socero suo salutem. Quesivisti naturam nocumentorum destruencium secundum omnen sensum temperatam naturam). The manuscript was described by H. O. Coxe, *Catalogus codicum manuscriptorum qui in collegiis aulisque Oxoniensibus hodie adservantur*, 2 vols (8+11 tomi) (Oxford, 1852), vol. 2 t. IV, pp. 101–2; J. M. Batista y Roca, *Catàlech de les obres lulianes en Oxford* (Barcelona, 1916), p. 44, n. 53; P. Bohigas, 'El repertori de manuscrits catalans. 2. Missió a Anglaterra', *Estudis Universitaris Catalans*, 11 (1926), pp. 121–30; reprinted in P. Bohigas, *Sobre manuscrits i biblioteques* (Barcelona, 1985), pp. 20–70 (28–36); D. W. Singer, *Catalogue*, vol. 1, p. 244. Cf. M. Pereira, *The Alchemical Corpus*, pp. 3, 8. I wish to thank the Assistant Archivist of Corpus Christi, Mrs Christine Butler, for her kind assistance during my work in the archives.

61. Cf. Pereira, *The Alchemical Corpus*, pp. 23, 29n; some years ago Andrew Watson published a preliminary note on Robert Greene de Welbe (A. G. Watson, 'Robert Green of Welby, Alchemist and Count Palatine, c. 1467–c. 1540', *Notes and Queries*, 32, 1985, pp. 312–13), but in a private conversation (January 1991) he regretted having received no new communications about Greene's manuscripts or biography.
62. Cf. *John Dee's Library Catalogue*, cited above, n. 60.
63. Cf. also the group of scientific and medical manuscripts studied by Linda Voigts ('The "Sloane Group"', cit. above, n. 9)
64. Oxford, Corpus Christi College, 244, f. 81r: 'Translatum fuit presens

Testamentum de lingua cathalonica in latinam anno gracie 1443 sexto Junii per Lambertum [blank space] apud Londonum in prioratu Sancti Bartholomei. Et quoniam predicta translacio mihi, Johanni Kirkeby, in multis non placuit, conscripsi manu mea propria capitulatim Testamentum in utraque lingua ad maiorem lucem veritatis percipiendam; et finivi anno gracie 1455 secundum computacionem Romane ecclesie mensis marcii die VII incompleto, hora quasi undecima ante meridiem.'

65. Cf. E. A. Webb, *The Records of St. Bartholomew's Priory and of the Church and Parish of St. Bartholomew the Great, W. Smithfield*, 2 vols (Oxford, 1921); N. J. M. Kerling, 'The Relations between St. Bartholomew's Hospital and the City of London, 1546–1948', *The Guildhall Miscellany*, 4 (1971), pp. 14–21; *Eadem*, 'The Foundation of St. Bartholomew's Hospital in West Smithfield, London', *The Guildhall Miscellany*, 5 (1972), pp. 137–48; *Eadem*, *Cartulary of St. Bartholomew's Hospital* (London, 1973). I wish to thank Mr Geoffrey Yeo, District Archivist of St Bartholomew's Hospital, for his kind assistance. He checked for me the index of personal names in the medieval records of the hospital, without finding any reference which would assist in identifying 'Lambertus' (letter, 14 January 1991).
66. The existence of two slightly different versions of the Latin *Testamentum* had already been stated by Dorothy Waley Singer (cf. her article cited above, n. 48), and by Lynn Thorndike (*History*, vol. 4, pp. 28–31).
67. That St Catherine was the place where the *Testamentum* (or perhaps, according to my hypothesis, an important copy of it) was written is commonly held by English scholars: cf. A. C. Ducarel, *History of the Foundation of St. Katherine by the Tower* (London, 1782), pp. 10–11, quoting T. Osborne's *Catalogue*: C. Jamison, *The History of the Royal Hospital of St. Katharine* (Oxford, 1952), p. 128. *The Registers of St. Katharine by the Tower* (London, 1945) start from 1584.
68. England and Northern Spain had important political and trading connections around the middle of the fifteenth century, as they had had during the first decades of the fourteenth.
69. Cf. Pereira, *The Alchemical Corpus*, p. 3n.
70. Cf. Ducarel, *History*, pp. 8–9; Jamison, *The History*, pp. 21–4.
71. CPR 3 May 1329; cf 2 September 1332 (if 'Jean le Rous of Raggelaie' is the same J. I. R. mentioned in the former letter). Cfr. Rymer, *Foedera*, vol. 2, 1, p. 24; D. W. Singer, *Catalogue*, vol. 3, App. II.
72. See G. E. Trease, 'The Spicers and Apothecaries of the Royal Household in the Reigns of Henry III, Edward I and Edward III', *Nottingham Medieval Studies*, 3 (1959), pp. 19–52; *idem*, *Pharmacy in History* (London, 1964), p. 60; L. G. Matthews, *The Royal Apothecaries* (London, 1967), with a list of French apothecaries at the English Royal Household, Appendix, pp. 175–6. The recent biography of Edward III by Michael Pack (*King Edward the III*, London, 1983) does not add further information on this matter.
73. Cf. especially W. L. Braekman, 'Queen Isabel's Dietary and its context', in his *Studies on Alchemy, Diet, Medicine and Prognostication in Middle English* (Brussels, 1986), pp. 43–82, esp. pp. 64–5; Isabel's interest in the rejuvenating elixir is also reported by Charles H. Talbot, 'The Elixir of Youth', in *Chaucer and Middle English Studies, in honour of R. H. Robbins*, ed. B. Rowland (London, 1974), pp. 33–4. For Isabel's link with St Katherine at the Tower see Jamison, *The History*, pp. 22–3.

74. Cf. above, n. 63.
75. Cf. Emeden, BRUO, p. 1078; cf. Voigts, 'The "Sloane Group"', pp. 34–7.
76. At folios 107rb, 124vb, 131rb, 131va.
77. E. H. Duncan, 'The Literature of Alchemy and Chaucer's 'Canon's Yeoman Tale: Framework, Theme and Characters', *Speculum*, 43 (1968), pp. 633–56.
78. Oxford, Corpus Christi College, 244, f. 19va: 'Et istud temperamentum debet eligi, sicut dicit Arnaldus de Villa nova in suo Rosario, in capitulo quod incipit: "Omnia sub termino diffinito", et in fine.' (cf. the Catalan text, f. 19ra). It should be noted, however, that this quotation occurs in a gloss added to the text of the *Testamentum* at an unknown stage of its diffusion before the time of Kirkeby's manuscript.
79. Cf. Voigts, 'The "Sloane Group"', pp. 35–7.
80. According to Faye Getz, the 1456 episode is 'the best indication that men of learning took Roger Bacon's writings about the restorative powers of the philosophers' stone seriously'. As for the reason, Getz points to the philosophical character of Bacon's remedies (Getz, *To Prolong Life*, p. 140; cf. also Pereira, 'Un tesoro inestimabile').
81. See Constantine of Pisa, *The Book of the Secrets of Alchemy*, cited above, n. 17.
82. C. Crisciani, 'La "Quaestio de alchimia" fra Duecento e Trecento', *Medioevo. Rivista di storia del pensiero medievale*, 2 (1976), pp. 119–69; *Eadem*, 'The Conception of Alchemy as Expressed in the "Pretiosa Margarita Novella" of Petrus Bonus of Ferrara', *Ambix*, 20 (1973), pp. 165–81; *L' arte del sole e della luna*, cited above, n. 24.
83. This is the interesting suggestion advanced by William Newman in his paper 'Technology and Alchemical Debate in the Late Middle Ages', *Isis*, 80 (1989), pp. 423–45.
84. 'Le Traité "Contre les Alchimistres" de Nicolas Eymerich', ed. and French translation by S. Matton, *Chrysopoeia*, 2 (1987), pp. 95–136.
85. Besides the obvious Arnald of Villanova, there are: Guillaume de Baufet, William Fabri de Dya, Jacques Albini, Jean Saulnier, Philippe Elephant, Thomas de Pisan, Valrand de Busrobert. Cf. D. Jacquart, *Le milieu médicale en France du XIIe au XVe siècle* (Geneva, 1981), p. 224. For three fifteenth-century physicians showing various degrees of interest in alchemy, see the article by the same Jacquart cited below, n. 103.
86. I. Rouaze, 'Un atélier de distillation du Moyen Age', *Bulletin Archéologique du Comité des Travaux Historiques et Scientifiques* (Ministére de l' Education Nationale, de la Jeunesse et des Sports) (Paris, 1989), reviewed in *Archives Internationales d' Histoire des Sciences*, 40 (1990), pp. 385–7.
87. C. A. Wilson, 'Philosophers, Iósis and Water of Life', *Proceedings of the Leeds Philosophical and Literary Society* (Literary and Historical Section), 19 (1984), pp. 101–219, esp. p. 73 and notes 531, 533.
88. Ibid., p. 84 and n. 618.
89. Ibid., p. 62 and n. 434; on Alderotti see N. Siraisi, *Taddeo Alderotti and his Pupils. Two Generations of Italian Medical Learning* (Princeton, 1981).
90. Wilson affirms that this was a means used by surviving Cathars to hide their sacred recipes ('Philosophers', pp. 85–6).
91. Wilson, 'Philosophers', p. 84.

92. Abuali Abincine *De Anima*, pp. 452–4: 'ad febres, ad vitium oculorum, et ad maculas corporis, scilicet morfeam'.
93. A copy is in MS Florence, Biblioteca Riccardiana, 119, ff. 142vb–166ra (XIV/XVth c.): cf. A. Pattin, 'Un recueil alchimique: le manuscrit Firenze, Bibl. Riccardiana, L.III.13 (119). Description et documentation', *Bulletin de la Société Internationale pour l' Étude de la Philosophie Médiévale*, 14 (1972), pp. 89–107.
94. Wilson, 'Philosophers', p. 81.
95. Diepgen, 'Studien', cited above, n. 34; recent works on Arnald and alchemy, in addition to those cited above, n. 34: A. Calvet, 'Les "alchimica" d'Arnaud de Villeneuve à travers la tradition imprimée (XVIe–XVIIe siècles). Questions bibliographiques', in *Alchimie. Art, Histoire et Mythes* (Paris and Milan, 1995), pp. 157–90; G. Camilli, 'Scientia mineralis e prolongatio vitae nel "Rosarius philosophorum"', *Micrologus. Natura, scienze e società medievali*, 3 (1995), pp. 211–25.
96. Pereira, *The Alchemical Corpus*, Catalogue I.6.
97. Yale, Beinecke Library, Mellon Collection MS 8; described in *Alchemy and the Occult. A Catalogue of Books and Manuscripts from the Collection of Paul and Mary Mellon Given to the Yale University Library*, eds I. Macphail, L. C. Witton II and R. Pachella (New Haven, 1968–77), vol. 3 (W. MacGuire, V. Pachella), pp. 54–6.
98. At f. 28v: 'bonam medicinam probatam contra pestilenciam' (Cf. *Alchemy and the Occult*, vol. 3, p. 56.)
99. *Alchemy and the Occult*, vol. 3, p. 56.
100. Book II, canon XIV; in Johannis de Rupescissa, *De consideratione*, p. 165.
101. *The Medical Renaissance*, Introduction p. xii.
102. When this chapter had already been written and revised, Chiara Crisciani and I made some research on the use of alchemical remedies to heal the plague: some writings documenting this use can effectively be found both in medical and alchemical literature, from the middle of the fourteenth century well into the fifteenth. These texts show a chain of connections and successive conceptual shiftings among remedies of traditional origin, such as gold and theriac, and alchemical ones: lapis philosophicus, quintessence, potable gold. All these are considered extraordinary medicines, more or less freely related to the idea of elixir and focused on gold and its powers, protecting the heart and expelling the poison from inside the human body. Cf. our forthcoming paper: 'Black Death and Golden Remedies. Some Remarks on Alchemy and the Plague', in *The Regulation of Evil*, edited by A. Paravicini Bagliani and F. Santi, *Micrologus Beihefte*, 2 (forthcoming).
103. D. Jacquart, 'Theory, Everyday Practice, and Three Fifteenth Century Physicians', in *Renaissance Medical Learning*, eds M. McVaugh and N. Siraisi (= *Osiris*, n. ser., 6) (1990), pp. 140–60.
104. On William Fabri see Thorndike, *History*, vol. 4, pp. 342–4; G. Carbonelli, *Sulle fonti storiche della chimica e dell' alchimia in Italia* (Roma, 1925), pp. 84–93; M. Pereira, *The Alchemical Corpus*, pp. 41–3; C. Crisciani, 'From the Laboratory to the Library: Alchemy according to Guglielmo Fabri', in *Renaissance Natural Philosophy and the Disciplines*, edited by A. Grafton and N. Siraisi (MIT Press, forthcoming).
105. William Fabri de Die, *De lapide philosophorum et auro potabile*, MS

Bologna, Biblioteca Universitaria, 138 (104), f. 245r: 'quid possit esse huius pestis angustia que manum adeo violenter detinet, ut moveri nequeat ad alta ... hanc medici curam impossibilem aiunt'.

106. Ibid.: 'Presul Italos aiebat medicos viam communem vulgarium medicorum sequi, quos sepe necessario fallacia experimenti eorum Ypocrate teste excusat. Addiciensque quod esset aliud medendi genus secretum perpaucis perpaucisque admodum medicis notum de quo Arnaldus de Ville Nova in sua Episola de retardanda senectute multum tetigerat, qui fuerat ultramontanus.'

107. Ibid., f. 245v: 'Successive post multos circuitos devenit ad aurum potabilem et ad artem transmutatoriam dicens: quid ais tu de illa medicina philosophorum quam Ixir dicunt?'

108. Ibid., f. 249v.

109. Ibid., ff. 250v–251r.

110. Ibid., f. 252r: 'Sicut sol celestis est sui luminis communicativus radiorum suorum ubique expansivus et diffusivus, sic et terrestris sol, scilicet aurum. Et quod sol celestis operatur in armonia celesti et toto macrocosmo, idem operatur terrestris in corpore in armonia terrestri et microcosmo minori in homine.'

111. According to John of Arezzo's, *Bistichius quidam florentinus faber argentarius atque homo litterarum ignarus repente summus in tota urbe evasit medicus*: MS Firenze, Biblioteca Medicea Laurenziana, (Plut. 77.22, f. 5r). Lorenzo was the son of Jacopo da Bisticci (who, in his turn, was one of the brothers of the more famous Vespasiano). See J. Hill Cotton, *Name-List from a Medical Register of the Italian Renaissance 1350–1550* (Oxford, 1976), p. 21: according to the unpublished Register by Hill Cotton (card index in the Wellcome Medical Library: sect. B 3–7) Lorenzo had some connection with Alessandro Sermoneta. Cf. also K. Park, *Doctors and Medicine in Early Renaissance Florence* (Princeton, 1985), p. 186; Park defines Lorenzo 'a physician' *tout-court*, whilst the polemical words by John of Arezzo stress his 'illiteracy', but give also some positive hint as to his job of silversmith (*faber argentarius*). Cf. M. Pereira, '"Medicina" in the alchemical writings attributed to Raimond Lull (XIVth–XVIIth centuries)', in *Alchemy and Chemistry in the 16th and 17th Centuries*, edited by P. Rattansi and A. Clericuzio (Dordrecht–Boston–London, 1994), pp. 1–15.

112. Venezia, Biblioteca Nazionale Marciana, lat. VI. 282, f. 77r: 'Et scias, candidissime lector, quod, quemadmodum mihi narravit scriptor huius operis, qui a Bistichio id ipsum furatus fuit, ipse Bistichius adhuc laborabat in aurificiis magisteriis cum has medicinas exerceret. Sed cum sibi omnia artis operative remedia bene ac feliciter successissent, animo alacriori sublimationes expertus, Christum secundum canones operis de philosophiae famulatu magnum, ac pene quidem divinum et nostris temporibus incognitum aggressus, enixe indagatus fuit et, Deo volente et favente fortuna, Christum rerum medicinalium contra omnes desperatissimas aegritudines na[c]tus est. Indeque nostrae tempestatis medicorum monarcha habetur.'

113. R. Palmer, 'Pharmacy in the Republic of Venice in the Sixteenth Century', in *The Medical Renaissance*, pp. 100–117: p. 110.

114. Charles Webster, 'Alchemical and Paracelsian medicine', in p. 303.

CHAPTER FOUR

Fascinating Women: The Evil Eye in Medical Scholasticism*

Fernando Salmón and Montserrat Cabré

> If he is young, delicate, of weak blood ... and you don't find another obvious cause for his illness, then you should be suspicious about the eye.

This is the advice that the Spanish physician Diego Alvarez Chanca gave in his *Tractatus de fascinatione* published in 1499. It was accompanied by a detailed description of the various signs that could appear in those young patients suffering the effects of an evil eye cast upon them.[1] The possibility that certain persons could harm others with the power of their sight, has been historically present in the circum-Mediterranean area.[2] Besides this broad and inclusive definition, the evil eye has taken in the past – as it is taking nowadays – different forms in the ways people identify it but also in how diverse social groups within a specific society relate to such a phenomenon. In contemporary Western institutional knowledge the evil eye has found a place as an object of study by folklorists, anthropologists and psychiatrists, who analyse it with the tools of the social sciences or as an epiphenomenal symptom of mental disorder.[3] In the late Middle Ages, theoretical discussions of the evil eye were given from inside dominant discourses and were the concern of academic natural philosophers, physicians and theologians, who identified its existence in society and gave to it plausible explanations within their epistemological frameworks. Since the evil eye implies a human agency in the production of sickness, accusations against its producers are significant for a history of blame.[4]

It is our aim in this chapter to analyse a scholastic attempt to place the evil eye in the arena of academic medical discussions in the Spanish kingdoms during the first third of the sixteenth century. In order to be changed from a *vulgi* belief into a proper *morbus, fascinatio* – as the evil eye was called in Latin[5] – needed to be explained with the tools provided by Galenism and natural philosophy. Following the standard scholastic pattern of inquiry – relying upon reason, authority and experience – the analysis of fascination allowed physicians to test the validity of a medical system by giving theoretical explanation and practical advice on a subject that, even if it was not new, had never been fully discussed before in university medical circles.

Bounding reality in a medical frame: authority, reason and experience

Medical concern about fascination appears scattered in Western Europe in various medical treatises from the fourteenth century onwards; however, it was not until the very end of the fifteenth century that it was singled out as a medical topic deserving a monographic approach. This was given expression with different fortuna in two treatises written in Latin by two Spanish university physicians. The first was the *Tractatus de fascinatione* composed by the royal physician Diego Alvarez Chanca.[6] Probably published in Seville in 1499, it seems to have had a very limited diffusion.[7] We have been unable to find a reference to Chanca's treatise in later works that deal with the topic. Thirty years later and without explicit acknowledgement of his immediate predecessor, a second attempt was taken by Antonio de Cartagena, a professor of medicine at the University of Alcalá[8] and author of a *Libellus de fascinatione*, published in the same city in 1530 alongside his *Liber de peste*.[9] The double bill presented by Cartagena proved to be more successful than Chanca's, and Cartagena's *Libellus* was widely quoted (sometimes in the form of bitter repudiations) in later works on fascination such as the lengthy *Opusculo de fascino* by Juan Lázaro Gutiérrez[10] or in treatises dealing with children's diseases such as the *Liber de affectionibus puerorum* by Francisco Pérez Cascales.[11]

Both Chanca and Cartagena presented fascination as a subject new to medical scholastic interests. In fact, in the discussions on particular diseases contained in the popular book three of Avicenna's *Canon* or in Rhazes's ninth book *Ad Almansorem*, the learned physician could not find fascination included among the diseases listed in these head-to-toe handbooks. At the end of the fifteenth century, fascination was not a well-defined disease in Latin Western medical thought and both Chanca and Cartagena used the rhetoric of social demand as justification for addressing the issue. The opening of Chanca's *Tractatus* re-created a conversation with a certain *doctus* that asked for his advice on *fascinatio*. Chanca referred his interlocutor to Socrates' opinion that one can only speak properly about what one knows properly. As the ancients[12] – Chanca's meditation continued – did not mention this subject, or, if they did, they did it rarely and in an ambiguous way, he preferred not to talk about it to talking about it wrongly. However, he had returned to the books of the ancients and he could not come back but sad. Because confusion reigned: some ancients denied the possibility of *fascinatio* and others accepted it; humble, but with the strength given by the belief that the desire to know is an intrinsic quality of man, Chanca announced his determination – with the help of the *Spiritus Sanctus* – of facing the enterprise. An enterprise that he described as only one step from which others could climb higher.[13]

The treatise was composed in Latin for physicians' use[14] and, significantly enough, the text began with the anecdote that opened Bernard of Gordon's *Lilium medicine*.[15] That was an expressive way of firmly claiming the value of his *Tractatus* in fortifying the Galenic tradition which he felt to be his heritage. By fitting into a medical framework a phenomenon that, although known since antiquity had never received a full medical explanation, Chanca was showing the validity of a medical system of thought – with respect to both its theoretical and practical sides – at a time when the physicians trained within the framework of Aristotelian natural philosophy and Galenic–Hippocratic medicine were being tested to give explanations of diseases perceived as new.[16] Chanca's commitment to defend the medical tradition to which he felt so close lies most clearly behind his best known work of 1514: the *Commentum in Parabolas Divi Arnaldi de Villanova*. Being involved in the new ways that Western Christendom developed to broaden its experience of the world,[17] Chanca was always faithful to the epistemological grounds on which his medical training had been based. Alongside his commentary on Arnau de Vilanova's *Parabolae medicationis*, he edited Arnau's text itself; a publication he justified by the usefulness of Arnau's aphorisms in the actual practice of medicine.[18]

Writing thirty years later, Antonio de Cartagena also pointed out the rarity of the topic. He saw his contribution as a step that others should build on and reminded his readers that progress in natural philosophy as well as in medicine was not the task of one single person because progress – according to Cartagena – was only possible by accretion. However, the Aristotelian orthodoxy of his conception of progress does not mean that Cartagena had to agree with his intellectual ancestors. And he did not.[19]

Our authors' claim for novelty in composing a treatise that dealt with fascination seems not to be historically accurate. At the beginning of the fourteenth century a work devoted to fascination is ascribed to Engelbert of Admont (*c.*1250–1331). Composed in a Benedictine monastery located in the present day Austrian Alps, Engelbert's *Tractatus de fascinatione* might have had a limited reception in southern Europe, and it is quite probable that neither Chanca nor Cartagena knew of its existence.[20] In fact, Engelbert's approach to the subject differs considerably from theirs as he is mainly concerned with exploring the body and soul relationship and the powers of the latter.[21] However, there was a closer precedent to Chanca's *Tractatus* and the reason why he did not refer to it might have not been just ignorance. Enrique de Villena (1384–1434), a learned aristocrat accused by his contemporaries of having more interest in natural philosophy than in the management of his properties, composed in Spanish a *Tratado de aojamiento* around 1420.[22] Villena justified his attempt to deal with fascination on the basis that many natural philosophers had dealt with the subject before, but none had explained its causes or its diagnosis and remedies.[23] The work begins with a display of all sorts of classical and medieval authorities to prove the evident reality of fascination. Later, Villena dealt with the prevention, diagnosis and cure of the disease. Although Villena's text does not reach the intellectual complexity of Chanca's, the parallels are evident in the use of authorities and the mention of particular examples. It has been argued that the common examples or authorities adduced by Chanca and Villena came from the same tradition and thus their similarity does not mean any direct connection.[24] But a close comparison of both texts hardly allows one to hold this view. It is clear to us that Chanca made extensive use of Villena's work. The description of the patient is strikingly similar, as is the method of diagnosis and some of the measures of prevention and treatment.[25] There was an obvious reason why Chanca should avoid mentioning Villena's name. After Villena's death, his library was inspected by inquisitor Fray Lope Barrientos with the Royal order of destroying all the books that dealt with magic and similar matters. Whatever the reality of the actual book-burning, what seems to be true is that, by the late fifteenth century, the name of Villena was associated with magic and secret books.[26] For this reason, Chanca's avoidance of mentioning his predecessor was a reasonable strategy to safeguard his text from an awkward situation. Similarly, Chanca was very cautious when approaching the second part of his treatise (*practica*). There, he made no reference to the remedies to prevent and cure fascination that Villena had included in his book[27] – such as the wearing of pieces of mirror or little hands near the head or neck – already labelling them as superstitious and against the faith.[28]

Cartagena does not mention either Villena's or Chanca's works. As we saw earlier, there was a specific reason to avoid mentioning Villena's treatise. However, we would suggest that Cartagena might not have known Chanca's treatise. If we compare the arrangement of the theoretical part of the treatises, their structures and contents do not bear any strong similarity. Chanca's theoretical part discusses ten questions. The first question asked if it was possible to find poison in the human body and if a human poisonous complexion could exist. After admitting that possibility, the second question tries to find out whether people of poisonous complexions are healthy. The third and fourth questions dealt with the mechanism of fascination and discussed whether fascination was something that could only be done by means of sight. The fifth to seventh questions were devoted to the recipient of fascination: humans, animals and plants. Questions eight and nine explained the characteristics of the fascinators and whether their action was a voluntary one or not. In his last question Chanca tried to account for why famous medical authors like Galen, Avicenna and Rhazes did not explain fascination. The theoretical part of Antonio de Cartagena's book comprises seven chapters where Cartagena proved – by means of authority, reason and experience – the reality of fascination (ch. 1) and refuted the explanations of the mechanism of fascination given by Avicenna (ch. 2), Thomas Aquinas (ch. 3), Gentile da Foligno (ch. 4) and Albert the Great (ch. 5). These chapters were written as a defence of emission theories as the only valid explanation of visual perception. In chapter six, Cartagena expounded his opinion about how fascination took place. Chapter 7 was devoted to different questions that Cartagena wanted to draw attention to, such as how anyone can become so venomous as to fascinate another person. He also asked if anyone could be fascinated, if any particular time was conducive to fascination, and which people had the power to fascinate (*vis effascinandi*). Cartagena went on to ask who were more subject to fascination, in which time of the year, why it was always the case that the fascinated are younger than the fascinators, and why fascination could only happen through the eye. The last question that Cartagena wanted to address in the first part of his *Libellus* was why he was writing on fascination given that nobody before him had done so.

Whatever the differences, however, both Chanca and Cartagena took the same point of departure. The special characteristics of fascination meant that to prove its existence was a necessary first step prior to its explanation. In order to do this, they employed the tools of scholastic orthodoxy – authority and reason – and a strong appeal to their own clinical experience.

The authorities they appealed to were not restricted to those of medical or philosophical character; theologians, poets and the Gospels were also taken into account.[29] Most of the time, these quoted authorities did not explicitly refer to fascination but to the possibility of the existence of a poisonous human body or to the dangerous nature of menstrual blood. But everything that served Chanca's or Cartagena's aims was welcomed. Chanca's use of Avicenna's *Sextus de naturalibus*, is very significant in this respect. Avicenna's idea of how fascination could be produced had been long ago rejected by Thomas Aquinas[30] and the opinion of the Church was quite consistent about the heresy implicit in Avicenna's idea that the human soul – through its imagination

– could affect other bodies.[31] Aware of this fact, Chanca quoted Avicenna's opinion, adding that, whatever Avicenna's opinion was, what is important is that he talked about fascination.[32] The use of authority as one of the main scholastic tools of inquiry leaves enough room for manipulation. An extreme example of this is Cartagena's refutation of Averroes: 'if Averroes would have spoken about fascination, he would have been of this opinion ...'. And obviously Cartagena would have disagreed.[33]

The various readings on the opinion of an author, alongside syllogistic reasoning and *questio* techniques, allowed Chanca and Cartagena to expound their views quite convincingly. Some of the authorities quoted to prove the reality of fascination did talk about some people producing harm to others by the power of their voice and sight, as Solinus held about certain African peoples[34] or (pseudo-) Alexander of Aprodisias did in the *Problemata*.[35] Others, such as Pliny in his *Historia naturalis*, referred to certain women from Scitia who, having a double pupil, can kill with their sight.[36] The Aristotelian tradition was also adduced as a proof of the reality of fascination, with the popular story contained in the *Secreta secretorum* of the young girl fed with napellus, whose sight and bite became poisonous.[37] An explicit reference to the Latin word *fascinare* as the production of harm through the eye, was included in a classical work, Virgil's *Eclogae*, when the author asked which eyes had fascinated their little sheep.[38] But, perhaps one of the most powerful direct mentions of fascination was contained in Saint Paul's letter to the Galatians ('*O insensati Galatae, quis vos fascinabit non obedire veritate, ante quorum oculos Iesus Christus praescriptus est, in vobis crucifixus?*').[39] The semantic extension of the term was developed in the *glossa ordinaria* that referred to certain people who are able to harm children with the power of their sight and in Thomas Aquinas's commentary on it, who specifically identified those people as old women.[40] Chanca used this quotation to create a parallel between the incredulity of the Galatians who did not believe in the Truth and Chanca's own contemporaries if they did not dare to believe in the reality of *fascinatio* after Chanca's advocacy of it.[41] Cartagena arranged the same material in a different way. In this case, the parallel – contained in Thomas's interpretation – was pointed out between those who after listening to Jesus's word threw it up, and the little children affected by fascination who vomited the milk they drink.[42] Aquinas's comment on Paul's letter was not the only place where he dealt with fascination in his lengthy work and our authors quoted explicitly two other works – *Summa Theologiae* and *Summa contra Gentiles* – where the Angelic Doctor refers to the production of fascination.[43] Within this tradition the opinion of Albert the Great was also referred to. Despite the fact that Albert had spoken on fascination in various places,[44] Cartagena choose Albert's *De motibus animalium*[45] to disagree with his opinions about the influence of imagination on the production of fascination.[46] Even if the disagreement was stronger with authors accused of false and heretical views, such as Avicenna or Algazel, yet both Avicenna's *Sextus de naturalibus* and Algazel's *Metaphisica* were widely quoted as important authorities that proved the reality of fascination.[47] The chronologically nearest author quoted was Gentile da Foligno. His opinion about the mechanism of production of fascination – contained in his commentary on the *Canon* – was analysed and rejected by Cartagena.[48] Chanca enlarged the list of the authorities brought into play with the views of wise men – Hebrews and Arabs – whose names he omitted due to the lack of familiarity of the reader with them.[49] Anonymous women's voices were also included as authorities in solving the problem of determining who are those more likely to be affected by fascination.[50]

Other quotations that did not refer explicitly to fascination were also utilized as a proof of its reality. The most common one was contained in Aristotle's *De sompno et vigilia* where it is said that if a women looked at a mirror when menstruating, the mirror would be misted.[51] From there to affirming that menstruating women could harm with the power of their sight was just a single step that both Chanca and Cartagena took.

Other texts were used to confirm prior assumptions that would be needed to discuss fascination, like the possibility of the existence of poison in a living human body. Apart from a large number of syllogisms that favoured this point, Chanca brought forward the authority of Averroes's *Colliget*, Avicenna's *Canon* and *De animalibus*, Galen's *Tegni, Commentarium in Hippocratis Aphorismos, De simplici medicina* and *De complexionibus*. To the same end he mentioned Arnau's *Parabolis medicationae* and Pietro d'Abano's *De venenis*.[52]

As we said before, all these quotations appeared in the context of a structure of discourse where the *questio* technique and all its paraphernalia of syllogistic reasoning were the main tools for the discussion and the validation of Chanca's and Cartagena's points of view.

But the reality of fascination could also be validated from experience. And Cartagena's opinion is conclusive: 'fascination is real because it does affect many children, and many of those die'.[53] Although from a modern perspective, Cartagena's clinical observation would be the strongest confirmation of the existence of the disease, it should be borne in mind that for Chanca or Cartagena, experience was just another way – neither better nor worse than authority and reason – to prove the reality of fascination. Thus, references to particular cases of fascination included the author's own experiences and trustworthy opinions.

The examples that Cartagena adduced from reliable sources included a case that took place in Guadalajara where a man broke mirrors with the power of a glance or the sad story that happened in Ocaña. There, a father fascinated his own children and killed his horses and, to avoid any human contact, he ran away to the desert.[54] Cartagena did refer to his clinical experience of diagnosis and treatment of fascinated children, but he does not tell us, as a proof of the reality of fascination, that he met any fascinator – male or female. Not much contact with fascinators was adduced by Chanca, although he suggested that he had met a fascinator, even if the case had happened a bit too late to test the fascinator's abilities. Chanca brought forward the example of a soldier who died, according to the Hebrew physicians that were treating him, from pestilential fevers. Chanca, who was also present during the last days of the process, thought that the soldier died from an excess of his own poisonous humours. This was confirmed by the choleric and dry complexion of the patient, his indecent morals and the reputation that he had as a fascinator among respectable people.[55] If fascinators were not often to be seen, personal experience (*nos observatione cernimus*) was taken into account when dealing with certain men who had the faculty to cure with their breath or saliva the effects of the bite of a rabid dog.[56] According to Cartagena, the example of the Spanish *salutatores* (literally, people who give health) was as valid as the observation of a fascinator in verifying the reality of fascination; because, he argued, if some people had a natural disposition to cure certain diseases, others could have the disposition to produce harm. The same parallel between people with natural powers to cure as guarantors of the existence of others with natural powers to harm, was adduced by Chanca. In the same line of reasoning and in addition to the mention of the *salutatores*, Chanca also explained that he had seen (*multi viderunt et ego ipse*) Alfonso V, King of Portugal (1438–81), curing *scrofulas* with his touch.[57]

Venomous bodies: sexing the agents

Sexual difference[58] is a crucial issue in the medical discourse about fascination. However, the disease was conceptualized in an apparently asexual framework. In the definition of fascination given by Chanca and Cartagena – a contagious disease in which certain venomous vapours came out from the eyes of one person, contaminated the air and entering a suitable body through the eyes or skin's pores produced the disease – the sex of the fascinator does not explicitly appear as a relevant matter.[59] Both men's and women's bodies could meet the requirements of a body with the power to fascinate; in fact, particularized examples of fascinators adduced by Chanca and Cartagena are sexed male. However, in the cultural frame where the disease was located, fascination was thought to be produced by a harmful power that women naturally possessed: a power whose origin was thought to be in either the potential or actual venomousness of women's bodies, based on the noxiousness of the menses.[60] This becomes clear when following the causality of fascination drawn by Cartagena. While discussing its causes, Cartagena stressed the influence of certain celestial constellations if someone was to acquire the power to fascinate; such a process could act upon either women or men. But there was one group of people which, defined by its sex and age, did not need any requirement of an astrological nature to acquire the power to fascinate. According to Cartagena, the natural process of ageing made women able to fascinate without any celestial help.[61] The same sexual ascription of a harmful power can be seen in Chanca's discussion of the characteristics of the fascinator, when he pointed out that under the same conditions – cold and dry complexions – women were more likely to fascinate than men.[62] Again, when considering and giving credence to the possibility of creating artificially (*per artem*) a poisonous human body, women's bodies were chosen to exemplify it.[63]

This view was certainly not limited to a medical reading of the evil eye. Contemporary theological literature showed its interest in fascination and women's agency over it. The evil eye was indeed one of the subjects dealt with in handbooks on superstitious beliefs and witchcraft practices, which flourished at the same time in Spain as guides for parish priests.[64] Theologians of the time had no doubt of the reality of fascination although for them, concerned as they were with the identification of religiously unorthodox practices, it was a borderline matter.[65] For them, it was important to determine whether the illness of the fascinated was due either to a natural disposition of the fascinators, to the agent's involvement with witchcraft or to a combination of both factors.

Martín de Andosilla (sometimes called Martín de Arlés), a regular canon trained in theology in Paris, wrote his *De Superstitionibus* in 1510, a work owing much to his previous experience while visiting the parishes of Valdeaibar, where he had been archdeacon.[66] Following Thomas Aquinas, he believed in a double causation for fascination. According to him, fascination was a natural process whose agents could be menstruating and old women whose wicked imagination set into motion the bodily spirits that, coming out through the eyes, would infect the surrounding air and cause sickness. However, it could be as well produced by a pact with the devil and in this instance, old women were more likely to be its agents since they were particularly wicked and prone to negotiate with the devil.[67] Pedro Ciruelo, a regular canon of Salamanca and professor of Thomist philosophy at the University of Alcalá where Antonio de Cartagena taught, published in 1538 his *Reprobación de las supersticiones y hechicerías*, a work which merited nine more reprints in the sixteenth century.[68] Even if he did not mention Cartagena's *Libellus*, Ciruelo's starting point is somewhat similar in acknowledging that many children died because of the evil eye. He saw a double causation for fascination, namely that naturally acquired and that produced by means of a demonic pact. He explicitly leaves its symptomatic treatment to physicians, but gives room for priests' intervention in those cases in which the disease was produced by witchcraft.[69] The division of labour between physicians and theologians envisioned by Ciruelo could be related to his silence in fully explaining fascination as a result of a natural process, particularly if it is considered that his professorship at the University of Alcalá could have given him familiarity with Cartagena's work. His reasoning on fascination seems to be apparently asexual. But neither Ciruelo nor most Renaissance and early modern theologians and inquisitors seem to have had any doubt about the proclivity of women to witchcraft.[70] A reading omitting devil intervention but focused on women's involvement in fascination as agents, can also be found in other contemporaries. Fray Martin de Castañega, a Franciscan theologian and preacher of the Inquisition, held a view on fascination that differs from Ciruelo and Andosilla. In his *Tratado de las supersticiones y hechicerías* published in Logroño in 1527[71] Castañega believed that fascination was a process due only to natural causes, thus leaving aside any demonic intervention. His reasoning, although only schematic, follows the lines of Chanca and Cartagena in maintaining that both menstruating and old women can inflict harm through the transmission of their corrupted humours helped by the air.[72]

The properties of menstrual blood

Women's menstruation was at the core of the identification of women's bodies with poisonous bodies in the medical tradition maintained by late medieval scholasticism. In the framework of fascination, after menarchy every women was potentially venomous when having the menses, and after losing her periods, every woman could in theory produce fascination. Only little girls were left without suspicion, but they would grow up to join the former groups.[73]

Menstruation, in medical thought, was considered to be the purgation that women needed to cleanse their bodies from excess moisture;

from a religious perspective, menstruation was the curse given to women after the Fall.[74] The conception of menstrual blood as a venomous substance, although it had its followers in antiquity,[75] does not seem to develop strongly in medical thought until the end of the thirteenth century, overlapping with a lively tradition of Salernitan origin which saw the properties of menstruation in a positive light, functioning as the way women's bodies developed to stay healthy.[76] The impact of Aristotelianism within scholasticism revived a misogynistic conception of women, in which female nature was despised to the extent of considering women poisonous beings,[77] and eventually found ways to usurp the medical tradition which had visualized female physiology without contempt.[78] The misogynistic position was built on a view of women as evil, popularized in a wide tradition of writings such as the *Secreta secretorum*[79] and the *Secreta mulierum*.[80] By the mid-sixteenth century the question of the noxiousness of menstruation had already become visible enough in medical literature to be the subject of debate.[81]

The venomous property of menstrual blood was widely used by Chanca and Cartagena as evidence of the possible coexistence of poison in a healthy body, and of the theoretical problems that the existence of fascination posed. The example of a misted mirror when looked at by a menstruating woman was constantly brought into play: when women are menstruating, some corrupted vapours from the boiling of menstrual blood ascend to the head and are eliminated through the pores of the eye. If a women then looks at a new mirror, a vaporous cloud will mist the mirror. The original version of the story contained in Aristotle's *De sompno et vigilia* (to be more accurate, in the *De somniis*) received different embellishments. In some the mirror is coloured with a bloody vapour, in others there are little red spots, but an uncoloured version was also available.[82] By mid-sixteenth century, some authors like the Spanish physician López de Corella added to the story his personal observation ('*and I have seen that*').[83]

If there was no doubt, according to Chanca and Cartagena, about the evil nature of menstruation, there were some inconsistencies about the danger of the sight of menstruating women. In some passages Cartagena defended their innocuousness, while in others he stated that, as they can infect the mirror, they can produce various sorts of harm.[84] The same can be said about Chanca's approach. When he explained that women were better able to fascinate than men, he based his assertion on the fact that women were more unstable than men, they ate more corrupted food – and so they generated more corrupted humours – and because every month in the days of their menstruation they expelled through their eyes corrupted vapours.[85] Neither Chanca nor Cartagena considered whether adult women who lacked their menses had power to fascinate – the best known examples of such people in this period being religious women and saints.[86]

However, there was agreement about the danger of menstrual blood itself. Chanca and Cartagena pointed to the generation of epileptics or lepers as the result of conception during menstruation, an idea shared by other university-trained medical authors of the fifteenth century,[87] which seems to have been extended by the mid-sixteenth to the possibility of generating monsters if conception takes place during menstruation.[88] Menstrual blood was also thought to be venomous if it was drunk, as was stated in the various treatises on poisons.[89] Its danger could also be tested by its actions on plants and metals.[90]

The conceptualization of menstrual blood as venomous was not confined to the theoretical framework that tried to explain the causation of the disease. It also had immediate practical consequences in the handling of the patient. Within a model of medical care dominated by Galenism, the care of a patient suffering from fascination would require the control of the six non-natural things. When dealing with the first of these non-naturals – the surrounding air – Chanca's recommendation was to keep the patient in a room of fresh air and, above all, not to allow visits by menstruating women because, Chanca argued, that would be to add poison to poison.[91]

When women grow up

The venomousness of menstrual blood did not decrease when the menses ceased. For if there was some ambivalence about the power to fascinate that menstruating women had, according to Chanca and Cartagena there was no doubt about the possibility that old women could inflict it. An analysis based on the physical changes of women's bodies after menopause was given by Cartagena to explain this fact. The menstrual blood that was expelled when the woman was young, could not be eliminated when she was old because her expulsive power had decreased and the tract for its elimination had been narrowed. Thus, Cartagena concluded, old women always carry menstrual blood in their veins.[92] And he added that the poisonous nature of the menstrual blood does not affect them because, while they were young, their bodies were used to it in every menstruation.[93] The vapours that came from this corrupted blood (Cartagena's explanation continues) ascended to the brain and they were eliminated through the eyes. If those venomous vapours met a proper recipient – children in Cartagena's opinion, children and weak adults in Chanca's view – they would have the effect of a poison on the patient's body.[94]

Despite their theoretical consistency in pointing out women as producers of fascination, Chanca and Cartagena also referred to the possibility of other agents. However, the image of the old women fascinating children prevailed in other medical works which, although including fascination, did not incorporate a theoretical argumentation comparable to that of Chanca or Cartagena. This image is the one chosen by the Spanish physician López de Corella to entitle a question he devoted to fascination in his *Treszientas preguntas de cosas naturales*: 'And why can old women fascinate children'.[95] This work is still in need of an accurate study, but its formal structure of short poems followed by a commentary, and the fact that it was written in Spanish, suggest that it was intended for a wide audience.

The view that old women possessed a potential harmful power to inflict on tender children also has its echoes in other medical genres. Damián Carbó, city physician of Majorca, took this fact seriously into account. In his book on midwifery, the first known work on this subject to be published in Spain (1541), Carbó openly warned that old women should not be allowed in the delivery room, except for those close to the mother-to-be, such as her mother or her mother-in-law.[96] Caution against old women in the delivery space is emphasized by Pavian professor of medicine Anthonius Guainerius who, acknowledging the presence of old women in the birthroom, recommends the physician to engage in prayerful words to cleanse the atmosphere from dangerous women who are old.[97]

The fact that Carbó does allow old women in the birthroom as long as they are closely related to the new-born may have a double significance. On the one hand, it suggests that women who are close to the new baby would avoid casting their glances directly upon him or her, and this precaution would restrain their potential danger. On the other, it reflects the importance that some authors gave to the role of an evil intention or imagination in the production of fascination. The influence of the soul over the body had been a current topic in medical scholasticism, which found enough space for discussion of its mechanism of production and to advise on its effects – from blushing to sudden death – in many treatises of the time, but mainly in the popular *Regimina sanitatis*. Various movements of the vital spirits and natural heat from or towards the heart could explain the physical effects of, for example, joy or anger.[98] This basic model was behind the belief that the effective danger of old women as fascinators increases if the glance is accompanied with a strong desire to produce harm. Hate or envy would produce a stronger boiling of the venomous blood and thus more subtle vapours and more effective poisonous glances. Chanca, although relying on this mechanism, offered an interesting variation where he emphasized the effect of the strong desire on the glance's object, without distinguishing the quality of the feeling, which could be hatred or love.[99] Even if they did not provide a theoretical explanation, most theologians, following Thomas Aquinas's teachings, believed in the influence of an evil imagination in the production of fascination. This is the position of Martín de Andosilla, who quoted Aquinas on this point, and it is also the view held by Castañega.[100] Extending Damián Carbó's suggestion, Martín de Castañega advised wet nurses to keep their babies away from old women's poisonous glances. But he also addressed old women directly, warning them about the potential harm of their glances and advising them not to look into the children's eyes or to kiss them on their mouths, because 'if in recalling it, they would have done it with wickedness, then the poison [of their glances] would be enhanced with the power of the imagination, and so they would fatally sin against the Fifth Commandment'.[101]

However, this view was a matter of debate. Cartagena insisted on the non-intervention of intention in the production of fascination.[102] In consonance with his idea of the celestial influence in the acquisition of the power to fascinate, he went further in advising no punishment for those who fascinated because they were just acting according to their nature. In fact, Cartagena states that legal prescriptions of his time did indeed follow this fair approach: 'because laws', wrote Cartagena, 'never established any penalty to punish those who do not fascinate under the control of their will but do it only through the celestial quality they have naturally'.[103] We have been unable to document historically specific cases where accusations against fascinators were made.[104] This could perhaps be explained if one takes into consideration how anthropologists see the evil eye nowadays. Drawing from their ethnographic data, they understand the evil eye to be a belief that fundamentally differs from witchcraft practices precisely in that it does not involve the search for and accusation of the producer.[105] Curative practices are straightforwardly related to the identification of the disease, hence the recognition of the gazer becomes unnecessary.[106] It is unclear whether Cartagena's view on intention extends to all procedures of fascination or only to those who acquired the *vis effascinandi* under celestial influence, leaving aside the old women who did not need this influence. Later in the century some medical authors found women not guilty, while evaluating their actions as due to their natural constitution.[107]

Men are neither menstruating nor old women

By the end of the fifteenth century and the first third of the sixteenth, learned discourses on fascination were set in a social climate where women had become a topic of debate, and the *Querelle des femmes* had acquired a cultural visibility unknown at earlier stages when women had not got involved in the controversy.[108] Fascination as a theme had grown within and in parallel with the strengthening of a misogynistic concept of women which from the mid-thirteenth century on had affected learned culture. The triumph of Aristotelian thinking in scholasticism was not unrelated to this phenomenon, since its theory of sex polarity – meaning that the sexes are significantly different and that men are superior to women – was central in the thirteenth-century Parisian faculties of theology, medicine and law. The popularity of misogynistic works ascribed to Aristotle are a sign of the extent and wide spread of his model.[109] That sex polarity is at stake in early modern Spanish conceptions of fascination becomes fairly clear when one considers not only the act of producing illness, but sets it side by side with contemporary views of healing.

The sexed approach of the medical discourse about fascination was stressed by bringing forward men with a natural power to heal. In the medical treatises that deal with fascination, a parallel is always made between the natural power that some persons (more likely women) had to inflict harm on others with their sight, and the natural capacity that some persons (men only) had to cure various diseases with their breath, the *saludadores*, literally, health givers. The causality – celestial influence – adduced by Cartagena to explain this positive power seems to be the same as for the acquisition of the power to fascinate. Indeed, as has already been said, the existence of the *saludadores* was pointed out by Chanca and by Cartagena as a proof of the reality of fascination. This opposition between the different capacities of men and women was widely adopted and held by other sixteenth-century Spanish medical authors. López de Corella's *Treszientas preguntas* clearly depicted the asymmetrical parallelism between fascinating women and healing men. When asking who the producers of fascination were, López de Corella had no hesitation in ascribing the power to old women. However, in his commentary on the question and without feeling the need to explain why the two topics run together, he referred to men (*saludadores*) of such a good star that they can influence positively the health of others.[110] The picture was shared both by contemporary natural philosophers and theologians. Martín de Castañega strongly asserted that there were men that 'due to the temperament of their complexional qualities' have a natural power to cure through their breath or their touch.[111]. Pedro Mexía, a humanist nobleman who wrote a compendium of knowledge first published in 1540, believed that harmful natural properties could be held by both women and men, but conceived the *saludadores* as male, ascribing to them the power of curing rabid dogs.[112]

The distribution of natural properties ascribed to women and men during the first third of the sixteenth century becomes, then, fairly clear. Women can naturally only inflict harm: old women were fascinators, menstruating women could or could not have such a power, but they would certainly grow up and lose their menses to enrich the number of the old ones. Finally, certain men can have the power to fascinate through celestial influence, an influence which could also be the cause of their ability to cure various diseases – with their touch or with their breath.

Fascination and the danger of women

Discourses on the production of harm and on the natural or acquired abilities to heal, were intricately intertwined and it is in their intersection where the danger of women can be fully perceived. Both Chanca and Cartagena re-elaborated as 'fascination' a current problem in which, among other outcomes of misfortune, the health of an individual suffered. The problem was generally being identified, treated and prevented within informal networks of care, mainly supported by women. Only sixty years before Chanca's treatise, Enrique of Villena was very precise in stating why physicians were not concerned with fascination in his own time. This illness was considered by doctors, according to him, a women's business, and being so it had been undervalued and left undiscussed by dominant medical discourses: 'Physicians nowadays know very little about this, because they dismiss the cure of this illness by saying that it is women's business, and they consider it beneath them, and that is why they do not reach its differences and secrets, which are reached by paying attention to it.'[113]

Signs of women's expertise on treating fascination are found among medical and theological authors, who incidentally explain what certain women thought about the cause of this illness and how it could be prevented and treated. Engelbert of Admont, in the first known treatise on fascination, stated that expert women (*mulieres expertae*) thought that both words and sight could inflict the illness on children.[114] Martín de Castañega recognized efficacy in a current practice in child-rearing – that of holding little pieces of mirrors to displace evil glances. And he recommended its use to wet nurses in order to keep their children safe.[115] Martín de Andosilla attributed to women the same practice of prevention and condemned it.[116] Condemnations frequently came with the recognition of women's command of a treatment. The efficacy of herbal remedies prepared by *sortilege et malefice* is not questioned, although it is stated that they work because of their natural powers, and not due to the words associated with them.[117] But women's authority and expertise were not only recognized on the practical side of the handling of the disease, and were extended to women's understanding of the mechanism of the production of fascination.[118] The acknowledgement of women's expertise did not imply its approval by an academic physician engaged in condemning women's healing practices. Without explicitly writing on fascination, Damián Carbó stated that women were responsible for the health of their children, and denounced the fact that women would seek the advice of midwives instead of that of the physicians not only regarding their health problems but also those of their children.[119] The rhetorical effort that Chanca and Cartagena made to prove their control over fascination was fully acknowledged by other university-trained authors who believed in the danger of women's involvement in healing practices. University-trained physicians had long been asserting their claims against empirics on the basis of the danger implicit in their practice. *Ydiote* and *illiterati* were identifying terms which did not point to any fundamental state in the constitution of human identity. The meaning of the exclusion from medical practice of groups such as *mulieres* and *vetule*, cannot then be dismissed with a general reference to empirics. For it is only this group of people who are specified by their sex and age, the ones who carry a medical discourse built on their natural capacity for producing harm.

The change of the epistemological status of *fascinatio* had important social consequences. By eliminating as superstitious others' ways of performing diagnosis and treatment of the evil eye, the university-trained physician placed fascination in his own domain of competence. Thus women, who had played the role of experts, were reduced from the double status of potential healers and producers of illness to just the latter. The shift was reinforced when discussing women's involvement in the treatment of fascination. According to Cartagena, those women who offer themselves as healers of fascination can only do it – if they do it at all – by establishing a pact with the devil.[120] The association between fascination and witchcraft was not made in any of the steps of Chanca's and Cartagena's explanation of the production of the illness; however, the connection was made when healing was concerned: women's involvement in a beneficial act of healing could only be made through the exercise of evil.

The danger implicit in their performing medical acts resulted in a triple bind for women: they were ignorant as practitioners, they are naturally potential producers of disease themselves, and they are prone to cure fascination by means of witchcraft.[121] Once this agenda had been established, a cultural setting for women's disempowerment had been drawn: but not all women bore the same danger.

The power to fascinate is consistently ascribed to old women, who possessed this property unless they avoided it by performing certain preventive practices. In this situation, danger does not come from an individual – as happens with witchcraft, since inquisitorial practices were developed to individualize witches – but it is ascribed to a particular group of women diffusely disseminated through social life.

The potential harmful effect of living together with old women could be prevented by others through segregation: so the safest way to keep fascination away would be to avoid eye contact with them. As was seen above, there are signs of this precaution against old women being implemented, and Chanca was certainly aware of the consequences of this agenda for social relations. He wondered with despair how it could be that nature, whose goal is human life, produces venomous human beings? Leaning on Aristotle's *Politics*, where it is stated that men are created by nature to live in society, Chanca wonders how nature can frustrate its own main goal?[122] This contradiction puts him in a difficult situation. He has no other resort but to acknowledge his inability to explain through intellectual reasoning something he knows through experience, i.e., nature's production of poisonous human beings.[123] Chanca faced what he perceived as a difficult intellectual contradiction – that of matching his experience of reality with Aristotle's thought – by avoiding naming that venomous social group. He certainly underlined the general inclination of women, young and old, towards the production of fascination, but in this context it is particularly significant that Chanca, who was familiar with Thomas Aquinas's commentary on Saint Paul's epistle to the Galatians, never mentioned Aquinas's direct opinion of old women as permanently potential producers of fascination.[124] In fact, it seems that his awareness of the consequences that naming agents had for social relations, may have stopped him from allocating direct blame.

Antonio de Cartagena did not perceive the existence of natural agents of fascination as a contradiction in the goals of nature. He takes a further step to clearly naturalize danger and to name a particular social group as producers of fascination. Thus, the *vetule*, who had not appeared in Chanca's test, take a prominent role in Cartagena's explanation. Cartagena's work on fascination translated into a medical frame a dominant trend across patriarchal cultures where old women have been the object of fear and the repository of social danger.[125] In the sixteenth century a particular increase in contempt for old women arose; cultural anxieties as well as social discriminations were directed against them as being the witches' prototype.[126] Fear of older women breaks what has been called the 'feminine genealogy', disempowering women from their social and symbolic potentiality.[127] It has been argued that changes in the gender system in sixteenth-century Spain were symbolically implemented through the suppression of the feminine from culturally dominant discourses.[128] The medical explanation of fascination contributed to this trend by stressing the harmful effects of women's nature.

Notes

* We deeply acknowledge particular help and general suggestions provided by Jole Agrimi, Rosa Ballester, Clive Cox, Monica Green, Harmke Kamminga, José Pardo Tomás, Juan Antonio Paniagua and Nancy Siraisi, as well as the rich discussion of the first version of the paper by the participants at the original conference. The editors, Jon Arrizabalaga, Andy Cunningham, Roger French and Luis García-Ballester, have been most supportive of our work throughout the research process.

1. 'Primum signum est cognitio dispositionis egroti, videlicet si sit infans formosus, graciosus et precipue si fuerit generosus vestitus ... vel si sit iuvenis et fuerit delicatus, levis sanguinis quemadmodum sunt colerici de colera rubea aut colerici sanguinei qui propter aperturam pororum et propter subtilitatem humorum faciliter pasciuntur a causis extrinsecis et cum in hiis non aparuerit alia evidens causa suspicandum est de oculo', Diego Alvarez Chanca, *Tractatus de fascinatione*, Seville, Petrus Brun, 1499, sig. c_3r. For bibliographical information on this edition see Juan Antonio Paniagua, *El doctor Chanca y su obra médica*, Madrid, Ediciones Cultura Hispanica, 1977, pp. 67–80.
2. For a map of the geographic distribution of the belief in the evil eye, see Clarence Maloney, 'Introduction', in Clarence Maloney (ed.) *The Evil Eye*, New York, Columbia University Press, 1976, pp. xii–xiii.
3. Enrique Perdiguero, 'El mal de ojo: de la literatura antisupersticiosa a la antropogía médica' *Asclepio*, 38 (1986), pp. 47–66; Anton Erkoreka, *Begizkoa. El mal de ojo entre los vascos*, Bilbao, Ekain, 1995; Marino Pérez Alvarez, 'El mal de ojo', in Marino Pérez Alvarez (ed.), *La superstición en la ciudad*, Barcelona, Siglo XXI, 1993, pp. 33–70.
4. Mary Douglas, *Purity and Danger. An Analysis of the Concepts of Pollution and Taboo*, London: Ark Paperbacks, 1984 [1st edn London, 1966]; *Eadem* 'Witchcraft and leprosy. Two strategies for rejection', in her *Risk and Blame. Essays in Cultural Theory*, London and New York, Routledge, 1992, pp. 83–101.
5. The broad semantic domain of the word *fascinatio* and its equivalents in different languages are listed in Jules Tuchman, 'La fascination', *Mélusine. Recueil de mythologie, littérature populaire, traditions et usages*, 2 (1884–85), pp. 169–73.
6. For a biography of Alvarez Chanca and an analysis of his work see, Juan Antonio Paniagua (above, n. 1). We are grateful to Professor Paniagua for sending us a photocopy of Chanca's treatise (being the copy from the library of the J. L. Galdiano Foundation, Madrid).
7. Paniagua (see above, note 1), pp. 66–8.
8. Antonio de Cartagena held the chair of *prima medicina* in Alcalá, at the

request of Cardinal Cisneros, from 1510 to 1532. There is no reliable biography of Cartagena and the scarce data available is often contradictory. See, Antonio Hernández Morejon, *Historia bibliográfica de la medicina española*, Madrid, Imprenta de la viuda de Jordán e hijos, 1942–45 (reprinted New York and London, Johnson Reprint Corporation, 1967), vol. 1, pp. 219–21; Luis Alonso Muñoyerro, 'Provisión de cátedras de medicina en Alcalá de Henares (1509–1641)', *X Congreso Internacional de Historia de la Medicina. Libro de Actas*, Madrid, 1935, vol. 1, fasc. II, pp. 72–199, and *idem, La Facultad de Medicina en la Universidad de Alcalá de Henares*, Madrid, Consejo Superior de Investigaciones Científicas-Instituto Jerónimo Zurita, 1945, pp. 198–9.

9. Antonio de Cartagena, *Liber de peste, de signis febrium et de diebus creticis. Additus est etiam huic operi libellus ejusdem de fascinatione*, Alcalá de Henares, Miguel de Eguía, 1530. For a description of this edition, see *Index Aureliensis*, vol. 7, p. 10, no. 132.686 (Aureliae Aquensis, Index Aureliensis Foundation, 1982); Julian Martin Abad, *La imprenta en Alcalá de Henares (1502–1600)*, Madrid, Arco/Libros S.A., 1991– , vol. 1– , pp. 400–401, no. 234.
10. Juan Lázaro Gutiérrez, *Opusculo de fascino*, Lyons, Ph. Borde, L. Arnaud, C. L. Rigaud, 1653, ff. 30–37.
11. Francisco Pérez Cascales de Guadalajara, *Liber de affectionibus puerorum, una cum tractatu de morbo illo vulgariter garrotillo appellato, cum duabus questionibus. Altera, De gerentibus utero rem appetentibus denegatum. Altera vero De fascinatione*, Madrid, Ludovicus Sanchez Typographus Regius, 1611, f. 123v. In fact, during the sixteenth and seventeenth centuries fascination became a theme in the growing literature on pediatrics, as has been observed by Rosa Ballester (personal communication, 13 September 1993). Francisco Núñez de Oria considered fascination in his *Libro de los casos, y enfermedades de los niños recién nacidos*, the section on children's diseases of his *Libro del parto humano*, published in 1580. Cf. José María López Piñero and Francesc Bujosa, *Los tratados de enfermedades infantiles en la España del renacimiento*, Valencia, Cátedra de Historia de la Medicina-Universidad de Valencia, 1982, p. 74.
12. We use 'ancient' as the equivalent of Chanca's use of *antiqui*, which includes medieval authors.
13. Alvarez Chanca (see above, note 1), sig. a_2r.
14. In the second part of his treatise, when Chanca deals with the treatment of fascination, he does not just consider certain remedies but makes clear that he is addressing those who have certain familiarity with it. The sophistication of his arguments and the fact that it is written in Latin suggest that he has a medical audience in mind: 'non curo explicare timore prolixitatis quia hunc tractatum non feci pro ignorantibus' Alvarez Chanca, (see above, note 1), sig. c_5v.
15. Bernardo de Gordon, *Opus Lilium medicinae*, Lyons, Gulielmus Rovilius, 1550, f. 4.
16. See the classic study by Juan Antonio Paniagua, 'Clínica del renacimiento', in Pedro Laín Entralgo (ed.), *Historia Universal de la Medicina*, Barcelona, Salvat, 1972, vol. 4, pp. 87–105. On the conceptualization of new diseases and its relation to professional battles, see Jon Arrizabalaga, John Henderson and Roger French, *The Great Pox. The French Disease*

in Renaissance Europe, New Haven and London, Yale University Press, 1997, pp. 252–77.

17. In the spring of 1493, Chanca got royal permission to accompany Columbus on his second trip to America (1493–94). From this experience Chanca wrote a letter to the Cabildo of Seville in which he explains in great detail his own fascination with the peoples, animals and plants of the new land. See, Juan Antonio Paniagua, 'Un médico europeo en el descubrimiento: Diego Alvarez Chanca', in José Maria López Piñero (ed.), *Viejo y nuevo continente: La medicina en el encuentro de dos mundos*, Madrid, Beecham, 1992, pp. 91–102; C. Varela, 'Carta del doctor Diego Alvarez Chanca al cabildo de Sevilla', in J. Gil and C. Varela *Cartas de particulares a Colón y relaciones coetáneas*, Madrid, CSIC, 1984, pp. 152–76.
18. See Paniagua (see above, note 1), pp. 99–123. A critical edition of Arnau's work is now available. See Juan Antonio Paniagua and Pedro Gil Sotres (eds), *Arnaldi de Villanova Opera Medica Omnia*, vol. 4.1, Barcelona, Publicacions de la Universitat de Barcelona, 1990.
19. The scholastic use of authority and reason as criteria to validate and develop medical knowledge based on the experience of an individual practitioner has been analysed by Chiara Crisciani, 'History, Novelty and Progress in Scholastic Medicine', *Osiris*, 6 (1990), pp. 118–39. Within medical scholasticism, the grounds for disagreement and open criticism of the opinion of the ancients from the late thirteenth century onwards are analysed by Fernando Salmon. 'The Many Galens of the Medieval Commentators on Vision', *Revue d'Histoire des Sciences*, 50 (1997), pp. 397–419.
20. On Engelbert's life and works, see J. B. Fowler, *Intellectual Interests of Englebert of Admont*, New York, Columbia University Press, 1947; for a list of manuscripts, see pp. 191–2. The work was attributed to Nicolo de Oresme in some MSS but his authorship has been dismissed. Nicolo had a chapter on fascination in his *Tractatus de configurationibus qualitatum et motuum* and its contents has nothing to do with Engelbert's. See Marshall Clagett, *Nicole Oresme and the Medieval Geometry of Qualities and Motions. A treatise on the Uniformity and Difformity of Intensities Known as Tractatus de configurationibus qualitatum et motuum*, Madison, University of Wisconsin Press, 1968, pp. 380–86.
21. For an analysis of Engelbert's ideas on fascination, see Lynn Thorndike, *A History of Magic and Experimental Science*, New York, Columbia University Press, 1934, vol. 3, pp. 434–5.
22. A critical edition of the treatise and an introductory study in, Enrique de Villena, *Tratado de aojamiento. A cura di Anna Maria Gallina*, Bari, Adriatica Editrice, 1978, (text on pp. 93–134).
23. Villena (see above, note 22), pp. 96–7.
24. Paniagua (see above, note 1), pp. 84–5.
25. Anna M. Gallina also held this view when she compared certain parts of Chanca's second part and Villena's. See Villena (see above, note 22), pp. 84–8.
26. Marcelino Menéndez Pelayo, *Historia de los heterodoxos españoles*, Madrid, CSIC, 2nd edn, 1965, vol. 1, pp. 615–20.
27. Villena explained the superstitious remedies but did not give the explanation of their functioning because that would be against the divine law:

'Prevention and cure of fascination can take place through three different ways as used by the ancients, and now by the moderns: through superstition, through virtue, through quality' ('por tres vias fue proveyda e usada de los antiguos, e agora los modernos: por stupesxisçion, por virtud, por qualitat'). Villena (see above, note 22), pp. 105–9.

28. ' ... et in practica multo minus suficienter repertum est; ideo cum timore ad eam accedo non nisi pauca que dispersim in antiquis reperi aducam. Veruntamen, omnia supersticiosa, que tam in remediando quam in cognoscendo morbum fascinationis a multis traduntur et ad hunc hodie in usu habentur, relinquam tanquam stem fidey repugnantia', Diego Alvarez Chanca (see above, note 1), sig. b_8v. For an overview on various remedies to prevent and cure the evil eye in South Spain during the Middle Ages see Alejandro García Avilés, 'Religiosidad popular y pensamiento mágico en algunos ritos del sureste español. Notas sobre el mal de ojo en la Edad Media', *Verdolay*, 3 (1991), pp. 125–39.

29. The various authorities referred to below, are repeatedly mentioned alongside Chanca's and Cartagena's treatises. We will merely give reference to those passages found to be more illustrative of the author's viewpoint.

30. Avicenna, *Liber de anima seu sextus de naturalibus IV–V*, ed. S. Van Riet; G. Verbeke, (introd.), Louvain and Leyden, Brill, 1968, IV pars, ch. 4, p. 65. Thomas Aquinas, *Summa Theologiae*. 1 pars, q. 117, a. 3 ('Utrum homo per virtutem animae possit corporalem materiam immutare'), Madrid, BAC, 1978, pp. 804–5.

31. Roland Hissette, *Enquête sur les 219 articles condamnés à Paris le 7 mars 1277*, Louvain, Publications Universitaires, 1977, pp. 116–17.

32. 'quidquid sit de opinione sua suficit quod concedit fascinationem', Diego Alvarez Chanca, (see above, note 1), sig. b_2v.

33. 'et huius opinionis esset Averrois, si de fascinatione loqueretur', Antonio de Cartagena (see above, note 9), f. 2vb.

34. Antonio de Cartagena (see above, note 9), f. 1rb. Solinus, *C. Ivlii Solini Collectanea Rerum Memorabilium*, ed. Theodore Mommsen, Berlin, Weidmann, 1958, pp. 13 and 26.

35. Diego Alvarez Chanca (see above, note 1), b_2v. *Problemata Aristotelis cum duplici translatione antiqua dupliciter et nova scilicet Theodori Gaze cum expositione Petri Aponi. Tabula secundum magistrum Petrum de Tussignano per alphabetum. Probemata Alexandri Aphrodisei. Problemata Plutarchi*, Venice, Bonetus Locatellus, 1501, sectio V, n. 52, f. 286rb. In several editions, Alexander's *Problemata* are cited together with (ps) Aristotle's *Problemata* and Pietro d'Abano's comment on it. One of Pietro d'Abano's commentaries is in fact a recollection of Avicenna's and Algazel's viewpoints on fascination. See ibid., f. 83vb.

36. Antonio de Cartagena (see above, note 9), f. 1rb (also 5va). The quotation of Pliny's position (contained in f. 1rb) is a long one and includes Cicero's opinion on the existence of people with the special powers of enduring the effect of fire. Pliny, *Natural History*, Cambridge, MA and London, Harvard Univesity Press, 1989, pp. 516–19 (The Loeb Classical Library, LCL 352, VII, ii. 16–19). Chanca refers to the same story as found in *Cosmogrofi*; see Diego Alvarez Varez Chanca (see above, note 1), sig. b_2v.

37. Diego Alvarez Chanca, (see above, note 1), sig. a_3v. For a comprehensive

analysis of this story, see Claude Thomasset, *Une vision du monde à la fin du XIIIè siècle. Commentaire du dialogue de Placides et Timéo*, Geneva, Librairie Droz, 1982, pp. 73–108.

38. Diego Alvarez Chanca, (see above, note 1), sig. b_2v; Antonio de Cartagena (see above, note 9), f. 1rb. Virgil, *Eclogues*, 3, l. 103 ('nescio quis teneros oculos mihi fascinat agnos'), edited by Robert Coleman, Cambridge, Cambridge University Press, 1977, p. 51.
39. *Epistola B. Pauli Apostoli ad Galatas*, Madrid, BAC, 1985, pars secunda, 3, p. 1130.
40. The glossa ordinaria and Thomas Aquinas's comment on it are in Aquinas (see above, note 30), pp. 804–5. See also Thomas Aquinas, *Commentarii in Epistolam ad Corinthios I (continuatio). Commentarii in caeteras omnes epistolas S. Pauli*, Paris, Ludovicum Vives, 1876, vol. 21, pp. 200–202.
41. Diego Alvarez Chanca, (see above, note 1), sig. b_2r–v.
42. Antonio de Cartagena (see above, note 9), f. 2rb.
43. Antonio de Cartagena (see above, note 9), f. 2ra–b. Thomas Aquinas, *Summa contra Gentiles*, Paris, Ludovicum Vives, 1874, lib. III, ch. 103, pp. 391–2. Aquinas (see above, note 29), pp. 804–5.
44. Albert's definition of fascination – as the action of the soul of one person over another through the means of sight or other senses – is quite consistent in his works. See Albertus Magnus, *Opera Omnia, vol. 9 (De somno et vigilia)*, Augustus Borgnet (ed.), Paris, Ludovicum Vives, 1890, lib. III, tract. 1, p. 185; *idem, Opera Omnia, vol. 27 (Commentarii in II Sententiarum*, Augustus Borgnet (ed.), Paris, Ludovicum Vives, 1894, dist. VII, F, art. 7, p. 153; *idem, De animalibus libri XXVI, vol. 2*, Hermann Stadler (ed.), Münster, Aschendorff, 1920, lib. XXII, tract. 1, ch. 5, p. 1353; *idem, Opera Omnia, vol. 17 (De fato)* Paulus Simon (ed.), Münster, Aschendorff, 1975, art. 2, p. 70; *idem, Opera Omnia, vol. 16 (Metaphysica. Libros quinque priores)* Bernhardus Geyer (ed.), Münster, Aschendorff, 1960, lib. IV, tract. 3, ch. 2, p. 187.
45. Albertus Magnus, *Parvorum naturalium (De motibus animalium)*, Augustus Borgnet (ed.), Paris, Ludovicum Vives, 1890, vol. 9, pp. 257–303.
46. Antonio de Cartagena (see above, note 9), f. 3rb.
47. Antonio de Cartagena (see above, note 9), f. 1vb y 1rb. Avicenna (see above, note 30), pp. 64–5; Algazel, *Metaphysics. A Mediaeval Translation*, J. T. Muckle (ed.), Toronto, Institute of Medieval Studies, 1933, pars II, tract. V, ch. 9, p. 194. Both texts were common quotations from the second half of the thirteenth century onwards when dealing with fascination and the power of soul over body, see Lynn Thorndike, 'Imagination and Magic. The Force of Imagination on the Human Body and of Magic on the Human Mind', *Mélanges Eugène Tisserant, vol. VII*, Città del Vaticano, Biblioteca Apostolica Vaticana, 1964, pp. 354–6.
48. Antonio de Cartagena (see above, note 9), f. 2vb; Gentile da Foligno, *Primus [et secundus] Avicennae Canononis ... una cum lucidissima Gentilis Fulginatis expositione*, Venice, Heirs of O. Scotus, 1520, Lib. 1, Fen II, Doctr. I, Suma I, cap. VIII, 102ra–102rb.
49. 'Cui veritati consonant multi alii doctores tam arabes quam ebraici quorum nomina hic non aduco quia non sunt noti apud omnes', Diego Alvarez Chanca (see above, note 1), sig. b_2v.

50. ' ... cuius oppositum contingit in corporibus debilibus et teneris quemadmodum sunt corpora puerorum et aliquorum adultorum habentium debilitatem compaginis et subtilitatem humorum a quo ortum habuit vulgare dictum a mulieribus dicentibus aliquem cito fascinari quia levem habet sanguinem et sic patet responsio ad dubium et eciam solutio ad argumentum', Diego Alvarez Chanca, (see above, note 1), sig. b_4v.
51. Diego Alvarez Chanca, (see above, note 1), sig. b_1r; Antonio de Cartagena (see above, note 9), f. 2rb. Aristotle, *On the Soul. Parva naturalia. On Breath*, London, Heinemann, 1986, [*On Dreams*, vol. 2, p. 357].
52. Diego Alvarez Chanca, (see above, note 1), sigs a_2v–a_3v.
53. 'Disserto ergo fascinationem veram esse, qua plurimi pueri inficiuntur plurimique fascinati moriuntur', Antonio de Cartagena (see above, note 9), f. 1rb.
54. 'Et nos, nostris temporibus, vidimus homines quoscumque inspexerint fascinantes; et relatam est mihi a fide dignis in civitate Guadalajara fuisse hominem qui solo intuitu minutatim specula frangebat; etiam in oppido in Ocaña relatum est mihi certissime fuisse hominem qui non modo extraneos, immo filios proprios oculis fascinabat et sepe perierunt equi aut pueri quos ipse inspexit quocirca affirmatum est ipsum conversationem humanam fugisse et in deserta se transtulisse', Antonio de Cartagena (see above, note 9), f. 1rb.
55. 'Erat vir iste complexione colericus, adustus, pravorum morum, difamatus apud vulgum et apud viros discretos pro maximo fascinatore, de quo multa referebuntur que ad sensum visa fuerunt in opere fascinandi, ex quibus concluditur quod in corpore humano reperitur venenum', Diego Alvarez Chanca, (see above, note 1), sigs a_3r–v.
56. 'Etiam nos observatione cernimuu salutatores in Hispania plurimos qui solo anhelitu liberant omnes eos quos momordis canis rabidus', Antonio de Cartagena (see above, note 9), f. 1rb.
57. 'Item per naturam reperitur homo habens virtutem sanandi aliquem morbum ut patet de rege Alfonso portugalense que habuit virtutem sanandi scrofulas solo tactu manuum et multi viderunt et ego ipse. Et eciam reperiuntur multi habentes virtutem sanandi rabiam sicut ubique reperitur per experientia', Diego Alvarez Chanca, (see above, note 1), a_4r. For a general account of the royal touch, see Marc Bloch, *The Royal Touch: Sacred Monarchy and Scrofula in England and France*, London, Routledge and Kegan Paul, 1973.
58. We use sex (and sexual difference) as the category which identifies the historical existence of women and men. In this regard, we take a position distinct from the unisex model which according to Thomas Laqueur prevailed in Western Europe until the eighteenth century: see Thomas Laqueur, *Making Sex: Body and Gender from the Greeks to Freud*, Cambridge, MA, Harvard University Pres, 1990. For an in-depth critique of Laquer's arguments, see Katherine Park and Robert A. Nye, 'Destiny is Anatomy', *The New Republic*, 18 February (1991), pp. 53–7. To us, the distinction between sexual difference and gender is important since we understood our sources as constructing gender upon sexual difference, that is, giving patriarchal meaning to a prior acknowledgement and particular explanation of sexual difference. On the political and historiographical implications of this stance, see Nancy Partner, 'No

Sex, No Gender', in Nancy Partner (ed.), *Studying Medieval Women*, Cambridge, MA, The Medieval Academy of America, 1993, pp. 117–41 (originally published in *Speculum*, April 1993).

59. 'Hiis dissertis probo effascinationem a manifesta qualitate evenire posse quoniam possibile est illum, cuius humores corrupti sunt vaporibus oculis emissis aerem inficere, et aerem pueros pre nimia teneritate modice resistentes', Antonio de Cartagena (see above, note 9), f. 4ra; 'Alio modo accipitur proprie prout ab omnibus communiter accipi solet et sic fascinatio solum fit per contagium factum per visum corporis humani in aliud corpus, Diego Alvarez Chanca, (see above, note 1), sig. b_3v.
60. Danielle Jacaquart and Claude Thomasset, *Sexuality and Medicine in the Middle Ages*, trans. Matthew Adamson, Oxford, Polity Press, 1988, pp. 74–8, and Helen R. Lemay, *Women's Secrets. A Translation of Pseudo-Albertus Magnus's "De Secretis Mulierum" with Commentaries*, Albany, New York, State University of New York Press, 1992, pp.34–49.
61. 'Vetule vim effascinandi habent, licet non necessario celestem', Antonio de Cartagena (see above, note 9), f. 5va.
62. 'Et ego per experientiam aliquando vidi homines difamatos hac pessima propietate fuissent predicte conplexionis. Credo eciam, ceteris paribus, in maiori numero reperiri mulieres hoc crimine lesas quam viros. Ideo quia ratione sexus fortiori lapsu a temperamento labantur et quia ut plurimum corruptibilioribus cibis vesentur quam viri, eciam quia quolibet mense ut menstruose superflucitates expellantur ebullit sanguis melanconicus menstruosus propter quam ebullitionem ascendunt vapores ad capud corrupti qui per oculum possunt exire ut apparet in exemplo de speculo', Diego Alvarez Chanca, (see above, note 1), sig. b_8r.
63. Diego Alvarez Chanca, (see above, note 1), sig. a_3v.
64. For a general overview see Luis S. Granjel, *Aspectos médicos de la literatura antisupersticiosa española*, Salamanca, Universidad de Salamanca, 1953.
65. For a historical account of theological attitudes towards witchcraft, see Julio Caro Baroja, *Las brujas y su mundo. Un estudio antropológico de la sociedad en una época oscura*, Madrid, Revista de Occidente, 1961. An English translation of this work is available as *The World of Witches*, trans. O. Glendinning, Chicago, Chicago University Press, 1965.
66. For his biography and a critical edition of his treatise, see José Goñi Gaztambide, 'El tratado "De Superstitionibus" de Martín de Andosilla', *Cuadernos de Etnología y Etnografía de Navarra*, 9 (1971), pp. 249–322.
67. 'Quod autem parvuli possint fascinari, hoc est, malo oculo infici et inde ledi, tenet Sanctus Thomas I parte, qu.CXVII, art.III ad II, ubi dicit, "quod ex forti imaginatione anime immutantur spiritus corpori coniuncti, que quidem immutatio spiritum maxime fit in oculis ad quos subtiliores spiritus perveniunt, oculi autem inficiunt aerem continuum usque ad determinatum spacium, per quem modum specula, si fuerint nova et pura, contrahunt quamdam impuritatem ex aspectu mulieris menstruate, ut ait Aristoteles libro *De sommnis et imaginibus* cap. II; sic ergo, cum aliqua anima fuerit vehementer commota ad malitiam, sicut maxime in vetulis contigit, efficitur secundum modum predictum aspectus eius venenosus et noxius, maxime pueris, qui habent corpus tenerum ac de

facili recipiunt talium impressiones. Possibile est etiam <quod> ex permissione divina vel etiam ex aliquo facto occulto cooperetur ad hoc malignitas demonum, cum quibus vetule sortilege aliquod fedus habent"', 'Martín de Andosilla' (see above, note 66), p. 287.

68. José Maria López Piñero, Francesc Bujosa Homar, et al., *Los impresos científicos españoles de los siglos XV y XVI Inventario, bibliometría y thesaurus*, Valencia, Universidad de Valencia-Cátedra de Historia de la Medicina, 1981, vol. 1, pp. 126–9 give the date of 1538 as its first edition; however, Alva V. Ebersole mentions that in 1872 an edition of this work had been catalogued as published in 1530. See Pedro Ciruelo, *Reprovación de las supersticiones y hechizerías*, Introduction and edition by Alva V. Ebersole, Valencia, Albatros, 1978, p. 9. An English translation has been published by Eugene A. Maio and D'Orsay W. Pearson, *Pedro Ciruelo's 'A Treatise Reprobing All Superstitions and Forms of Witchcraft'*, New Jersey, Fairleigh Dickinson University Press, 1977.
69. Ciruelo, (see above, note 68), pp. 94–6.
70. Ciruelo, (see above, note 68), section II, chapter I, pp. 48–52. This was understood by Ciruelo's later commentators, cf. Granjel (see above, note 64), p. 31. For interesting analysis of the historiography of witchcraft, see Anne Llewellyn Barstow, 'On Studying Witchcraft as Women's History: A Historiography of the European Witch Persecutions', *Journal of Feminist Studies in Religion*, 4 (1988), pp. 7–19, and Elspeth Whitney, 'The Witch "She"/The Historian "He": Gender and the Historiography of the European Witch Hunts', *Journal of Women's History*, 7, Fall (1995), pp. 77–101.
71. The treatise was reprinted again in Logroño two years later; see José Maria López Piñero, Francesc Bujosa Homar, et al., (see above, note 68), p. 100. In this paper we use the modern edition prepared by the Sociedad de Bibliófilos Españoles, Fray Martín de Castañega, *Tratado de las supersticiones y hechicerías*, Madrid, Sociedad de Bibliófilos Españoles, 1946 (based on the 1529 edition).
72. Martín de Castañega, (see above, note 71), pp. 71–4.
73. Medieval medical literature is far from consistent at giving menarche and menopause ages. Menstruation starts between 12 to 15 years, while the time span given to menopause is from 35 to 65, although Hildegard of Bingen thought some women menstruate up to 80, *Causae et curae*, Paulus Kaiser (ed.), Leipzig, B. G. Teubner, 1903, p. 105.

J. B. Post, 'Ages at Menarche and Menopause: Some Mediaeval Authorities', *Population Studies*, 25 (1971), pp. 83–7, thinks 45–48 as the average age for menopause – considering it more likely that the lower and not the higher figure that the sources present would have been met, due to general trends in women's life expectancies; Darrel W. Amundsen and Carol Jean Diers, 'The Age of Menarche in Medieval Europe', *Human Biology*, 45 (1973), pp. 363–9, propose 12 to 14 as the average age of menarche.

A fourteenth-century Middle English manuscript entitled 'The Nature of Wommen' puts menarche between 12 and 14, and menopause in the forties; Muscio gave 14 and 40 to 50 as normal menarche and menopause ages, see Monica Green, 'Obstetrical and Gynecological Texts in Middle English', *Studies in the Age of Chaucer*, 14 (1992), p. 85, n. 76.

It is difficult to interpret the wide time span given to menopause, which was also given by some authors of late antiquity like Oribasius, Aëtius and Paulus Aegineta, who give 35 to 60, with 50 as the average age; Darrel W. Amundsen, and Carole Jean Diers, 'The Age of Menopause in Classical Greece and Rome', *Human Biology*, 42 (1970), pp. 79–86.

74. Charles T. Wood, 'The Doctor's Dilemma: Sin, Salvation and the Menstrual Cycle in Medieval Thought', *Speculum*, 56 (1981), pp. 710–27.
75. For a complex study of the ways medicine and natural philosophy constructed sexual difference and gender in the middle ages, and their uses of ancient authors, see Joan Cadden, *Meanings of Sex Difference in the Middle Ages. Medicine, Science and Culture*, Cambridge, Cambridge University Press, 1993.
76. To evaluate the importance and intricate development of this tradition, see Monica H. Green, 'The Development of the "Trotula", *Revue d'Histoire des Textes*, 26 (1996), pp. 119–203; and Monica H. Green, 'A Handlist of the Latin and Vernacular Manuscripts of the So-Called "Trotula" Texts, Part I: The Latin Manuscripts', *Scriptorium*, 50, (1996), pp. 137–75. The Anglo-Norman verse translation of the 'Liber de sinthomatibus mulierum', one of the texts identified by Monica Green, has been edited by Tony Hunt, *Anglo-Norman Medicine. Volume II: Shorter Treatises*, Cambridge, Brewer, 1997, pp. 68–128, who provides a working edition of the Latin text.
77. In the popular *Breviarium practice* ascribed to Arnau de Vilanova, gynecological diseases are directly related to those due to the bite of a poisonous animal: 'In hoc, meo deo auxiliante, de egritudinibus que proprie mulieribus accidunt tractare intendo et quia mulieres ut plurimum sunt animalia venenosa de morso animalium venenosorum consequenter tractabo', *Opera Arnaldi de Villanova*, Lyons, F. Fradin, 1504, 217vb.
78. Monica H. Green, '"Traittié tout de meçonges": The *secrés des dames*, "Trotula" and Attitudes Towards Women's Medicine in 14th- and early 15th-century France', Marilyn Desmond (ed.), *Christine de Pizan and the Categories of Difference*, Milwaukee, University of Minnesota Press, forthcoming. We thank Monica Green for allowing us to use her work prior to publication.
79. W. F. Ryan and Charles B. Schmitt (eds), *Pseudo-Aristotle The Secret of Secrets. Sources and Influences*, London, The Warburg Institute, 1982.
80. An explanation of menstruating and old women as producers of fascination is given in Helen Rodnite Lemay, *Women's Secrets. A Translation of Psuedo-Albertus Magnus's 'De secretis mulierum' with commentaries*, Albany, State University of New York Press, 1992. For the textual history and the history of its reception, together with a list of manuscripts, see Margaret Schleissner, 'Pseudo-Albertus Magnus: "Secreta mulierum cum commento": Deutsch critical text and commentary', PhD, Princeton University, 1987.
81. Ian McLean, *The Renaissance Notion of Woman. A Study in the Fortunes of Scholasticism and Medical Science in European Intellectual Life*, Cambridge, Cambridge University Press, 1980, pp. 39–40.
82. Aristotle (see above, note 51), p. 357.
83. 'Anssi veras en el espejo como una tela de sangre despues que se vuiere mirado en el alguna mujer al tiempo que le viene su purgación y esto yo

lo e visto, mas claramente lo veras cuando el espejo es nuevo', Alonso López de Corella, *Treszientas preguntas de cosas naturales*, Valladolid, Francisco Fernández de Córdova, 1546, question 49, sig. c_7r.

84. 'Patet hoc, nam sanguinis menstruus qui de venis in matricem expellitur potest cum evaporat per oculos sicut inficit speculum inficere alia', Antonio de Cartagena (see above, note 9), f. 4ra.
85. Diego Alvarez Chanca (see above, note 1), sig. b_8r.
86. In the gynecological literature of the late Middle Ages it appears incidentally acknowledged that certain religious women would not have the need to purge their bodies through menstruation because of the activities and duties of religious life – a reinterpretation of an ancient explanation in Christian terms, see Monica Green, 'Obstetrical and Gynecological Texts in Middle English', *Studies in the Age of Chaucer*, 14 (1992), p. 86, n. 78.
87. Helen Lemay, 'Women and the Literature of Obstetrics and Gynecology', in Joel T. Trosenthal (ed.), *Medieval Women and the Sources of Medieval History*, Athens and London, University of Georgia Press, 1990, p. 196.
88. Ottavia Niccoli, '"Menstruum quasi monstruum": parti mostruosi e tabú mestruale nel '500', *Quaderni Storici*, 44 (1980), pp. 402–28.
89. Petrus Abano, *Conciliator ... Libellus de venenis, eodem auctore. Petri Carrarii Questio de venenis ad terminum. Symphoriani Champerii Lugdunensis in Conciliatorem cribrationes*, Venice, Junta, 1565 (Facsimile edition. Padua, Antenore, 1985), f. 267rb.
90. 'Patet eciam a simili de muliere menstruosa cuius sanguis cadens super plantas viridadiorum eas marcescit et arescit ut plerumque per experientiam contum est', Diego Alvarez Chanca, (see above, note 1), sig. b_5v.
91. '... teneantur infirmi in aere claro et super omnia custodiatur ne visitetur a muliere menstruosa quoniam hoc esset addere venenum veneno', Diego Alvarez Chanca, (see above, note 1), sig. c_3v.
92. 'Dico quod sanguis menstruum quem in iuvenia poterant extra corpus deponere, nunc in senecta pre nimia virtutis debilitate in venis retentus, cum venenosus est inficit pueros, quippe si vetule menses non habeant id non evenit quod sanguine illo careant, sed quia vie strictissime sunt et expulsiva debilis, quo fit ut sepe sanguinem menstruum in venis habeant,' Antonio de Cartagena, (see above, note 9), f. 4ra.
93. 'Et si quis querat quare ergo vetule iste venenose non sunt, et non nimium male valent; respondeo quod venenum vipere ei non est venenum. Respondeo secundo quod tanta est consuetudo sanguinis illius menstrui in venis femelle, quod dum vetule sunt, membra earum non offenduntur a sanguine facto venenoso', Antonio de Cartagena (see above, note 9), f. 5ra.
94. Antonio de Cartegena (see above, note 9), f. 4ra.
95. 'Y porque pueden las viejas a los niños aojar', Alonso López de Corella, Alonso, (see above, note 83), question 133, sig. e_6v. Each of these questions was divided into two parts: a small poem (eight or nine verses) in a characteristic popular style and a commentary on it. The commentary, which is generally not much longer than the poem, was written in prose in a much more learned style and it usually alluded to various medical or natural philosophical authorities.
96. Damián Carbó, *Libro del arte de las comadres o madrinas y del regimiento*

de las preñadas y paridas y de los niños, Majorca, Hernando de Cansoles, 1541, sig. e_6r, 'Sean todas familiares guárdense de algunas viejas estrañas que no sea madre o suegra o su muy propincua'.

97. '... et in presentis bonum est ut legenda beate margarite legatur sanctorum reliquas super se habeat et breviter quas sciveris cerimonias ut infirme tue ac vetulis applaudas facito tamen quo si sortilegicam mulierem aliquam ibidem esse suspicio sit ea pellenda foris erit.' Cf. Helen Lemay, (see above, note 87) p. 197, 206.

98. *Arnaldi de Villanova Opera Medica Omnia, vol. X.1 (Regimen Sanitatis ad Regem Aragonum)*, L. García-Ballester and M. R. McVaugh (eds), Introduced by P. Gil-Sotres, J. A. Paniagua and L. García Ballester, Barcelona, Universitat de Barcelona, 1996. For a study of the passions of the soul and its influence on the body, see pp. 803–27. See also Luis Garcia Ballester, 'Soul and body. Disease of the soul and disease of the body in Galen's medical thought', in Paola Manuli and Mario Vegetti (eds), *Le opere psicologiche di Galeno*, Naples, Bibliopolis, 1988, pp. 117–52.

99. ' ... ut ulterius non faciliter ascendant (*the vapours*) propter cranei soliditatem a quo faciliorem habent exitu per oculum quam per aliam viam multis de causis ... tertio quia in aprehensione rei vise precipue si cum odio aut amore considerantur fit conamen virtutis visive et impulsus versus rem visam mediantibus radiis visualibus exeuntibus ab oculis in quo conaminem et impulsu violenter expelli possunt fumositates et vapores existentes in oculo et in cerebro,' Diego Alvarez Chanca, (see above, note 1), sig. b_4r.

100. Martín de Andosilla (see above, note 66), p. 287.

101. Martín de Castañega (see above, note 71), p. 73. The moral responsibility of the individual in certain acts committed against Catholic morality which were due to natural causes, was a matter of debate among sixteenth-century Spanish theologians. See Melchor Bajén Español, 'Sexo, moral y medicina en la España de la contrareforma. Un informe inédito del jesuita Miguel Pérez (1550–1605) sobre la polución', *Dynamis*, 15 (1995), pp. 443–57.

102. 'Effascinator naturaliter agit nullo voluntatis imperio, ideo etiam si velit aliquem effascinare non poterit si indispositus ille sit, et etiam si aliquis dispositus sit, effascinabit eum invite. Nam ut apertis oculis si res luce aut lumine illuminata sit et spiritus splendore illustrata, non possumus eam non videre, sic postquam aer venefica qualitate spiritus effascinantis infectus est, non potest offendere res aptus ut offendi possit, nec vice versa', Antonio de Cartagena (see above, note 9), f. 5rb.

103. 'Ergo abnegandum non est quod sicuti animalia aliqua sunt que aliis sunt venefica et inimica, sola coelesti qualitate, sic sint nonnulli homines qui constellatione maligna aliis hominibus adversentur, et effascinatores sint, quo fit quod tales homines etiam licet effascinent, et interimant, nulla digni sunt poena. Ideo leges nunquam disposuerunt poena aliqua hos punire, ratio est quia isti nullo voluntatis imperio effascinant sed sola qualitate coelesti qua inviti naturaliter agunt', Antonio de Cartagena (see above, note 9), f. 3va.

104. Maureen Flynn, 'La fascinación y la mirada femenina en la España del siglo XVI', *Historia silenciada de la mujer española desde la época medieval hasta la contemporánea*, edited by Alain Saint-Saëns, Madrid,

Editorial Complutense, 1996, pp. 22–37, documents some Inquisitorial processes against women who diagnosed and cured fascinated children, but it does not mention any prosecution against a fascinator. The same lack of interest in identifying fascinators can be drawn from María del Carmen García Herrero and María Jesús Torreblanca Gaspar, 'Curar con palabras (oraciones bajomedievales aragonesas)', *Alazet*, 2 (1990), pp. 67–82.

105. Josep Marti I Pérez, 'El "mal de ojo" en L'Alguer (Cerdeña)', *Lares. Rivista trimestrale di studi demo-etno-antropologici*, 54, 2, April–June (1988), pp. 211–26, p. 220.
106. Vivian Garrison and Conrad M. Arensberg, 'The Evil Eye: Envy or Risk of Seizure? Paranoia or Patronal Dependency?', in Clarence Maloney (ed.), (see above, note 2), pp. 286–328, p. 315.
107. Elvira Arquiola, 'Bases biológicas de la feminidad en la España moderna (siglos XVI–XVII)', *Asclepio*, 40, 1, (1988), pp. 297–315, esp. p. 305.
108. Maria-Milagros Rivera Garretas, 'El cuerpo femenino y la "querella de las mujeres" (Corona de Aragón, siglo XV)', in Georges Duby and Michelle Perrot (general editors), *Historia de las mujeres. vol 2. La Edad Media*, edited by Christiane Klapisch-Zuber and Reyna Pastor, Barcelona, Taurus, 1992, pp. 593–605.
109. Prudence Allen, *The Concept of Woman. The Aristotelian Revolution, 750 BC–1250 AD*, Montreal, Eden Press, 1985, pp. 413–68.
110. López de Corella (see above, note 83), question 133, sig. e_6v.
111. 'Cap. XII. Que los saludadores no son hechiceros y qué virtud sea la suya: ... Desta manera podría ser que algunos hombres fuesen así complexionados que tuviesen virtud natural oculta en el aliento o resollo y en la saliva, y aún en el tacto, por razón del temperamento de las cualidades complexionales', Martín de Castañega (see above, note 71), p. 62.
112. Pedro Mexía, *Silva de varia lección*, edited by Antonio Castro, Madrid, Cátedra, 1989, vol. I, p. 411.
113. 'E los fisicos de agora saben en esto poco, porque desdeñan la cura de tal enfermedat, diziendo que es obra de mugeres, e tiénenlo en poco, e por eso non alcançan las diferençias e secretos dello, que se alcançan parando en ello mientes.' Anna Maria Gallina, the editor of Villena's text, interprets this paragraph as if Villena were saying that scholastic medicine was not considering the evil eye as an illness in the first half of the fifteenth century; she acknowledges that later medical prominent authors will. Enrique de Villena (see above, note 22), p. 129.
114. 'Ita et multa mulieres experte dicunt et tenent quod aspectos et verba aliquorum horum noceant pueris in cunis per impressionum atque passionibus in ipsorum puerorum corporibus consequenter ex aspectibus illorum propter quod eciam ab antiquo inducta est consuetudo nutricibus frequenter velatio facies puerorum ... ', Engelbert of Admont, *Tractatus de fascinatione*, Bayerische Staatsbibliothek, Munich, CLM 18225, f. 324rb.
115. Martín Castañega (see above, note 71), p. 73.
116. 'Similiter superstitiose sunt quedam mulieres affligentis humeris parvulorum quedam fragmenta speculorum vel frustula vel peciolas ex corio vulpis vel melote, credentes per hoc tales parvulos non infici ab oculis infectis. Hoc vanum et superstitiosum est et sine ulla ratione,

scilicet naturali aut astrologica aut theologica, ut supra dictum est', Martín de Andosilla (see above, note 66), p. 287.

117. 'Nec tamen negare debemus illas herbas habere virtutem medicinalem ad fumationes faciendas contra infirmitates puerorum et etiam iuvamentorum; non tamen hoc provenit ex collectione precise talis diei, nec ex collectione ante solis ortum vel post solis ortum, ut quidam fatue credunt, sed ex virtute naturali earum herbarum, quam etiam eo tempore iam attingunt', Martín de Andosilla, (see above, note 66), p. 276.

118. ' ... cuius opositum contingit in corporibus debilibus et teneris quemadmodum sunt corpora puerorum et aliquorum adultorum habentium debilitatem compaginas et subtilitatem humorum a quo ortum habuit vulgare dictum a mulieribus dicentibus aliquem cito fascinari quia levem habet sanguinem et sic patet responsio ad dubium et etiam solutio ad argumentum', Diego Alvarez Chanca, (see above, note 1), sig. b_7v.

119. 'Y porque tenemos oy una platica que las mujeres preñadas y paridas en sus necesidades y para las criaturas a las comadres antes que a los medicos piden consejo', Damián Carbó, (see above, note 96), sigs 2_1v–$_2$r.

120. 'Et in nostra Hispania sunt vetule que demonibus potius quam creatori morem gerunt, que nituntur quibusdam figuris et characteribus pueros ab effascinatione absolvere, hec iudicio meo videtur Galenus detestari, quoniam postquam pueri effascinati sunt, eisdem auxiliis curari debent quibus solent egritudines prave et venenose amoveri', Antonio de Cartagena (see above, note 9), sig. 8rb.

121. Jole Agrimi and Chiara Crisciani, 'Medici e 'vetule' dal duecento al quattroento: problemi di una ricerca', *Cultura popolare e cultura dotta nel seicento*, Milan, Franco Angeli Editore, 1983, pp. 144–59; *Eaedem*, 'Immagini e ruoli della "vetula" tra sapere medico e antropologia religiosa (secoli XIII–XV)', *Poteri carismatici e informali: chiesa e societá medioevali, A cura di Agostino Paravicini e André Vauchez*, Palermo, Sellerio editore, 1992, pp. 224–61; a French version was published as 'Savoir médical et anthropologie religieuse. Les representations et les fonctions de la *vetula* (XIIIe–XVe siécle)', *Annales ESC*, September–October, (1995), pp. 1281–308.

122. 'Quia alias natura frustraretur fine quam intendebat, sed hoc est imposibile quia natura semper operatur propter finem. Igitur imposibile videtur quod venenositas reperiatur in complexione humana et sic nullius complexionis et nullius etatis erit homo venenosus cum talis non sit. Quoniam est nota, antecedens probatur quia cum natura intendit producere hominem, intendit producere illum sociabilem quia homo est animal sociabile ut vult Aristoteles primo *Politicorum*; sed si illum produceret venenosum talis esset incomunicabilis et separabilis a consortio humanorum quod non intendebatur a natura et sic esset frustata suo fine', Diego Alvarez Chanca, (see above, note 1), sigs b_6v–$_7$r.

123. 'Licet ad hanc questionem respondere sit dificile propterea quia ut supra dictum est ut plurimum venefici sunt tales per individuales propietates que non per discursum rationis, sed per via experimentali cognoscuntur quare dificile erit de eis ratiotinare. Sed ut intelectus audientium fiat sollicitus et curiosus ad maiorem investigationem aliquod proposse dicam petendo veniam de insuficientia, quia inhertia ingenii proprii et dificultas materie condignam percendi facultatem merentur', Diego Alvarez Chanca, (see above, note 1), sig. b_7r.

124. Thomas Aquinas (see above, note 40).
125. Françoise Héritier-Augé, 'Older women, stout-hearted women, women of substance', in *Fragments for a History of the Human Body, Part Three*, edited by Michel Feher with Ramona Nadaff and Nadia Tazi, New York, Zone Books, 1989, pp. 281–99.
126. Georges Minois, *History of Old Age: From Antiquity to the Renaissance*, translated by Sarah Hanbury Tenison, Cambridge, Polity Press, 1989, pp. 230–32, 254–6. For a general overview of the anxieties surrounding old age in the Middle Ages, see Shulamith Shahar, *Growing Old in the Middle Ages*, London, Routledge, 1997.
127. Luce Irigaray, 'Le mystère oublié des généalogies féminines' in *eadem, Le Temps de la Différence*, Paris, Minuit, 1989, pp. 103–23.
128. Ruth Anthony El Saffar, *Rapture Encaged. The Suppression of the Feminine in Western Culture*, London, Routledge, 1994; Ann J. Cruz, 'La búsqueda de la madre: Psicoanálisis y feminismo en la literatura del Siglo de Oro', in Alain Saint-Saëns (ed.), *Historia silenciada de la mujer española desde la época medieval hasta la contemporánea*, Madrid, Editorial Complutense, 1996, pp. 39–64. We thank María-Milagros Rivera and Ana Vargas for bringing these works to our attention.

CHAPTER FIVE

Medicine at the German Universities, 1348–1500: A Preliminary Sketch

Vivian Nutton

Within the German-speaking areas of Europe universities were, with the single exception of Prague (founded in 1348), creations of the period after the Black Death.[1] Hence they offer an excellent opportunity to examine the development of medicine and medical education in what is still a relatively obscure period and, in most textbooks, unexplored territory. Historians without German must have recourse to Puschmann's classic *A History of Medical Education*, now more than a century old, in order to gain a basic overview.[2] Even German medical historians, when they deign to consider developments in the later Middle Ages, rarely go beyond individual texts, individual practitioners and individual universities.[3] A general survey, even one based largely on secondary material, is thus of value, not least in pointing to a tradition of learned medicine outside the charmed circle of Bologna, Padua, Montpellier and Paris.[4]

The German universities and their foundations fall neatly into four chronological groups.[5] The first is very closely linked with the aspirations and needs of the Holy Roman Emperor, his court, and his administration; Prague, established by the Emperor Charles IV, 1348; Vienna, founded by the Hapsburg Duke Rudolf IV in reaction to Prague, 1365; Heidelberg, the university of the Palatine Elector, 1386. Cologne, 1388, and Erfurt, approved by the Elector of Mainz in 1379 but not properly set up until 1392, were both civic foundations, dependent at first on the wealth of their towns as centres of trade and commerce. A rather disparate and not uniformly successful trio follows: Würzburg, which enjoyed a precarious existence from 1402 to 1411; Leipzig, the university of Saxony, in 1409, following an exodus of German students from Prague; and tiny Rostock, the university of Mecklenburg in 1419. There is then a gap of almost forty years until a veritable spate of new foundations; Greifswald in Pomerania, 1456, following a secession from Rostock; Freiburg in the Hapsburg-ruled Breisgau, 1457; Ingolstadt in Bavaria, 1472; Trier, 1473; Mainz, 1476/77; Tübingen in Württemberg 1477, to which one might add Louvain, 1425, and Basle, 1460. Two later universities should also be mentioned; Wittenberg, founded in

1502 at the behest of, and, in its initial stages run by, a medical man, Martin Pollich von Mellerstadt (1450–1513), and Frankfurt an der Oder, the university of Brandenburg, 1506. This pair shows neatly the effects of political change on the creation of universities; the founding of Wittenberg reflects the political division of Saxony after 1464, that of Frankfurt the great increase in the power and authority of the dukes of Brandenburg.[6] Subsequent foundations, beginning with that of Marburg in 1527, reveal the impact of the Reformation and confessionalism, but that is another story.

All these seventeen or so universities were conceived from the start as teaching the full range of academic subjects, including medicine, although frequently the evidence for actual instruction taking place is severely limited. At Prague, for example, before 1409, when the students of the German Nation, and many professors, left for Leipzig, the name of only one professor of medicine is known, Balthasar de Marcellinis de Tusia (Tuscany?), who lectured in his own home. However, a handful of medical men, notably Magister Gallus de Monte Sion (active 1350–1360) and Christian von Prachatitz (active 1386–1409), lectured on related themes of astronomy and *physica* within the Arts faculty. From 1409 to the end of the century organized medical education seems to have ceased. A few names of medical men active in the university are recorded, a very occasional promotion to MB, and, in 1460, a solitary MD, Johann von Krcina.[7] Medical activity at Trier is equally obscure. In 1475 there was a Dean and an assistant, who were present at the audit of the Rector. The Dean was probably Peter von Viersen, who participated in the first election for Rector in 1473 and who helped to prepare the statutes of 1474. He may have left Trier in 1477, at the end of his year as Rector of the university, to go to Mainz, where in 1480 he was appointed Rector of that university and doctor to the Elector of Mainz. The names of two other medical professors are known; Wilhelm von Menningen was apparently Dean of medicine in 1485, and Petrus Hernsheimer was Rector of the university from 1499 to 1501. But the provision of posts does not signify activity, and there is no reference to teaching or of the medical faculty attempting to control lesser practitioners or apothecaries until the late seventeenth century.[8] At Freiburg, the first holder of the ordinary chair of medicine, Matthaeus Hummel (1425–77), was notorious in both city and university for not lecturing at all during the first years of the university's existence, beginning only in 1471. But Hummel had a good excuse: he was the university's first Rector, a universal scholar with doctorates in law, arts, and medicine, and he was heavily occupied in sorting out the problems of the young university. As he wrote in 1470, 'I have planted a vine, which has turned to bitterness' (cf. *Jeremiah* 2:21), and his assumption of his academic teaching duties may have come as a welcome relief from his administrative labours.[9]

For the most part, too, the earliest surviving statutes and regulations for a medical faculty are considerably later than the university's foundation charter, which points to the relative unimportance of the medical professors within the university structures. Even at Erfurt, where a member of the medical faculty was chosen as Rector twenty times between 1394 and 1500 (a much higher percentage than the faculty's numbers might suggest) this may have been much more because of the doctor's contacts with the rulers of Saxony and Thuringia and his small teaching commitments than because of any faculty power-base or respect for medicine.[10] Indeed, the numbers of medical graduates were rarely great enough to demand the immediate creation of a specific medical faculty. At Mainz and Tübingen there was a gap of some twenty years after the university's foundation, while at Greifswald, where the teaching of medicine for the first 103 years was entrusted to a single professor, promotions 'according to university statute' required the presence of doctors of other faculties since no other MD was available in the town to act as witness.[11]

Greifswald was not alone in having only one medical professor, although most universities had two, as at Leipzig, dividing medicine into theory and practice. Only Vienna had three professors, the third lecturing on 'Introductory texts'. None the less, even when the statutes demanded two professors, the posts were not always filled. According to one contemporary source, Heidelberg was 'empty of physic' in the middle years of the fifteenth century, when the university's annalist reported that 'medicine does not flourish in our university'.[12] Nor were numbers of members of the faculty, i.e. those doctors, licentiates and bachelors with the right to teach, any more numerous. Seven medical men (out of 46 masters) took the oath when the university of Leipzig was founded in 1409, and the number had risen to nine by the time of the creation of the medical faculty in 1415, but in 1438 there was a general complaint that there had been a lack of lectures and poorly organized lectures for several years.[13] Between 1392 and 1524 at Erfurt there were usually between three and five resident members of the faculty; the most was eight in the 1450s, but in 1395 and 1421 there were none at all. Cologne in 1389 had five doctors of medicine in the faculty, and fourteen in 1477. Between 1388 and 1558 the names of 115 teachers of medicine are known there, distinguished above all, as their most recent historian admits, for their mediocrity.[14]

Numbers of medical students were correspondingly small. At Cologne, the German university with the highest student population, between 1389 and 1558 some 167 students matriculated in medicine, and 241 graduated, substantial numbers compared with the 44 students who gained a medical licence or doctorate at Erfurt between 1392 and 1500, or the 29 names recorded as graduating at Leipzig between 1447 and 1500.[15] At Ingolstadt between 1472 and 1500 there were no more than five medical students at any time, and 31 in all. No wonder that an elderly professor there was allowed to teach at home, 'because the number of medical students is not great, indeed is usually tiny'.[16] In the whole of Germany there may have been no more than twenty or thirty medical students beginning their course in any one year, around 0.4 per cent of the total student population.[17] Even allowing for the fact that the medical course would last for some five or six years after graduation in arts, the total numbers studying medicine in any single university would have been very small. No wonder that there was rarely any specific auditorium or a college assigned to the medical faculty.[18]

The official statutes of the medical faculties of all the universities were very similar. Indeed, those of Cologne in 1393 became the model for those of Heidelberg in 1425, and of Ingolstadt in 1472; those of Vienna in 1389 were used for those of Freiburg and Basle in 1460. They lay down the authors to be studied, and, frequently, a precise order of study. The staple authors were Galen, especially the *Tegne*, Hippocrates, especially *Aphorisms*, Johannitius, Rhazes, and Avicenna's *Canon*. At Cologne, although the statutes makes no mention of Avicenna, there is evidence for lectures on the *Canon* taking up a large proportion of medical teaching. The same statutes also mention the poem on urines of Giles de Corbeil, the *Viaticum* of Constantine, and Galen's *Method of healing*, books 7–14. In many of the statutes provision is made for a period of supervised medical practice, lasting from six months to two years, before the candidate is allowed to proceed to a licence or the doctorate. There is also much about the methods of examination, the various disputations and lectures necessary at each stage of a progression to the MD, and an oath which lays down properly moral practice and appropriate respect for one's seniors.[19]

None of this is in any way unusual or typical only of Germany; indeed, a German medical student would have found himself studying the same set books in Italy, Spain, France or England. This concentration on the solid standard authors of a Graeco-Arab past continues into the later years of the sixteenth century, and is only slightly modified by the appearance, in a decision of the Leipzig faculty in 1502 and in the Wittenberg statutes of 1508, of 'more modern' commentators such as Giovanni Arcolano (*c.*1390–1458) and Jacques Despars (*c.*1380–1458), both long enough dead to be counted as classic.[20] Only in the Wittenberg statutes is there even a hint of teaching developments elsewhere: Hippocrates' *Aphorisms* are to be read in the new, humanist translation of Laurentianus, and the sections on fevers from Galen's *Ad Glauconem* are also recommended.[21] This does not mean that the medical teachers themselves were out of touch with what was going on elsewhere. The thirteen books owned by Professor Bernhard von Loen which came after his death to the Cologne faculty in 1461 included the *Consilia* of Gentile de Foligno, and works by Marsiglio di Santa Sofia, and probably others by Tommaso del Garbo and Guglielmo da Varignana, albeit authors dead more than half a century.[22] Far more impressive in both number and quality were the holdings of the two libraries at Erfurt, that of the *Collegium maius*, probably dating from around 1400, and the Bibliotheca Amploniana, given in 1412 to the university by Amplonius Ratingk the Elder, Professor of Medicine and, in 1394, Rector. By 1524, at least 1598 works of medicine were available there, 277 in the *Collegium*, 1321 in the Amploniana, with multiple copies of the standard works, and some of more recent commentators, like Gerardus de Solo (d. *c.*1360). There were also several works on surgery, like that of Henri de Mondeville (*fl.* 1310), the *Anatomy* of Mondino dei Liuzzi (d. 1326), and a variety of writings on medical astrology, including a copy of the *Aggregationes de crisi*.[23] Erfurt is exceptional in being a university with a major collection of medical books. Yet, even here, the impression that one gets is of a slightly outdated package of information, better, admittedly, than in many other places, but not as good as one would like.[24]

Against this background the Tübingen statutes of 1497 look positively revolutionary.[25] As well as laying down a specific teaching plan (not uncommon in the fifteenth century), they provided for instruction in botany, surgery and anatomy. In the holidays, the professor was to arrange for the students to spend two months learning about the 'campestria simplicia', herbs, roots etc., how to recognize and use them. A surgical course was laid out, based on Avicenna's *Canon*, book IV, fens 3–5, Albucasis, or some other approved antique author. Book IV, fen 7 of the *Canon* was also recommended as very useful. A doctor wishing to graduate in surgery as well as in medicine had to attend the surgical lectures for one year and have some practical experience; one who wished to graduate only in surgery had to have two years of lectures and surgical disputations, and attend a formal anatomy. The anatomy display, for which permission had been earlier granted to Tübingen in 1482 by Pope Sixtus IV, was to take place every three or four years, at Christmas-time, on the corpse of an executed criminal.[26] During the demonstration, the relevant chapter of Mondino was to be read and commented upon, and afterwards the MDs and, unusually, the *Magistri* and students from the Artists, were to attend the burial. Mondino survived here until 1538, when his tract, 'stuffed with errors and innumerable mistakes', was replaced by sections from Galen, 'that most expert dissector (*in consectionibus exercitatissimus*)'.[27]

Botany, anatomy and surgery; here are the first echoes of developments taking place in northern Italy, in Bologna, Padua, and Ferrara, but they were not always so welcome. Although in many ways the statutes of Wittenberg reflect those of Tübingen, this was not true of medicine. Botany, anatomy, and surgery are all omitted from the statutes of the medical faculty, which is perhaps surprising to those who have seen their promoter, the Rector Martin Pollich von Mellerstadt, as a champion of the new medical humanism in his previous post at Leipzig and who recall that he had in 1493 himself produced an edition of Mondino's anatomy at Leipzig.[28] Indeed, there is far more evidence for an interest in anatomy at the older university than at Wittenberg. In 1502 and again in 1511 there were unsuccessful proposals for the introduction of a public anatomy at Leipzig, either every three years or for students in their final year. The 'unanimous and universal wish' of the faculty for an annual dissection was finally granted in 1519, seven years before the earliest record of a dissection, of a human head, at Wittenberg, and seventeen years before the creation of a chair there specifically devoted to anatomy.[29] Although provision for an annual anatomy was made at Ingolstadt in the 1507 plans of reform, and later on by other German universities, the Tübingen example for botany was not followed up elsewhere until perhaps the middle of the century.[30] At Frankfurt an der Oder, the Dean of the medical faculty was to organize twice a year in early and late summer an outing to visit the hills, woods and valleys to look at medicinal plants. One or more apothecaries was to be invited along to help identify the plants and, in autumn, the roots, and the students were to form their own collections 'as is customary'.[31] No German university in the sixteenth century repeated Tübingen's surgical course, and it is not clear if that university itself followed its own regulations for surgery or for botany.[32]

The Tübingen statutes and the introduction of anatomy are regularly viewed by medical historian as proofs of modernity, 'the most progressive of all German medical statutes' in Klaus Pielmeyer's phrase.[33] But three caveats need to be entered. First, and most obvious, is that statutes tell us what ought to be done, not what is being done. Historians have concentrated, *faute de mieux*, on them, and on tracking down the 'first' anatomies, and have said very little, if anything, about what then followed. In Vienna, the example of Galeazzo di Santa Sofia, who organized a dissection in February 1404 in the hospital of Vienna, was not repeated until 1418.[34] In 1435 student demand led to a decision to hold an anatomy and to appoint Johannes Aygel in 1436 'Lector anatomiae'. There was a similar student request in 1440, which, alas, could not be fulfilled, for the condemned criminal in 1441 survived his hanging and recovered in hospital. The next anatomy would appear to have been in 1444, and from then on an anatomy was held on average every four or five years, a disappointment to those students and bachelors who in 1435 had demanded a male and female dissection in alternate years.[35] In 1478 the students of the Cologne medical faculty approached the authorities with a request for an anatomy, appealing to the common good and to practice elsewhere. The next year, following a unanimous decision of the faculty, the request was forwarded to the emperor, who allowed them to claim two corpses a year for dissection. The first dissection of a criminal took place in February 1480, to which doctors from Bruges, Leiden, Delft, Münster and places closer to hand were invited. Later evidence for human dissection at Cologne is hard to find, and Erich Meuthen supposes that until the seventeenth century there was a general reliance on animal anatomy. Other universities show a similarly sporadic pattern, which at the very least requires a certain scepticism towards the demands of the statutes and even the fulfilment of faculty decisions to hold a dissection, should a corpse become available.[36]

Secondly, since many of the medical teachers had spent some time in Italy, they can hardly be suspected of ignorance of developments there.[37] Numbers are hard to come by; but over 80 per cent of professors in the second half of the fifteenth century had visited Italy, usually Padua, Bologna and, at the end of the century, Ferrara. The numbers are somewhat fewer for the first half but, even so, several professors had also studied at Vienna, the German university most in touch with developments south of the Alps. If human dissection took place in Italy as often and as regularly as is usually assumed (an assumption that is far from easy to prove), then the failure of the Italian-trained Germans to bring the anatomical habit with them on their return requires explanation.[38] At the very least it suggests that the benefits of dissection were not as convincing to them as they appeared to nineteenth-century historians of medicine. Besides, the very careful preparations insisted on by the civic authorities in Vienna for the anatomy of 1452, and the faculty discussions about the need to restrict attendance at anatomies (for fear of disturbance) and to hold them in private show that public support for dissection was hardly enthusiastic.[39] The introduction of university anatomy in Europe is far from being a simple story; to transform a single dissection into a regular, structured series is far more complex than many historians have heretofore believed.[40]

Nor need one suppose that this relative neglect of anatomy, botany or surgery was the result of a generally theoretical orientation of university teaching. Both statutes and what remains of the literary productions of professors tell a very different story, one that emphasizes a commitment to medical practice. Most statutes lay down qualifications for practical experience before a licence or degree is to be granted; the Wittenberg professors were told to bring along their students with them on their visits to the sick, so that 'what they teach in theory may be demonstrated in practice'. The Leipzig faculty insisted three times in the fifteenth century that their medical degree was to be gained only after two year's practical experience with a recognized medical teacher, whether in Leipzig or elsewhere. The same provision also held true for Erfurt. Cologne, Heidelberg and Ingolstadt went even further by including a section in the statutes *De modo practicandi*. This enjoined upon students and faculty the duty of respect; one should not abuse colleagues, or steal patients from them; a doctor who left the town without officially entrusting his patients to another doctor, however, could have no redress if, on his return, he found another had taken over – but, even so, his patient should be returned to him as soon as possible.[41]

The Cologne and Ingolstadt statutes also forbid any association with empirics, especially if they were Jewish; an exception might be made for surgery, provided that the empiric was a good Christian.[42] Here two common regulations are conflated, one against empirics, the other against the practice by the doctor of surgery, defined in some statutes as using iron and fire. This was to be left to surgeons, with whom the German medical faculties seem to have had reasonably good relations. Those physicians who did go in for surgery do not appear to have attracted the scorn of their physician colleagues or the resentment of the surgeons. Peter von Ulm (*c.*1390–*c.*1440), doctor to the Elector Palatine, was famous for his skill in both medicine and surgery. In his *Chirurgia*, written in German at the end of his life, he provided surgeons in general with a major collection of recipes drawn from his own practice and from older texts in both Latin and German. His Heidelberg colleague, Heinrich Münsinger (1397–1476), enjoyed a similar reputation for his skills in medicine and surgery. His own book on surgery incorporated recipes of both physicians and surgeons, and some of his own remedies circulated equally widely among surgeons and barbers.[43]

Against the empirics, however, there seems to have been a constant battle. The 1476 statutes at Erfurt established firmly that, in the eyes of the town council, the university faculty was to have charge of medical licensing; surgeons, stone-cutters, and the like were to be examined by them and were only to be allowed to practise if the faculty approved.[44] In the official letter of foundation of the university of Freiburg in 1457, Archduke Albert of Austria specifically mentioned the medical faculty. The city council must see to it that only those approved of by the faculty should be allowed to heal. Surgeons, barbers, physicians, even apothecaries, rootcollectors and 'those who are called empirics' could only be allowed to ply their skills in the territory of Freiburg if they had first been approved by the faculty.[45] This close relationship of town and university was fostered here (unlike at Ingolstadt) by the appointment of one of the medical professors as *Stadtarzt* and, also, by the similar appointment of local practitioners to university chairs.[46]

In a small town like Freiburg, the alliance between town and university against lesser healers might have been effective. In Vienna, where in 1454 eleven MDs served a population of around 50 000, the task was as vain as that in London in the next century. Quacks, healers, Jews, baptized and unbaptized, priests and old women were all pursued with varying degrees of ineffectiveness. Sometimes a surgeon or a doctor with a foreign degree correctly approached the faculty for permission to practise; others, like Sebald of Ravensburg, were threatened with prosecution for decades, albeit ineffectively. When an energetic Dean and local authorities collaborated, then the drive against quackery could be successfully maintained. In 1409, the quack Johannes Delphinus was prosecuted at the instance of Dean Nicholas von Hebersdorf, with the approval of the official of the Bishop of Passau and the local Benedictine Abbot, excommunicated, and publicly burnt in Bohemia. Katherina Gruner, 'a cursed old woman', 'unlearned and certainly inexpert', was finally forced under pain of excommunication to a public confession of her incapacities – but only after a long process and appeals to the Roman Curia, the costs of which had to be borne by the faculty, as she had no money herself. More often, however, powerful patrons intervened to protect their own healers. In 1422 Duke Albert V ordered the faculty not to interfere with the medical activities of Caspar the Jew. In November 1438 the mayor of Vienna dealt scornfully with a faculty petition against empirics, 'neophytes', Jews and old women. In 1454 King Ladislaus refused to act against Jewish physicians when asked by the faculty on grounds both of its own rights and statutes and of the decisions of the church forbidding such use of Jewish medicine. Others claimed to be surgeons, hence outside the jurisdiction of the faculty, or simply continued in practice, defying all bans, fines and excommunications. From the point of view of patients, the faculty might be almost as bad as a quack – and much more expensive. Two Viennese poems sum this up neatly. Both begin with the same couplet:

> Fingit se medicum quiuis idiota prophanus
> Judaeus, monachus, histrio, rasor, anus.
> (Any layman, heretic, Jew, monk, actor, barber or old woman can claim to be a doctor.)

The first continues with a denunciation of the alchemist, soap dealer, dyer, forger or oculist who becomes a doctor; the second, much longer, delivers an attack on the *medicus*, for his devilish ways with his fees –

and ends with a preference for mountain herbs over vain words, and a warning never to make a doctor one's heir.[47]

Control of apothecaries was another aim achieved only in part. While the Vienna faculty and the apothecaries at times collaborated to inspect shops, regulate the quality of drugs, and stamp out empirics, the apothecaries succeeded in avoiding total submission, and plans for a faculty dispensary were never implemented.[48] By contrast, at Heidelberg in 1471 the faculty with the approval of the Elector Frederick succeeded in imposing an official pharmacopoeia, listing the drugs to be used, official prices, and the antidotaries (Nicolaus, Mesue, Avicenna, Arnald of Villanova in that order) which were to act as guides. No laxative was to be given without medical approval, and no compound drug was to be prepared save in the presence of a doctor.[49] Similar procedures seem to have been adopted earlier at Cologne, where in 1470 a jar of theriac was ordered to be burnt after having been rejected by the medical professors. Eight years later a joint commission of the medical faculty and the town was set up to oversee the apothecaries, but no official pharmacopoeia was enacted until 1565.[50] At Leipzig, the Elector empowered the doctors in 1474 to inspect the drugs on sale in the apothecaries' shops to see that they were of good quality, and still in good condition, but a complaint in 1502 suggests that even an annual inspection had not been carried out for some time.[51]

University authorities also were occasionally involved in examinations for leprosy.[52] At Cologne the task was originally in the hands of a civic official, the Leper-master, but by 1477 the medical faculty had gained the right also to carry out the test. The rivalry continued for a further century at least, with both sides endeavouring to gain exclusive rights.[53] At Heidelberg, the university professors may have participated from early on in the examinations for leprosy, and the same may have been true at Erfurt, where the town and university authorities worked closely together.[54] In Vienna and at Mainz in 1493, the medical faculty joined in the examination with a surgeon or barber-surgeon.[55] Elsewhere, e.g. at Ingolstadt and Leipzig, university control of the leprosy examination may have been a development of the sixteenth century.[56]

The impression that the medical professors in Germany in the fifteenth century were heavily involved in medical practice rather than in theory is borne out by their literary productions. Copies of their lectures are almost non-existent – Knab's many volumes of commentary on Aristotle and Mellerstadt's lectures on Aristotle are rare survivals – and annotations, like those made by Ulrich Ellenbog (*c.*1435–99), very briefly a professor at Ingolstadt, give only a fleeting impression of their quality.[57] What remains is very much at a practical level; plague tractates, *regimina*, advice on syphilis, recipe collections (e.g. that of Heinrich

Münsinger at Heidelberg), *consilia* and the like.[58] The work of a fifteenth-century professor that enjoyed the widest circulation, *Ein guts nützlich büchlin von den ausgeprennten Wasser*, by Michael Puff aus Schrick (*c*.1400–73), a member of the Vienna faculty from 1433 to his death, nicely exemplifies this. This composite work gives individual descriptions of some 82 herbal distillations along with directions for manufacture and use. Its kernel is a genuine work of Puff, a book on *Distilled Waters*, written in 1455 and revised in 1466, supplemented by an anonymous tract on distilled waters that circulated also under the name of Ortolf von Baierland, and by two other short pieces. This 'useful little book' went through 38 printed editions between 1476 and 1601, to say nothing of at least fourteen copies in manuscript.[59] A similar concern with a practical problem marks the more famous tract *Von der gifftigen besen tempffen und reuchen der metal* (*On bad and poisonous fumes and vapours of metal*) written by Ulrich Ellenbog in 1473 for the Augsburg goldsmiths and arguably one of the classics of occupational medicine. In its organization and advice it is a long medical *consilium*, relating the standard medical Galenism to the particular concerns of his patients.[60]

Another area of practical expertise in which medical professors specialized was that of medical astrology.[61] The activity of its most skilled representative, Georg Tannstetter or Collimitius, who began lecturing in mathematics at Vienna in 1503, falls into the sixteenth century, but he continued a tradition of complex mathematical and medical learning that was already existing in Vienna a century earlier, e.g. in Jacob Engelin's *Tractatus de cometis* of 1402.[62] The production of almanacs including medical, meteorological, and political predictions for the coming year was not confined to Vienna. Examples of similar activity can be found in almost all universities, from Louvain (where 'Louvain prognostics' became a shorthand name for the whole genre) to Leipzig. Erhard Winsberger, who was called to Ingolstadt in 1476, had studied law, theology, and astrology as well as medicine in Paris. His *In exhortatione recepta et iudicium contra vennena turcorum* (1476) mixes astrology and medicine with classical reminiscences and examples.[63] At Leipzig, where a series of distinguished medical astrologers taught both medicine and mathematics, Mellerstadt produced a series of *Prognostica* between 1482 and 1490 (except for 1485) that went through some 22 printings in both German and Latin.[64] Similar publications continued to be the staple of many German authors for many more years, including not least Paracelsus.[65] They displayed their authors' command of some complex technical reasoning, as well as their ability to relate the individual patient and his or her ills to the macrocosm. Information so gained from the heavens was essential for a proper conduct of life on earth; one needed to take precautions against a predicted onset of conflict or political catastrophe just as much as against that of plague or dysentery.

The practical abilities of the members of the German university faculties were rewarded highly with canonries, prebendaries, and the like, and with the income from attending on bishops and princes, or wealthy citizens. If the academic ladder was long and costly (not least its degree costs which, claim German historians, were even higher than those of Italy), the profits to be gained were enormous, once one became established.[66]

Increasingly, the medical training of a German university teacher came to involve some time spent in Italy, and it is possible to investigate the influence of Italian humanism on the medical faculties. Indeed, given that most medical historians have concentrated on the Greek humanism of Leoniceno and his followers, a brief survey of the effects of the earlier Latin humanism is not without value.[67] For many universities not enough information survives for even a guess at the intellectual activities of both teachers and students; in others, as at Cologne, the medical faculty and its members seem to have been remote from the activity of the humanists in neighbouring faculties. In 1481, one humanist complained, there was only one doctor in the town who could be described as educated.[68]

Elsewhere, more can be said. Vienna, for instance, had maintained close links with Italy since the days of Alberto di Cremona (d. 1370) and of Galeazzo di Santa Sofia in the early years of the fifteenth century. The royal physician in the 1450s, Jacobus de Castro Romano, was a friend of many of the Italian humanists, notably Pius II, and exchanged letters with many of them. Specific humanist interests among the professoriate, however, appear somewhat later, with Johannes Tichtel (active 1482–1503) and Barthomäus Steber (active 1490–1506). Tichtel was a friend of the poet and physician Conrad Celtis, and made his home available to him for lecturing on Greek and on literature. Steber, who had studied in Italy, was keen on anatomy. In 1491, when the city council refused permission for a human dissection, only allowing a pig to be anatomized, he intervened personally with the council and was promised the corpse of a criminal. To universal surprise, the convict survived his hanging, and was granted his freedom. Steber's book on syphilis, printed in Vienna in 1498, shows his abilities nicely, not least in its elegant Latin.[69]

Both Steber and Tichtel belonged to the *Societas Danubiana*, a literary society, whose leading light was another faculty member, the imperial physician Cuspinianus (1473–1529). Their interests and activities show the strengths and weaknesses of the new Latin humanism.[70]

All were stylists, whose Latin, replete with classical allusions, was far removed from that of the early years of the century.[71] Cuspinianus, poet, humanist and historian, lectured on poetry as well as on medicine to the university, and was seen as the leading humanist of the day.[72] What this meant for medical teaching is less clear. That some saw this new classicism as a threat is clear from the protest made in 1511 by Martin Steinpeis (active 1490–1527 and eight times Dean) against changes introduced by Cuspinianus, the new Dean, in which Steinpeis publicly declared in German that some of his colleagues ought to be expelled from Vienna for incompetence. He was suspended for a while from his university teaching, and later compiled his own *Student's Guide to Medicine* (1520), in which he proclaimed his faith in the old, solid authorities, Avicenna and their Italian commentators.[73]

It is tempting to see a similar debate taking place at Leipzig at the end of the fifteenth century and revolving around the controversial figure of Martin Pollich von Mellerstadt, from whom the Leipzig circle of followers of Conrad Celtis took their title, the *sodalitas Polliciana*. He was involved in two notorious battles with colleagues: with Simon Pistoris in medicine over the origins of syphilis and the role of medical astrology, and with the theologian Konrad Wimpina over the status of theology and its relationship to poetry. But although many have seen Mellerstadt as a hero for his vigorous rejection of medical astrology and for his championing of Leoniceno, as well as for defending the poet's right to freedom of speech, the situation is far more complex than this.[74] As Sudhoff and, more recently, James Overfield have pointed out, all parties to the argument have claims to being considered humanists, although Mellerstadt certainly exploited his acquaintance with the very latest of Italian fashions.[75] His own later activities at Wittenberg, however, do not suggest a great desire for change, and a case can be made for Leipzig, not Wittenberg, as showing, in the early sixteenth century greater receptivity towards humanism. Leipzig, for instance, used the elder Pliny as a text for lectures in natural philosophy some years before its rival university, and the teaching of classical Latin and Greek was more advanced there than elsewhere.[76] As has already been argued, demands for anatomy were both made and satisfied at Leipzig some years before they were at Wittenberg.

A similar interest in the new humanism as a literary manifestation can be found at Ingolstadt, where in 1477 Erhard Windsberger was allowed to lecture on poetry ('to improve our good students') as well as on medicine, and above all at Erfurt, where in the early years of the sixteenth century a veritable chorus of poets and literary figures was formed, including Eobanus Hessus (1488–1540), Ulrich von Hutten (1488–1523) and Georg Sturtz (1490–1548).[77] The influence of the revival of the classics can here be seen to have an effect on the content of medical teaching; Rhazes, Isaac Israeli, Johannitius, staples in the collection of Amplonianus in the first half of the fifteenth century, are replaced by appeals to Hippocrates, Dioscorides, Asclepiades (!), Pliny and Celsus. The list of portraits of physicians, according to Eobanus Hessus, hanging in the museum of Georg Sturtz in the 1520s included ones of Herophilus, Asclepiades, Critobulus, Galen, Celsus, Paul of Aegina and Antonius Musa. Between 1524 and 1531, their number had been increased by likenesses of Prodicus, Creon (i.e. Acron of Acragas), Critias (i.e. Crinas), Charmis, Thessalus, Avicenna, Vettius Valens, Serenus, and Macer, a far cry, save for Avicenna, from the medieval authorities.[78] The leading proponent of this new Erfurt humanism would appear to have been Georg Eberbach (*c.*1450–1508), who after studies at Erfurt, Freiburg, and Ferrara, became a member of the medical faculty of Erfurt in 1489. Four times Dean, twice Rector of the university, and from 1492 Ordinarius of Medicine, he also owned a pharmacy in the town. He was a friend of several leading humanists, notably Johannes Trithemius and two Erfurt colleagues Nicolaus Marschalk and Conrad Mutianus. He was responsible for the printing by Wolfgang Schenck at Erfurt in 1499 of the Latin version of Psellus's *De victus ratione*, translated from the Greek by Giorgio Valla and first published at Venice in the previous year.[79] This was the first time a classical Greek medical author was printed as such in Germany, and it is interesting for not being Galen or Hippocrates.[80] Soon afterwards, Marschalk published a '*Small Commentary*' to accompany this translation, in which he explained the new 'humanist' technical terms for the benefit of medical students and others, giving German equivalents for the names of some of the herbs and parts of the body. Marschalk cites in his preface as authors familiar to Eberbach, Hippocrates, Galen, Dioscorides, Asclepiades, Celsus and Pliny, a list that need not have included any direct acquaintance with Greek on the part of Eberbach, but which is firmly classical in its orientation.

The Erfurt Psellus marks a beginning, but only a very small one, for it shows the weakness, as far as medicine was concerned, of the new humanism. Only Celsus counted as a rediscovered author,[81] and his prescriptions, although written in Ciceronian Latin, were duplicated by Galen, by later medieval authorities, and above all by Pliny. Despite the assault on Pliny's authority as a medical source delivered by Leoniceno and others, he remained a necessary conduit of classical information. Whether as the quarry for literary allusions (for Pliny is Marschalk's source for his reference to Asclepiades) or for remedies, Pliny continued to be used and respected. Joachim Vadianus, the Swiss humanist and Vienna-trained doctor, announced in 1522 that Pliny was still his favourite author, although 'he was a man, and hence could slip and fall into error'.[82] Nor had the humanists much to put in the place of the standard texts, for few in Germany knew Greek and only a few humanist translations of a handful of Hippocratic and Galenic writings had appeared in printings of the *Articella*, the corpus of standard university set texts. Only by the 1520s, when the new tri-lingual schools were beginning to turn out students who knew enough Greek to go with their better Latin was there the possibility of a humanistic Greek medicine with a wide following.

In 1500, however, this was still some way off. A few names can be given of university teachers of medicine with Greek – perhaps Eberhard; Peter Burchard, professor at Ingolstadt, whose *Parva tabula Hippocratis* (Wittenberg, 1520), a portion of *Epidemics* VI in Latin with commentary and with a preface by Melanchthon, served as a clarion call in Germany for the new Greek medicine;[83] and Theodoricus Ulsenius (*c.*1460–1508), the holder very briefly of chairs in 1502 and 1504 in medicine at Mainz and Freiburg. Poet, astrologer, physician, and moralist, Ulsenius is best known for his *Speculator* (1497? or 1501), a versification of many of the traditional *Salernitan Questions*, as well as for his writings on syphilis.[84] Where he learned his Greek is not clear, but he resided in Nuremburg from 1492 to 1501, and also knew the Augsburg physician Adolphus Occo and his important collection of Greek medical manuscripts.[85] Ulsenius had certainly enough Greek for him to publish in 1496 a version of the *Aphorisms* of Hippocrates, probably based on that of Laurentianus, accompanied by a poem *Clinicus pharmacandi modus* which was dedicated to Mellerstadt. The translation is unusual in that it rearranged the *Aphorisms* into an order Ulsenius thought more appropriate for practice, beginning with the recognition of disease, and continuing with discussions of possible therapies, before concluding in book II with the aphorisms concerned with disease.[86] Seven years later, in 1503, he brought out at Augsburg an edition of the famous Hippocratic letter in which Hippocrates reported his treatment of the philosopher Democritus.[87] Ulsenius used the humanist Latin translation by the Italian Rinuccio Aretino, which he probably knew from a manuscript copy made in 1498 for his friend, the Nuremberg doctor and book-collector Hartmann Schedel.[88] He appended to it some of his own poems, but he did not include, probably because it was not yet finished, his *Lumen vitae*, in which he expounded the moral and philosophical significance of this famous story.

With Ulsenius, Occo, and Schedel we have moved largely outside the university to the prosperous cities of Augsburg and Nuremberg, rivals to Vienna in their claims to be the German centres of the revival of humanism. Neither city had a university as yet, but it was in them that the new literary humanism, civic power and medical wealth came together.[89] Both Schedel and Occo had enormous collections of manuscripts copied in Italy, and both were in touch with the latest developments in Italy and elsewhere in Germany. Compared with the intellectual activity taking place here, and in such courts as that of the Tyrol, even what was happening at Erfurt or Leipzig appears insignificant – a warning to university historians not to overestimate their subject.[90] Yet it is possible to argue that, without the institutional base provided by the universities in the second and third decades of the sixteenth century, the second wave of humanist, and more robustly Hellenic, medicine could not have gained a strong hold in Germany or flourished outside a few aristocratic urban centres. Moves to reform the medical faculties on the Italian model took time; it is perhaps not until the 1550s that one can see a wholesale reorganization of German universities along Italian lines, but there is also evidence, from the 1520s, of individual teachers bringing back from Italy at least the rhetoric of the new Hellenic humanism and trying to impose it on their students and on their fellow faculty members. But to think of humanism solely in terms of Greek and the introduction of the new Galenism is, as the second part of this chapter has tried to show, to miss the earlier, mainly literary humanism. It undoubtedly produced a change in the language of medicine – although whether the poems of Ulsenius made a more satisfying alternative to a medieval commentary on Hippocrates is an open question – and, as some have argued, by its insistence on individuality and on new, humanist values, it may have prepared the way for a realignment in medicine as well as in theology and literature. But such a realignment was long in coming, and, even when it arrived, there were many who were prepared to defend stoutly the older, more solid medical learning that had been the staple of the German medieval universities.[91]

Notes

1. The following will be referred throughout by the name of the author: Horst Rudolf Abe, *Die Erfurter medizionische Fakultät in den Jahren 1392–1524*, Erfurt, 1973–74; Harry Kühnel, *Mittelalterliche Heilkunde in Wien*, Graz, 1965; Leonore Liess, *Geschichte der medizinischen Fakultät in Ingolstadt von 1472 bis 1600*, Munich, 1984; Erich Meuthen, *Kölner Universität, Band 1: Die alte Universität*, Cologne, 1988; Klaus Pielmeyer, *Statuten der deutschen medizinischen Fakultäten im Mittelalter*, Bonn, 1981; Eduard Seidler, *Die medizinische Fakultät der Albert-Ludwigs-Universität Freiburg im Breisgau*, Berlin, 1991; Eberhard Stübler, *Geschichte der medizinischen Fakultät der Universität Heidelberg 1386–*

1925: Karl Sudhoff, *Aus dem ersten Jahrhundert der Leipziger medizinischen Fakultät*, Leipzig, 1909.

2. E. T. A. Puschmann, *A History of Medical Education*, London, 1891; see also C. D. O'Malley, *The History of Medical Education*, Berkeley, 1970, pp. 79–96; and Gernot Rath, 'Medical Education at the S. German Universities in the 15th and 16th Centuries', *Journal of Medical Education*, 35 (1960), pp. 511–17. A substantial amount of valuable information lurks in the entries in *Die deutsche Literatur des Mittelalters, Verfasserlexikon*, 2nd edn, 9 vols, eds K. Ruh, G. Keil, W. Schröder, B. Wachinger, F. J. Worstbrock, Berlin, 1978– (hereafter cited as VFL).
3. Even such excellent surveys of medieval medicine as G. Baader and G. Keil, *Medizin im Mittelalterlichen Abendland*, Darmstadt, 1982, pp. 1–44, and H. Schipperges, *Der Garten der Gesundheit: Medizin im Mittelalter*, Munich and Zurich, 1985, say little or nothing. Schipperges, pp. 289–91, has no entry in his list of 'medico-cultural developments' between the death of Guy de Chauliac in 1368 and Paracelsus around 1520.
4. Nancy Siraisi's chapter, 'The Faculty of Medicine', in Hilde de Ridder-Symoens, *A History of the University in Europe*, vol. 1, Cambridge, 1992, pp. 360–87, is excellent in its coverage of Italy and France, but omits the German side entirely except for a reference to anatomy teaching in Vienna.
5. Details are most accessible in F. H. Rashdall, *The Universities of Europe in the Middle Ages*, Oxford, 1936; and in L. Boehm and R. A. Müller, eds, *Universitäten und Hochschulen in Deutschland, Österreich und der Schweiz*, Düsseldorf, 1983. Meuthen, pp. 1–40, provides an excellent recent survey, concentrating on the German universities.
6. For a broad discussion of these later groups, see P. Baumgart and N. Hammerstein eds, *Beiträge zu Problemen deutscher Universitätsgründungen der frühen Neuzeit*, Nendeln, 1978.
7. Pielmeyer, p. 12; M. Cierny, *Medizin und Mediziner an der Prager Karls-Universität*, Zurich, 1973, pp. 15–31. Details of individuals with medical interests can be found in Renate Bickerl, *Die Magister der Artistenfakultät der Hohen Schulen zu Prag und ihre Schriften im Zeitraum von 1348–1409*, dissertation, Erlangen, 1971, and Lothar Schletz, *Die Magister der Artistenfakultät der Hohen Schulen zu Prag und ihre Schriften im Zeitraum von 1409 bis 1550*, dissertation, Erlangen, 1971. I have not seen Renate Dix, *Frühgeschiche der Prager Universität, Gründung, Aufbau und Organisation, 1348–1409*, dissertation, Bonn, 1988. For Gallus, see VFL, vol. 2 (1980), cols. 1065–9; for Christian, VFL, vol. 1 cols 1222–3.
8. Pielmeyer, p. 43, with refs.; a more detailed account is given in an as yet unpublished Cologne dissertation of Michael Trauth, 'Die Triere Universität zur Zeit der Aufklärung', pp. 52–60 (information from Dr Hort, who kindly obtained xeroxes for me).
9. Seidler, pp. 24–5.
10. Abe, pp. 250–52.
11. Pielmeyer, pp. 44, 46, 35. On the creation of faculties and faculty statutes, see E. T. Nauck, *Zur Geschichte des medizinischen Lehrplan und Unterrichts der Universität Freiburg i. Breisgau*, Freiburg, 1952, which ranges far more widely than its title suggests.
12. Stübler, p. 4, Herman Weisert, 'Die ältesten Statuten der Medizinischen Fakultät Heidelberg 1425', *Ruperto Carola*, 33 (1981), pp. 57–71, and

'Universität und Heiliggeiststift', *Ruperto Carola*, 33 (1981), pp. 72–87, argues that a medical faculty existed in 1390, was given new statutes in 1425, and enjoyed a greater success in teaching than these comments might suggest.

13. Sudhoff, p. 8. It was decided to create two posts specifically for medical teachers, with special stipends.
14. Figures from G. Erler, *Die Matrikel der Universität Leipzig*, Leipzig, 1897, vol. 2, p. 70, with Sudhoff, pp. 5–7; Abe, p. 48; Meuthen, pp. 120, 124.
15. Meuthen, p. 120; Abe, p. 66 (cf. plates 69–70 for the actual entries in the graduation book for doctors); Erler, *Matrikel*, pp. 69–73.
16. Liess, p. 50.
17. Abe, p. 26, suggests this figure; at Erfurt, 82 per cent were enrolled in the faculty of arts, 15 per cent as jurists, 2.5 per cent in theology. The figures for Cologne and Leipzig show similar balances.
18. At Heidelberg, the medical faculty shared the building with the jurists, and the *Dionysianum*, one of whose founders was Gerhard Hohenkirche, a member of the medical faculty from 1420 to 1448, was in part intended to house medical students, and included a library made up largely of Gerhard's books, Stübler, pp. 13, 23; VFL vol. 4, 1983, cols 99–100. Gerhard was clearly influenced in this by his former Erfurt colleague Amplonianus Ratingk (1365–1435), who gave money for a *Collegium* there and endowed it with his magnificent medical library, Abe, pp. 144–7. At Leipzig *c.* 1509, the medical faculty complained at having to share premises with the lawyers, Sudhoff, p. 45.
19. Pielmeyer provides a handy summary of most of the statutes. Meuthen, pp. 121–2, describes the Cologne statutes in detail. Gundolf Keil and Rudolf Peitz, '"Decem quaestiones de medicorum statu". Beobachtungen zum Fakultätenstreit und zum mittelalterlichen Unterrichtsplan Ingolstadts', in Gundolf Keil, Bernd Moeller and Winfried Trusen, *Der Humanismus und die oberen Fakultäten*, Weinheim, 1987, pp. 215–38, provide evidence (from MS Kahrsruhe, Badische Landesbibliothek, unbekannter Herkunft 5) of the actual texts used in medical instruction at Ingolstadt in 1476, eighty or so years before the first detailed Studienplan of that university.
20. K. Sudhoff, *Die medizinische Fakultät der Universität Leipzig im 1. Jahrhundert der Universität Leipzig*, Leipzig, 1909, p. 13; W. Friedensburg, *Urkundenbuch der Universität Wittenberg 1*, Magdeburg, 1926, pp. 46–50.
21. Both may represent aspiration far more than reality. Laurentianus's translation, first published at Florence in 1494, did not become at all widely available until the Venice, 1523, printing of the *Articella*. (But Mellerstadt knew of Ulsenius's edition, see below, note 75, which was based on Laurentianus.) Although the *Ad Glauconem* was available in the 1490 and subsequent printings of the Latin *Opera Omnia Galeni*, these were beyond the pocket of most medical students. Had Mellerstadt heard of the Greek 1500 edition of the *Ad Glauconem*, and was assuming that new translations would swiftly follow?
22. Meuthen, p. 122. The list of books was published by Friedrich Moritz, 'Aus der medizinischen Fakultät der alten Universität Köln', in *Festschrift zur Erinnerung an die Gründung der alten Universität Köln*, Cologne,

1938, pp. 242–8. Identification of some of the works is by no means certain. The only extant manuscript from his collection, Wiesbaden, Staatsbibl. 61, contains, among other works, 'Recipes of Master de Varignana' (Guglielmo or Bartolommeo?); see G. Kricker, 'Ein medizinisches Kollegbuch aus Köln im Angang der 15. Jh.', *Zentralblatt für Bibliothekswesen*, 43 (1926), pp. 73–8.
23. Abe, pp. 87–92, gives a useful survey.
24. Cf. the list of medical books given to the Great College at Leipzig in 1459 and that of books in the Small College in 1507, Sudhoff, pp. 16–19. The books owned by Eberhard Knab (*c.*1420–80), who was associated with Heidelberg as student and later professor from 1439 to his death, are perhaps even more traditional (the latest authority included is Bartolommeo da Montagnana, *fl.* 1430); his own university lecture notes concentrate heavily upon Avicenna's *Canon*. But Knab had not been to Italy. See Colette Jeudy and Ludwig Schuba, 'Erhard Knab und die Heidelberger Universität im Spiegel von Handschriften und Akteneinträgen', *Quellen und Forschungen aus italienischen Archiven und Bibliotheken*, 61 (1981), pp. 60–108.
25 Pielmeyer, pp. 46–52; based on J. Haller, *Die Anfänge der Universität Tübingen*, Stuttgart, 1827, pp. 301–9.
26 The papal letter is published with a good translation and discussion by Bernard Schultz, 'A fifteenth-century Papal brief on human dissection', *Medical Heritage*, January (1986), pp. 50–56. Sixtus IV had given permission in 1476 for the foundation of the university.
27. Pielmeyer, p. 76.
28. *Anathomia Mundini emendata per doctorem Melerstat*, Leipzig, [1493], discussed at length by Sudhoff, pp. 122–5, and by V. Nutton, 'Hellenism postponed: some aspects of Renaissance medicine, 1490–1530', *Sudhoffs Archiv*, 81 (1997), pp. 159–60, who argues that Mellerstadt's contribution was only stylistic. The frontispiece is reproduced in N. G. Siraisi, *Medieval and Early Renaissance Medicine*, Chicago, 1990, p. 87. For a discussion of the statutes and of Mellerstadt's role in them, see, above all, W. Friedensburg, *Geschichte der Universität Wittenberg*, Halle, 1917, caps 1 and 2.
29. For Leipzig, Sudhoff, pp. 44–5, 48 (note also the complaint, p. 43, of a lack of teaching in botany); H. Helbig, *Die Reformation der Universität Leipzig im 16. Jahrhundert*, Gütersloh, 1953, pp. 18–31; O. Clemen, *Kleine Schriften zur Reformationsgeschichte*, Leipzig, 1982–86, vol. 3, pp. 34–7; vol. 8, pp. 30, 100. For Wittenberg, Friedensburg, *Geschichte*, pp. 62–4, 136–9, 181. Sudhoff, pp. 113–21, describes anatomical publications by Leipzig authors not in the medical faculty.
30. Liess, pp. 60–61; pp. 69–71 (botany, introduced by Leonhard Fuchs in 1526).
31. Pielmeyer, p. 57, noting that the Frankfurt statutes cannot easily be dated; they fall between 1524 and 1550. Injunctions to would-be doctors to collect their own plants go back a long way; cf. G. Keil, VFL, vol. 5, 1985, cols 346–8 s.v. Kräuter-sammel-kalender. In the late fourteenth cenury, Prague had a small herb garden, the creation of a royal apothecary, see Cierny, *Medizin und Mediziner*, p. 24.
32. In its demand for botany as an official part of the course, the Tübingen statutes were institutionalizing what was now fashionable within Italy

(especially at Ferrara and Venice in the wake of the great controversy over the identification of the herbs in Pliny's *Natural History*) but, as yet, no Italian teaching on botany was required by statute. For possible Italian influence on a fifteenth-century German's rules for medical botany, see Werner Dressendörfer, 'Hartmann Schedels Angaben zur Aufbewahrung von Arzneimittein in Apotheken', in Gundolf Keil, ed., *Festschrift zum 70. Geburtstag von Willem F. Daems*, Pattensen, 1982, pp. 543–50.

33. Pielmeyer, p. 46.
34. Kühnel, p. 41. In December 1416, the faculty met 'pro anathomia celebranda', but their decision on the proper way to advertise a future dissection implies that no actual anatomy took place then, see Karl Schrauf, *Acta facultatis medicae universitatis Vindobonensis*, 1, Vienna, 1894, p. 34, and that the next dissection took place in 1418, ibid., p. 38. For Galeazzo, see also VFL, vol. 8, cols 582–4.
35. VFL, vol. 1, p. 92; vol. 2, pp. 2, 21, 29–31, 40, 55–58 (the first anatomy of a woman). Kühnel, pp. 66, 74, 75. L. Schönbauer, *Das medizinische Wien*, Vienna and Urban, 1947, p. 50, calculates that only fourteen dissections took place between 1404 and 1498. G. Baader, 'Medizinische Theorie und Praxis zwischen Arabismus und Renaissancehumanismus', in Gundolf Keil, Bernd Moeller and Winfried Trusen, eds, *Der Humanismus und die oberen Fakultäten*, Weinheim, 1987, pp. 200–205.
36. Meuthen, p. 123, also referring to some anatomy teaching in Prague *c.* 1460, but this appears to be instruction from a book, not by dissection. Cf. also the exhibition catalogue, *Älteste Stadtuniversität Nordwesteuropas*, Cologne, 1988, p. 20, for a photo of the imperial letter.
37. Cf. the demand at Leipzig in 1509 for the introduction of dissection 'in the Italian manner', Sudhoff, p. 48. For three examples of Germans with Italian training, see Bernhard Schnell, 'Arzt und Literat. Zum Anteil der Ärzte am spätmittelalterlichen Literaturbetrieb', *Sudhoffs Archiv*, 75 (1991), pp. 44–57.
38. Cf. Wellcome Institute, MS 5265, *c.*1464, a letter of the University of Pavia requesting the body of a witch for an anatomy, and admitting that, contrary to the statutes (which prescribed an annual anatomy), none had taken place for five or six years.
39. Schrauf, *Acta facultatis medicae, II*, pp. 30–31, 57–8, 181, 196.
40. Siraisi, *Medieval and Renaissance Medicine*, pp. 88–9, notes the Vienna anatomy, but concentrates on Italy.
41. Pielmeyer, pp. 20, 22, 25–6, 42, 44, 52, 55, lists the various statutory requirements for practical experience. For Heidelberg, see Weisert, 'Die ältesten Statuten', pp. 68–9.
42. Liess, pp. 12–13, 52–3. The Ingolstadt section is taken verbatim from that of Cologne.
43. For Peter, see VFL, vol. 6, 1987, cols 783–90; for Münsinger, VFL, vol. 7, 1989, cols 458–64, with refs.
44. Abe, pp. 40–43.
45. Seidler, p. 22.
46. Liess, pp. 52–3, noting occasional exceptions. Cf. also Gundolf Keil, 'Chirung, Chirurgie', in *Lexikon des Mittelalters*, vol. 2, 1983, col. 1854.
47. Schrauf, *Acta facultaties medicae*, vol. 2, pp. x, gives the many references; Kühnel, pp. 47–53. Cf., for London, Sir George Clark, *A History of the Royal College of Physicians of London*, vol. 1 (Oxford, 1964), pp. 107–

24, and Margaret Pelling and Charles Webster, 'Medical Practitioners', in Charles Webster, ed. *Health, Medicine, and Mortality in the Sixteenth Century* (Cambridge, 1979), pp. 168–89. For similar problems in Leipzig, Sudhoff, pp. 92–3; and for the career of Jörg Radendorfer, driven out as a quack from Frankfurt am Main in 1499, and from Nuremberg in 1502/3, despite enjoying occasional official support and protection, see VFL, vol. 7, 1989, cols 966–8. The old article by Karl Sudhoff, 'Kurpfuscher, Ärzte und Stadtbehörden am Ende d. 15. Jh.s', *Sudhoffs Archiv*, 8 (1915), pp. 98–124, is still useful.

48. Kühnel, pp. 53–9. Cf. also Kurt Ganzinger, 'Apotheke und Universität', *Beiträge zur Geschichte der Pharmazie*, 28 (1976), 1–4; Gundolf Keil, 'Zur Frage der kurativ-konsilierischen Tätigkeit des mittelalterlichen deutschen Apothekers', in Peter Dilg, ed., *Perspektiven der Pharmaziegeschichte. Festschrift für Rudolf Schmitz*, Graz, 1983, pp. 181–96.
49. Stübler, pp. 15–17.
50. Meuthen, p. 125.
51. Sudhoff, 89–91; 43, for the accusation of laziness.
52. Alois Paweletz, *Lepradiagnostik im Mittelalter und Anweisungen zur Lepraschau*, dissertation, Leipzig, 1915; Friedrich Lenhardt, *Blutschau*, Pattensen, 1986, pp. 146–50.
53. Johannes Asen, *Das Leprosenhaus Melaten bei Köln*, dissertation, Bonn, 1908, 67–70, referring to statutes from the end of the 16th century relating to examinations by the Leper-master. This would seem to contradict the view expressed, e.g. by Meuthen, p. 125, that the medical faculty gained dominance, if not exclusive control in 1491. I have not seen O. von Bremen, 'Leprauntersuchungen der Kölner medizinischen Fakultät', *Westdeutsche Zeitschrift für Geschichte und Kunst*, 18, (1899), pp. 65–77.
54. Meuthen, p. 125.
55. Siegfried Reicke, *Das deutsche Spital und sein recht im Mittelalter*, Stuttgart, 1961, pp. 268–9.
56. Liess, pp. 74–5; Sudhoff, p. 36, quoting a faculty decision of 1490 claiming the right of the faculty alone to examine lepers.
57. Knab's books are the subject of a major study by Colette Jeudy and Ludwig Schuba, 'Erhard Knab und die Heidelberger Universität im Spiegel von Handschriften und Akteneinträgen', *Quellen und Forschungen aus italienischen Archiven und Bibliotheken*, 61 (1971), pp. 60–108; cf. also VFL, vol. 4, 1983, cols 1264–73. The library of his Heidelberg colleague Konrad Schelling, VFL, vol. 8, 1991, cols 631–2, is also relevant. For Ellenbog's annotations, see V. Nutton, 'Ellenbogiana', *Würzburger medizinhistorische Mitteilungen*, 8 (1990), pp. 221–4; and for his writings, Liess, 114–15; VFL, vol. 2, 1980, cols 495–501. A (teaching?) commentary on Hippocrates, *On Ancient Medicine*, is said to exist in Melk, Stiftsbibl. 999 (cf. VFL, vol. 6, 1989, col. 906).
58. For Münsinger, Stübler, pp. 27–9; J. Telle, 'Mitteilungen aus dem "Zwölfbändigen Buch der Medizin"', *Sudhoffs Archiv*, 52 (1968), pp. 310–40; Gerhard Eis, *Forschungen zur Fachprosa*, Bern, 1971, pp. 81–90; VFL, vol. 6, 1987, cols 783–90; vol. 7, 1989, col. 459. Sudhoff, pp. 100–112, 185–208, gives an excellent selection from the medical writings of Leipzig physicians. For Prague, see VFL, vol. 1, cols 154–5 (Sigmund Albich); cols 1222–3 (Christian von Prachatitz); and vol. 2, 1980, cols

1065–9, Gallus. For Vienna, VFL, vol. 2, cols 561–3 (Jacob Engelin); vol. 4, cols 1150–54 (Johannes Kirchheimer [or Ketham]).

59. Kühnel, p. 73; VFL, vol. 7, 1989, cols 908–9; and cols 80–81 (pseudo-Ortolf). A version of the book preserved in a Zurich manuscript has been edited by L. Welker, *Das 'iatromathematische Corpus'*, Zurich, 1988, pp. 226–49. Cf. similar books on distillation by another colleague of Puff aus Schrick, Kaspar Griessenpeck (VFL, vol. 3, 1982, col. 257, teaching 1458–77), discussed by Eis, *Forschungen*, pp. 28–34; and by Johann Tollat von Vochenberg, Kühnel, p. 73.
60. Ellenbog's book, first printed in 1525, was edited by Frank Koelsch and Friedrich Zoepfl, *Elrich Ellenbog*, Munich, 1927. See also Edwin Rosner, 'Ulrich Ellenbog und die Anfänge der Gewerbehygiene', *Sudhoffs Archiv*, 38 (1954), 101–10.
61. K. Grossmann, 'Die Frühzeit des Humanismus in Wien bis zu Celtis Berufung 1497', *Jahrbuch für Landeskunde von Niederösterreich*, 22 (1929), esp. pp. 220–54, is fundamental.
62. Kühnel, pp. 91–2; VFL, vol. 2, 1980, cols 561–3; K. Sudhoff, *Iatromathematiker*, Breslau, 1902, pp. 44–60; B. Milt, *Vadian als Arzt*, St Gallen, 1959, pp. 114–16, for Tannstetter's influence; Franz Stuhlhofer, 'Georg Tannstetter (Collimitius); Astrononom, Astrologe und Leibarzt bei Maximilian I. und Ferdinand I', *Studien zur Weiner Geschichte. Jahbruch des Vereins für Geschichte der Stadt Wien*, 31 (1981), pp. 7–49; *idem, Humanismus zwischen Hof und Universität*, Vienna, 1996; Conrad Bonorand, *Personenkommentar II zum Vadianischen Briefwechsel*, St Gallen, 1983, pp. 249–53, a useful summary; Welker, *Iatromathematische Corpus*, summarizes earlier German medical astrology.
63. Liess, pp. 117–20.
64. Sudhoff, pp. 128–31 (Mellerstadt), and for Leipzig medical astrology in general, pp. 40–42, 47, 125–27. Further details of Mellerstadt's publications are given by Helmut Schlereth, 'Opera Pollichiana', *Würzburger medizinhistorische Mitteilungen*, 4 (1986), pp. 185–202.
65. For Cologne in the later sixteenth century, see Meuthen, p. 124; for Prague, see Cierny, *Medizin und Mediziner*, pp. 16, 18, 22, 29. For Paracelsus, see W. D. Müller-Jahncke, *Astrologisch-magische Theorie und Praxis in der Heilkunde der frühen Neuzeit*, Stuttgart, 1985, pp. 67–89; cf. also pp. 134–50, for a survey of medical astrological writers from 1450 to 1550.
66. The topic is treated at length by Abe, pp. 55–71.
67. The most useful survey of the impact of (literary) Italian humanism on Germany is perhaps H. O. Burger, *Renaissance, Humanismus, Reformation*, Bad Homburg, 1969, which has a good geographical range.
68. Meuthen, p. 124 (citing Rudolphus Agricola, hardly an unprejudiced witness in questions of 'Bildung'); it is possible that this is an allusion to the departure of the physician Balthasar von Bingen, who left that year to become Dean of the Faculty of Arts at Greifswald, but his subsequent activities show no sign of humanist influence, ibid. p. 177.
69. Kühnel, pp. 33 (Albert), 39–43 (Galeazzo), 96 (Jacobus), 79–82 (Tichtel), 82–83 (Steber), with further references. See in general, Peter Uiblein, 'Bezienhungen der Wiener Medizin zur Universität Padua im Mittelalter', *Römische historische Mitteilungen*, 23 (1981), 271–301.
70. The best study of humanism in Vienna in this period is K. Großmann,

'Die Frühzeit des Humanismus in Wien', *Jahrbuch für Landeskunde von Niederösterfeich*, 22 (1929), pp. 313–27; Burger, *Renaissance, Humanismus, Reformation*, pp. 283–380, is still useful.

71. A nice example of the stylistic influence of Italian humanism can be seen in the *regimina* of Vincent Schwoffheim of Leignitz, who after his MB at Leipzig in 1432, went to study in Italy, Sudhoff, pp. 185–91. Written *c.*1450 in fine humanist Latin, they contain elegant classical allusions to Homer and Hippocrates's cure of the plague of Athens (taken from Pliny), and the preface, p. 185, shows the influence of the new Latin rhetorical teaching in its structure and vocabulary.
72. Hans Anckwitz-Kleehofen, *Der Wiener Humanist Johannes Cuspinian*, Graz, 1959; Bonorand, *Personenkommentar II*, p. 267; Milt, *Vadian*, pp. 114–15.
73. R. J. Durling, 'An Early Manual for the Medical Student and the Newly Fledged Practitioner'; Martin Steinpeis, 'Liber de modo studendi seu legendi in medicina (Vienna, 1520)', *Clio Medica*, 5 (1970), pp. 7–33; Kühnel, pp. 84–6. I have not seen Christian Panulik, *Martin Stainpeis:<Liber de modo studendi seu legendi in Medizin>. Bearbeitung und Erläuterung einer Studieneintleitung für mediziner im ausgehenden Mittelalter*, dissertation, Munich, 1980.
74. Literature on these debates is substantial. The major documentation is given in G. Bauch, *Geschichte des Leipziger Frühhumanismus*, Leipzig, 1899; Sudhoff, pp. 134–52; and *Aus der Frühgeschichte der Syphilis*, Leipzig, 1912; Friedensburg, *Wittenberg*, caps 1 and 2; Clemen, *Kleine Schriften*, vol. 3, pp. 253–5; Schlereth, *Pollichiana*. An overview of the syphilis controversy in Germany, from an interesting perspective, is by P. A. Russell, 'Syphilis, God's Scourge or Nature's Vengeance? The German Printed Response to a Public Problem in the Early Sixteenth Century', *Archiv für Reformationsgeschichte*, 80 (1989), pp. 286–307. Roger French, 'The Arrival of the French Disease in Leipzig', in *Maladie et société (XIIe–XVIIe siècles)*, Paris, 1989, pp. 133–41, repeated in J. Arrizabalaga, J. Henderson and R. French, *The Great Pox*, New Haven, 1997, pp. 91–7, adds little.
75. J. H. Overfield, *Humanism and Scholasticism in Late Medieval Germany*, Princeton, 1984, pp. 173–85, on the controversy with Wimpina; note Sudhoff's warnings, p. 151, that to associate Mellerstadt with the 'new spirit' is a very uncertain procedure; 'Gerade diese Syphilisauffassung zeigt uns recht deutlich, wie schwach es im positiven Sinne mit dieser ganzen medizinischen Renaissance bestellt war'. Cf. also Catrien Santing, *Geneeskunde en Humanisme*, Rotterdam, 1992, pp. 201–4, for a discussion of his friendship with Ulsenius (*c.*1460–1508).
76. In the second decade of the sixteenth century, Johannes Lange of Lemberg was lecturing on Pliny and the historian Quintus Curtius, see V. Nutton, 'John Caius und Johannes Lange; medizinischer Humanismus zur Zeit Vesals', *NTM*, 21 (1984), pp. 81–7; Clemen, *Kleine Schriften*, vol. 1, pp. 110–12.
77. Liess, pp. 117–20; Abe, pp. 93–140. On Sturtz, Clemen, *Kleine Schriften*, vol. 3, 51–7.
78. Abe, p. 98, with comments on the changes between the two editions. For the dates, see C. Krause, *Helius Eobanus Hessus. Sein Leben und seine Werke*, Gotha, 1879, vol. 1, pp. 389, 397; vol. 2, p. 102. The information

on which the poems are based is largely derived from Pliny. In the second version, Avicenna asks why, when his Arab birth did not prevent him from being the 'great glory of medicine', the barbarity of his translation should stop him being read; he was clever enough (*disertus*) in Arabic. See also V. Nutton, 'Hellenism postponed'.

79. Eberbach's responsibility is made clear by Marschalk's preface to his *Leve interpretamentum*, Erfurt, 1499, sig. a1v. The author is not Psellus, but another Byzantine author Theophanes Chrysobalantes, see J. A. M. Sonderkamp, *Theophanes Chrysobalantes*, Bonn, 1987, pp. 1–6, and V. Nutton, 'Hellenism postponed'.

80. Professor Keil drew my attention to the portions of Hippocrates *Aphorisms* 1.1 and *Prognostic* 2 included in early printings of Ortolf von Baierland from 1472 on, see Franz-Josef Worstbrock, *Deutsche Antike-Rezeption 1450–1550*, Boppard, 1976, p. 76 f. (and not recorded in Hippocratic bibliographies); in the Augsburg, 1479, edition, they are found on fols xvr and xvii v–r respectively.

81. His rediscovery in 1425 attracted great humanist interest, see the edition of *Celsus* by F. Marx, Leipzig, 1915, pp. xl–lxv. The medical poet Serenus, first printed around 1474, also gained admirers. Marschalk also cites the agricultural writer Columella, but far less often than Pliny, or even Martial, the epigrammatist. Only one medieval author is named, Rhazes's *Ad Almansorem*, on the last page, fol. c. iv. verso.

82. J. Vadianus, *Loca aliquot ex Pomponianis commentariis*, Basle, 1522; his comment on Pliny's fallibility (and much else), he took from Leoniceno's *De Plinii et plurium aliorum medicorum in medicina erroribus* (probably in the edition of Ferrara, 1509), see V. Schenker-Frei, *Biblioteca Vadiana*, St Gallen, 1973, n. 586.

83. Liess, p. 124. Where he learned his Greek is uncertain but, after his return from Wittenberg in 1521, he produced a notable series of pupils, including Johann Agricola (1496–1570, on whom see Liess, pp. 131–5 and Peter Dilg, 'Johann Agricola Ammonius' Kommentar zu Galens *Methodus medendi*', in F. Kudlien and R. Durling, *Galen's Method of Healing*, Leiden, Brill, 1991, pp. 190–98), and Leonhard Fuchs (1501–66, Liess, pp. 127–30).

84. Catrien Santing, *Geneeskunde en humanisme. Een intellectuele biografie van Theodoricus Ulsenius (c. 1460–1508)*, Rotterdam, 1992.

85. Adolphus Occo (1447–1503) makes a fleeting appearance in many studies of Southern German humanists and some of his manuscripts, now in Munich, are familiar to editors of Hippocrates and Galen, but there is no modern study of either him or them, cf. *Allgemeine deutsche Biographie*, 24 (1887), pp. 126–7; Santing, *Ulsenius*, pp. 87–93.

86. Santing, *Ulsenius*, p. 160, is not entirely clear on the extent to which Ulsenius is indebted to Laurentianus; she lists the changes in order on pp. 251–5.

87. On this letter, see now Thomas Rütten, *Demokrit lachender Philosoph und sanguinischer melancholiker. Eine pseudohippokratische Geschichte*, Leiden, 1992, pp. 152–4, who dates the edition to *c.*1480, but cf. Santing, *Ulsenius*, pp. 235–41, for an argument for the later date.

88. For Schedel, see R. Stauber, *Die Schedelsche Bibliothek*, Freiburg, 1908; O. Meyer, 'Hartmann Schedel', *Medizinhistorisches Journal*, 4 (1969), pp. 55–68; VFL, vol. 8, 1991, cols 609–21; cf. also cols 621–5 (Hermann

Schedel), and Bernhard Schnell, 'Arzt und Literat', *Sudhoffs Archiv*, 75 (1991), pp. 44–57.

89. Cf. for introductory surveys of these cities as centres of humanism, R. Pfeiffer, *Ausgewählte Schriften*, Munich, 1960, pp. 222–34; N. Holzburg, *Willibald Pirckheimer*, Munich, 1981; I have not yet seen R. Kiessling, 'Das gebildete Bürgertum und die kulturelle Zenträlität Augsburgs im Spätmittelalter', in B. Moeller, H. Patzer and K. Stackmann, eds, *Studien zum städtischen Bildungswesen des späten Mittelalters und der frühen Neuzeit*, Göttingen, 1983, pp. 553–84.
90. For the court of the Tyrol, see Peter Assion, 'Der Hof Siegmunds von Tirol als Zentrum spätmittelalterlicher Fachliteratur', in G. Keil, P. Assion, W. F. Daems and H. U. Roehl, eds, *Fachprosa-Studien*, Berlin, 1982, pp. 37–75.
91. I am grateful to the members of the Cambridge conference on late medieval medicine for their comments on this paper, as well as to Nancy Siraisi, who drew my attention to several Italian parallels; Irmgard Hort, who criticized a first draft and provided me with xeroxes of some of the rarer German articles and theses; and Gundolf Keil for his bibliographical assistance. They are not responsible for my errors and misinterpretations.

CHAPTER SIX

Stones, Bones and Hernias: Surgical Specialists in Fourteenth- and Fifteenth-Century Italy

Katharine Park

> From what I have said, you can see how wrong people are who call anyone who performs operations to treat illnesses a surgeon. For we should not call just any lay practitioner [*operator idiota*] or little woman [*muliercula*] a surgeon, even though they lance abscesses, stitch up wounds, and do similar work. We should rather utterly bar them from these operations, wherever they practise, and flee their treatments, for they operate wrongly and inappropriately, and if occasionally they perform successful cures, it is not due to their competence but to luck ... A great host of these ignorant people and empirics flourishes at present – and not only at present, but also in the time of Albucasis and Avenzoar, as is clear from their writings – especially in the treatment of broken bones and dislocated joints.*

> Whereas [Maestro Antonio and Maestro Francesco of Norcia] are staying voluntarily in Florence and out of consideration for the welfare of its citizens are disposed to practise in the service of the inhabitants of the city and its subject territories; and whereas they have no property and cannot live from their work and trade if they must also pay taxes; and whereas tax exemptions have been granted to other foreign medical specialists [*habentibus aliquid singulare in exercitio medicine*], especially bone surgeons; and whereas that speciality is no more important than their own [hernia surgery], given the importance of the parts affected: ... let the said Maestro Antonio and Francesco be exempt and immune from all taxes of any description for their entire lives.[1]

These two early fifteenth-century Florentine texts offer contrasting perspectives on an important sector of medical practice in late medieval and Renaissance Italy: the large and flourishing world of surgical practitioners who specialized in the treatment of a particular condition, most notably hernias, fractures, dislocations, bladder stones and cataracts. For Niccolò Falcucci, trained in the text-based university disciplines of physic and surgery and author of an influential Latin treatise on practical medicine, those practitioners were a blight and a public menace, as can be seen from the first extract above; ignorant of anatomy and of the principles of medical theory, they relied on a combination of experience, luck and nerve, often causing irreparable harm to their patients. For the patrician members of Florence's advisory and legislative councils, on the other hand, the same practitioners – or at least an important subset of them – were an important community resource, whose presence in the city was worth one of its extremely rare lifetime tax exemptions, as evidenced in the second extract. The discrepancy was not uncharacteristic: there are many other instances in which empirically trained surgical specialists were extravagantly lauded and courted by municipal governments,[2] at the same time that their kind were being reviled by university-educated physicians and surgeons like Falcucci.[3] Indeed, in the early fourteenth century, Henry of Mondeville had already commented explicitly on the gap between learned and lay perceptions of surgical competence, noting that

> it is the habit of all princes, prelates, and ordinary people these days in all the western lands ... not to trust any medically learned surgeon [*medico cyrurgico scientifico*] very far, for they say that a surgeon ought not to be a cleric because, while a cleric is in the schools, the layman [*laicus*] is learning the technique of manual operation.[4]

How do these two competing perceptions relate to one another? Who were these surgical specialists and how did they fit into the complicated world of medical practice in late medieval and Renaissance Italy? Historians of medicine have traditionally tended to take the invectives of Falcucci and his learned colleagues more or less at face value – as description rather than polemic – and to dismiss these practitioners as, at worst, 'quacks' or 'charlatans' or, at best, 'irregular' or 'marginal' healers, unlicensed by the authorities and catering to a gullible popular clientele unable to afford the luxury of what Falcucci called 'noble and most honoured doctors [*medici*]'.[5] Although more recent scholars, sensitive to the pressures on and interests of Latinate physicians and surgeons attempting to establish themselves as a learned profession, have offered a much more nuanced view, many of them have none the less persisted in ignoring surgical specialists altogether, lumping them with or subordinating them to barbers, or describing them as representatives of 'illicit', 'unofficial', or 'popular' medicine – as they indeed later seem to have become.[6]

Such confusions are understandable, given both regional variations in the evolution of surgical practice – Michael McVaugh notes that there is very little evidence of surgical specialization in the Crown of Aragon before the fifteenth century[7] – and the paucity of written sources. The men and women who engaged in this kind of practice produced no literary legacy of their own, at least until the later sixteenth century, so that they are known principally through the hostile accounts of Latin medical writers such as Falcucci or (to a lesser degree) through judicial records reflecting their prosecution for unlicensed practice. Furthermore, they often came from social groups poorly represented in the surviving archival documents. None the less, it is possible to assemble these sources into a discernible, if fragmentary picture of an important, dynamic, and often well-respected group of medical practitioners.[8]

This chapter aims to sketch the outlines of specialized surgical practice in fourteenth- and fifteenth-century Florence, supplemented by material collected by other scholars for other Italian cities. In it, I will begin by arguing that surgical specialists constituted a sizeable, well-established and relatively well-defined group of medical practitioners, clearly distinguished from both general surgeons and barber-surgeons on the one hand, and from itinerant sellers of charms and nostrums on the other, and I will end by pulling together what evidence I have been able to assemble concerning the most visible and coherent branch or 'school' of the empirical surgical tradition in Italy: the families of hernia surgeons native to the territories of the isolated Umbrian town of Norcia.[9]

The books of the Florentine *catasto* of 1427 yield a preliminary sense of the size and contours of this group of practitioners in a prosperous Italian urban centre. The *catasto* was a comprehensive wealth tax, and the officials in charge of its administration collected declarations and compiled detailed summaries of assets, obligations and dependents for every household in the city, including those of men like Maestro Antonio and Maestro Francesco of Norcia – 'Maestro' was the doctor's standard honorific – who were tax exempt, as we saw above. These records provide a comprehensive picture of the male medical practitioners active in the city at that time, though for various reasons – women's legal incapacity, the fact that they were much less likely to be heads of household, the tendency not to identify them by occupation – they obscure the significant, if smaller, numbers of women also engaged in healing activities of this sort.[10] In the Kingdom of Naples, for example, all the women who appear in the lists of officially licensed medical practitioners were surgical specialists, and their sex was frequently cited among their qualifications; given the demands of female modesty and the physical intimacy required for many surgical operations, the licensing officials considered it in the public interest to have female surgeons available to treat female patients.[11]

The books of the Florentine *catasto* contain the records of 37 (male) heads of household and their dependents identifiable as doctors in 1427.[12] From these and other municipal documents, I have been able to ascertain the type of practice engaged in by 32 of these men: eighteen physicians, five men referred to in general terms as surgeons (*chirurghi*) and nine identified in these or other records by a surgical speciality. The last group consisted of the following:

1.–4. Maestro Antonio di Giovanni of Norcia, with his brother (see 6. below) the beneficiary of the legislative tax exemption with which I began this chapter. Aged 60, he lived with his three adult sons, Maestro Luca (30), Maestro Bartolomeo (28), and Maestro Giovanni (24). All four appear in these and other documents as hernia doctors ('*medici de' crepati*'). The raw wealth of their composite household, fully itemized in their declaration, was calculated at a respectable 1 668 florins.[13]

5. Benedetto di Francesco, shoemaker and eye doctor ('*chalzolaio e medico d'occhi*'), aged 52, with raw wealth of 147 florins.[14]

6. Maestro Francesco di Giovanni of Norcia, hernia doctor, aged 48, 599 florins.[15]

7. Maestro Simone di Pacino of San Martino, tooth doctor ('*maestro di denti*'), aged 45, 101 florins.[16]

8. Maestro Stefano di maestro Lodovico, called Scappuccino, poultice doctor ('*medico degl' impiastri*'), aged 40, 758 florins.[17]

9. Maestro Domenico di maestro Giovanni, 'bone doctor [*medico d'ossa*] and physician', aged 48, 923 florins.[18]

To these one may plausibly add one of the men described generally as a surgeon:

10. Maestro Giovanni di maestro Piero of Norcia, aged 60, 23 florins. Maestro Giovanni immigrated from Norcia in the late fourteenth century, together with his father, and probably belonged to the Norcian tradition of empirical surgeons, which I will discuss below, although I have to date found no explicit reference to the nature of his practice.[19]

This group of practitioners seems to have been fairly representative of the surgical specialists active in fourteenth- and fifteenth-century Florence. In the first place, their listed competencies – hernias, bones, teeth, eyes and poultices – exhaust the most commonly found specialties in the period.[20] (In Florence, as elsewhere, hernia doctors seem also to have treated what contemporaries called the 'stone disease', or *male della pietra*.[21]) I have also found occasional references to practitioners with other specialities – e.g., a (female) 'ringworm doctor', who appeared in the *estimo* of 1359,[22] and a Betto di Tieri di Betto of Castelfranco Superiore, whose 1426 matriculation entry in the Guild of

Doctors, Apothecaries and Grocers identified him with the phrase, 'medet de morbo clancli'[23] (presumably referring to the condition called *cancro*) – but either these were uncommon types of practice, or they did not constitute the practitioner's primary occupation and therefore appear less often in the records.

In the second place, as far as I have been able to determine from other tax distributions – unfortunately less detailed and complete than the 1427 *catasto* – the relative number of surgical specialists in the *catasto* is also roughly typical: they seem to have made up about 25–30 per cent of the men identifiable as doctors practising in the city in any given year.[24]

Finally, this particular group of practitioners demonstrates a characteristic pattern of occupational inheritance by family. Although physicians and other surgeons had some tendency to cluster within families,[25] this tendency was far more pronounced for surgical specialists, who seem to have transmitted their knowledge from – in the case of these male practitioners – father to son. Thus of the nine identifiable surgical specialists in the 1427 *catasto*, all five hernia doctors (the brothers Maestro Antonio and Maestro Francesco of Norcia, together with Maestro Antonio's three sons) belonged to a single lineage. Two other specialists, Maestro Stefano and Maestro Domenico, had had fathers skilled in the same kind of practice as their own (poultices and bones respectively), and the fact that these two men's grandfathers had also been doctors – to judge by their fathers' patronymics – suggests that those specialties may have been in the family for some time.[26] The same was probably also true for the tenth hypothetical surgical specialist I listed above, Maestro Giovanni di maestro Piero of Norcia. I have found no information about the training or the fathers of the dentist and the eye surgeon, Maestro Piero di Feo and Benedetto di Francesco, but Benedetto's other occupation of shoemaker suggests that he may have begun with shoes and only later turned his needle to couching cataracts.[27] Some of these men may, like Benedetto di Francesco, have combined their surgical practice with other occupations, as appears to have been common at the time.[28]

In these respects, the evidence from the *catasto* confirms – or at least does not contradict – the standard view of the empirical surgeon as an artisanally trained specialist. In other respects, however, these men belie the traditional stereotype of the empiric as a marginal and illegitimate practitioner, catering to the uncritical poor. To begin with, all were matriculated as doctors in the Guild of Doctors, Apothecaries and Grocers and were therefore fully licensed and legally qualified to practice.[29] (This situation may have reflected Florence's unusually lax matriculation procedures; Venetian documents from the early fourteenth century refer to the convictions of some practitioners of this sort for unlicensed practice, though in many such cases, licence was eventually granted by special act of the Great Council.)[30] Furthermore, all had stable practices in the city, often of many years duration, and other evidence also suggests that they were well established and well respected – not only Maestro Antonio and Maestro Francesco's desirable tax exemption, which was not unique, but also Maestro Domenico's much coveted continuing contract as staff surgeon to the hospital of Santa Maria Nuova, largest and wealthiest hospital in the city, which he had inherited from his father, together with his knowledge of the treatment of fractures and dislocations.[31] Finally, there is the evidence of their wealth, as registered in the detailed inventories of property in the *catasto* records. Of the ten surgical specialists in the *catasto*, three (Maestro Simone di Pacino, Maestro Giovanni di maestro Piero, and Maestro Benedetto di Francesco) were frankly poor, though no poorer than several of the men matriculated as general surgeons; their raw household wealth placed them in the bottom half of the city's population. But the others fell above the seventieth percentile,[32] and their declarations show a solid if modest patrimony; most owned their own houses in the city and several pieces of land in the Florentine countryside.

Other documents and earlier tax distributions yield similar results, showing that surgical specialists varied considerably in their financial security; although some were nearly indigent, others – for example, the eye doctor Maestro Falcone di maestro Falcone di maestro Rinuccio, in the hearth tax of 1352, or the bone doctor Maestro Stefano di maestro Iacopo dell'Ossa, in the *prestanza* of 1369 – were men of great personal wealth.[33] Furthermore, a number of these specialists came from families that had already established themselves socially and economically, or were in the process of doing so. For example, the eye doctor Maestro Lionardo di maestro Iacopo di ser Tignoso Tignoselli came from a family of some note in Volterra, where he was salaried by one of the local hospitals; he served as ambassador to Florence in 1385, an experience that may have encouraged him to immigrate to the capital, which he did shortly afterwards, receiving not only immediate Florentine citizenship for himself and his sons, but also one of the much rarer and more coveted lifetime tax exemptions. One son, Rinieri, obtained a university degree, became a physician (appearing as such in the *catasto* of 1427), and married into the aristocratic Guicciardini family.[34] This pattern, whereby sons of immigrant empirical surgeons became university-educated physicians and married into established Florentine families, was not uncommon: Maestro Niccolò, son of Maestro Giovanni di maestro Piero of Norcia, did so, as did Maestro Domenico, son of the immigrant bone doctor Maestro Giovanni di maestro Ciuccio of Civitavecchia. Maestro Domenico continued to identify himself simultaneously as bone doctor and physician, which indicates that the practice of physic and empirical surgery, like that of physic and general surgery,[35] were not necessarily as one might ordinarily assume.[36] Surgical specialists might also come from native Florentine families of some standing; the poultice doctor Maestro Zanobi di Iacopo Mangani qualified as eligible for the priorate in the scrutiny of 1382 and was captain of the prestigious Parte Guelfa at his death in that same year.[37]

Thus one should not assume that empirically trained surgical specialists necessarily came from socially and economically marginal families; while this is certainly true of some, others made a handsome living and were solidly, if not brilliantly, established in Florence's social hierarchy. In the same way, one cannot necessarily conclude that practitioners of this sort were hired only by those who could not afford another kind of doctor or that they were viewed with suspicion not only by academic physicians and surgeons, but also by the civil authorities. The reality appears considerably more complicated: communal governments were among the principal clients of surgical specialists and were willing to go to considerable lengths to attract them and to support their work.

Consider, for example, the Florentine practice of granting empirics lucrative tax exemptions of the kind obtained by the hernia doctors Maestro Antonio and Maestro Francesco di Giovanni of Norcia in 1405. As the text of the decree I cited at the beginning of this chapter indicates, such privileges were extremely rare and tended to be reserved exclusively for surgical specialists, among all doctors, on the grounds of public interest. This tradition seems to have begun in the 1330s, with the grant of a blanket tax exemption to Maestro Iacopo dell'Ossa of Rome, publicly salaried bone doctor to the city's poor,[38] but it was soon widened to include other empirics: Maestro Leonardo di ser Tignoso of Volterra, eye doctor (in 1388);[39] Maestro Niccolò di Bartolino of Parma or Pavia, bone doctor (in 1401);[40] Maestro Antonio and Maestro Francesco di Giovanni of Norcia; and Maestro Luigi, a converted Jew from Ostia 'experienced in the treatment of bones and hernias' (1416).[41] During this same period, only two other practitioners (both physicians) received similar privileges, and one of these was Maestro Luigi's brother Maestro Diamante, who seems to have ridden in on his specialist sibling's coat tails.[42]

Why were the city authorities so eager to attract surgical specialists to the city? Part of the answer lies in the commune's record of employing just this kind of practitioner to serve particular segments of its dependent local population, notably its military forces, its prisoners and condemned criminals, and its poor. The first salaried position of this sort was the post of communal bone doctor, appointed 'to treat and heal the people of the city and countryside of Florence as required, especially the poor and those without resources, without taking any fee from them' – a lucrative position filled for over fifty years after 1320 by Maestro Iacopo dell'Osso of Rome and his three sons, Maestro Niccolò, Maestro Giovanni, and Maestro Stefano.[43] The second was the post of doctor to the Stinche (the communal jail) and to those condemned to 'have a member amputated or extracted at the [Gate of] Justice' (site of the city gallows), as the appointment typically read.[44] Either the municipal bone doctor or the municipal prison doctor might be temporarily assigned to the battlefield, as in the case of the war against Pisa in the early 1360s.[45]

It is easy to see why the army and the judicial system required surgical specialists – practitioners specially trained in the treatment of wounds and broken bones. It is less obvious why Florence would also have drawn its publicly salaried poor doctors exclusively from this group, yet this was in fact the case. Examples include not only the dell'Ossa dynasty of bone doctors, but also two other specialized practitioners employed by the commune in the 1350s and early 1360s: the eye doctor Maestro Beltrame di maestro Neri of Cortona, previously hired by the city of Lucca, and Maestro Gregorio di Neri of Pisa, whose act of appointment explained that 'the city of Florence needs capable surgeons, especially those skilled in the treatment of eyes, hernias, abscesses or boils [*antracis sive malarum bullarum*] and in the restoration of broken and dislocated bones'.[46] Maestro Beltrame's appointment was equally explicit, noting that the city 'lacks a good doctor expert in the treatment of diseases of the eyes'.[47]

Florence was not unique in drawing its *medici condotti*, or publicly salaried doctors, from among the ranks of surgical specialists; the statutes of Lucca adopted in 1308 specified that the city treasurer should appoint a 'doctor who knows how to treat broken arms and legs and other members of the poor'.[48] Other fourteenth-century Italian towns hired both physicians and surgeons in this capacity, often in tandem,[49] but even these often included empirical specialists. Thus the panoply of doctors on the Venetian public payroll included practitioners such as Maestro Domenico of Chioggia, 'a surgeon with special experience in hernias and the stone disease' (1322); Maestro Pellegrino of Padua, 'expert in the stone disease' (1329); and Maestro Bonaventura, 'a person of great utility to the city, because he is the only one specially trained in fractures and dislocations of bones' (1319).[50]

The wording of Maestro Bonaventura's appointment, like Maestro Beltrame's in Florence, suggests one reason why communal governments may have wished to attract surgical specialists to their cities by grants of citizenship and public contracts: the conditions treated by surgical specialists (fractures and dislocations, hernias, wounds, cataracts) were not only extremely common and debilitating, but also highly treatable, so that skilful practitioners of this sort might acquire impressive reputations for producing results. The situation must have been exacerbated by the fact that many general or academically trained surgeons were unwilling to assume the marked risks of operating for hernia, cataract or stone, preferring to leave it to specialists. For example, after losing three hernia patients, Bartolomeo of Montagnana, professor of medicine at the University of Padua, noted in his *Consilia* (comp. 1428–48), 'I decided from then on not to treat this illness, and I sent many who came to me away, fleeing both the work and its meagre profits',[51] while his colleague Leonardo of Bertipaglia prefaced his own description of cutting for stone by remarking, 'I never wanted to get involved with this operation, although in my time I have seen it performed by many men experienced in it [*experimentatores in tali arte*]'.[52]

Finally, such operations, as Michael McVaugh has graphically described, could be extremely painful, even when not life-threatening.[53] In the days before anaesthesia and transfusions, the most successful surgeons might well have been those specialized in a single procedure, performed several hundred times a year with the utmost speed. Medical faculties such as that at the university of Bologna offered their students specialized instruction in fractures and dislocations[54] but, as academic medical writers themselves repeatedly acknowledged, no amount of book learning could substitute for clinical experience.

For all these reasons, cities such as Florence and Venice sought to attract surgical specialists to treat not just the poor, but also its more prosperous citizens. Thus of the various empirics granted Florentine citizenship or lifetime tax exemptions, only Maestro Iacopo dell'Ossa found himself in the public employ. The rest – Maestro Antonio and Maestro Francesco of Norcia, Maestro Lionardo di ser Tignoso of Volterra, Maestro Niccolò di ser Bartolino – presumably relied in large part for their livelihood on private practice, working out of their shops or homes and treating patients of various social ranks. One of Maestro Niccolò's clients may well have been the young Ser Giovanni di Gherardi of Prato, budding author and future lecturer on the works of Dante at the university of Florence; after slipping on a cucumber peel in the Via Calimala in 1392, Ser Giovanni recorded, he went immediately to the bone doctor, who 'set it for me with excruciating pain'.[55]

As this reference suggests, the more established surgical specialists, whose operations would presumably have required appropriate tools and furnishings, worked in their houses or rented shops, which appear among the lists of assets and obligations in their *catasto* declarations.[56]

There is evidence, however, that there was a peripatetic element even to the practice of these men and that the specialized nature of their skills required them to travel at least within the near countryside in order to have access to a reasonable pool of patients. The contracts of Florence's communal bone doctors in the fourteenth century included an allowance to support a horse, since, in the words of one of Maestro Iacopo dell'Ossa's early contracts, 'Maestro Iacopo is often required to go and treat poor people in the countryside and district of Florence and ... he cannot conveniently go to them on foot'.[57] The same pattern appears in documents concerning surgeons without public obligations; for example, the hernia doctor Maestro Giovanni di maestro Piero of Norcia in 1427 declared 'a mule on which he goes to treat patients'.[58]

In addition to these more established practitioners, there were also surgical specialists who spent at least part of their careers (or part of each year) as true itinerants, travelling from town to town in search of work. In 1396, for example, Maestro Antonio di Giannetto da Castelfranco petitioned the Florentine councils for tax relief for himself and his family of seven children, noting that he was 'constrained by necessity to practise his art both in the city and in the countryside, and sometimes outside the countryside of Florence'.[59] A notice from 1346 sheds considerable light on this otherwise almost invisible sector of medical practice, announcing the arrival in Lucca of two brothers specialized in the treatment of hernia and stone:

> Announcement and notification on the part of Maestro Francesco and Maestro Bonagratia degli Scolli of Parma, master surgeons. If there is any one of any status who is afflicted with rupture, hernia or stone and who wishes to be treated for these infirmities or illnesses, or for any other illness that can be treated by surgery, let them appear tomorrow at the inn of Ugolino of Beverino by the gate of San Donato. The said masters will treat anyone who come to them for the said infirmities and illnesses at their own expense, without receiving any payment until [their patients] have fully recovered, in accordance with the contracts they have made with them – the rich [to pay] according to their infirmity and their resources, and the poor to be treated for the grace and love of God.[60]

This document points to a number of things that seem to have been generally characteristic of specialized surgical practice. One was the tradition of treating the poor free. Although some cities required this of all medical practitioners, almost all of the actual references I have found to it concern surgical specialists; thus the Florentine *condotte* of Maestro Iacopo dell'Ossa of Rome, Maestro Andrea di Bartolo, and Maestro Gregorio of Pisa all indicate that they had been treating the poor without compensation on their own initiative – something that, together with their preferential treatment by tax officials and city councils, may explain some of the hostility of the physicians and academically trained surgeons.[61]

Another common practice of surgical specialists, also referred to in the Lucca announcement, was the use of a notarized contract between doctor and patient specifying the services to be performed, the results to be expected, the fee to be collected, and the payment schedule. I have not yet found any Florentine examples, but a document of this sort from Bologna appears to be typical. Drawn up in 1476, it proclaimed that

> I, Maestro Giovanni of Ragusa promise of my own free will to cure Antonio, nephew of Maestro Annibale di fu Michele de' Malpighi of Bologna of ringworm [*tigna*], without trickery or fraud, within the next month, and I promise that his illness will not return. Furthermore, I promise to restore his hair, in the same quality and quantity that he used to have. And the said Maestro Annibale promises to give me three ducats, which are being held by Maestro Domenico of Loro, citizen of Bologna ... And once it is assured that the said illness will not come back, ... he must have the said Maestro Domenico give me the three ducats.[62]

Although in this case Maestro Giovanni's fee was put on deposit, it was also common for surgical specialists to receive partial payment ahead of time – something that was in general prohibited to physicians.[63]

Such contracts seem to have been particularly suited to this kind of practice, with all of its insecurities: on the one hand, they guaranteed the surgeon his fee, often fronted him money with which to pay for the medicines and assistants required by such operations, and documented the patient's consent to the procedure; on the other hand, they reassured the patient about to embark on an uncertain, expensive, and often painful and dangerous course of treatment – sometimes at the hands of an otherwise unknown itinerant – that he or she had legal recourse in the event of negligent treatment or an unsuccessful outcome.[64] In addition, however, as Gianna Pomata has recently argued, the contract between doctor and patient, in which payment was contingent on successful treatment, had broader historical significance: it reflected a pre-professional medical order that saw the exchange of payment and treatment as a mercantile transaction, governed by the assumption of 'equity' between patient and practitioner, rather than a professional order in which the value of therapy was judged according not to its efficacity but its 'canonicity'.[65] Common even in the practice of physicians in the thirteenth century, the use of the contract gradually fell from favour in élite practice, as learned physicians and master surgeons began effectively to claim a specialized medical judgement inaccessible to their lay clients and to demand to be paid for their professional learning and services rather than for the outcome of their treatment. From this point of view, the prevalence of the contract among surgical specialists and their patients may reflect the inability of this group to lay claim to such privileges – or perhaps the fact that they did not need to make such a claim, given the widespread faith in their services.

How did these fourteenth- and fifteenth-century Italian surgical specialists relate to the general spectrum of medical practitioners in Florence and other cities of the period? Although historians have to date identified them with two principal groups of practitioners, barber-surgeons and so-called 'charlatans', both of these identifications are problematic. In all the cities about which I have any hard information, the more established surgical specialists whose work I have been describing were clearly distinct from and of higher status within the profession than the 'barber-doctors' (*medici barbitonsores, medici della barba, barbitonsores sive/et medici*) found in the fourteenth-century Venetian documents collected by Stefanutti or matriculated in the books of the Florentine Guild of Doctors, Apothecaries and Grocers.[66] Barber-doctors performed completely different kinds of operations from the demanding and sometimes dangerous surgery of the specialists, confining themselves for the most part to relatively simple procedures such as cupping, bleeding, applying leeches and pulling teeth. By the same token, the matriculation lists of the guild did not confer on barber-doctors the honorific title of 'maestro', which the empirical surgeons shared with physicians and general surgeons.[67]

More complex is the relationship of surgical specialists to the group of practitioners usually referred to in histories of medicine as 'charlatans' (*ciarlatani*, a word dating to the fifteenth century and apparently of Italian origin). As some historians have repeatedly emphasized, the term 'charlatan' is a slippery one; polemical rather than descriptive from the outset, it tells more about the assumptions of the writers who use it than to people to whom it is applied.[68] It began to assume its modern sense in the late sixteenth and seventeenth centuries, when physicians started to use it to discredit their non-academically trained competitors by associating them with the itinerant showpeople who were also called *cantambanchi* or *montambanchi* from their custom of performing on benches; these men (and less commonly women) frequented urban markets and fairs, and they made their living by juggling, performing magic tricks, singing, dancing, telling stories or peddling various medicinal preparations for which they made false and extravagant claims.[69]

In the fourteenth and fifteenth centuries, however, both the philological and the social situation were less clear-cut. As I have already argued, it was surgical specialists rather than itinerant peddlars or the relatively lowly barber-surgeons that offered the most serious competition to physicians and more generally trained surgeons bent on consolidating their professional authority and their control over the practice of medicine. It is for this reason that they were singled out for attack by writers such as Falcucci, particularly in the period immediately after the Black Death, which ushered in a subtle but extended crisis in the authority, confidence and reputation of the traditional medical élites.[70] But this hostility was not universal, and other academic doctors, such as Bartolomeo of Montagnana (himself the son of an empirical surgeon) viewed their skills and experience with considerable respect.[71] Those medical writers such as Falcucci who did fulminate against the surgical specialists did not tend to emphasize their fraudulence and itinerancy; the great social campaign against vagabondage and itinerant poverty did not begin until the early sixteenth century, and the most serious competitors of university-educated physicians and surgeons were, after all, not occasional travelling practitioners, but those with established shops and practices next door.

On the surface, empirical surgeons had little in common with the itinerant pedlars of nostrums known most commonly in the fifteenth century as *cerretani*. There may, however, be more to their association than at first meets the eye. Although *cerretano* seems to have been used generally to refer to travelling scoundrels (including, but not restricted to, friars and preachers), its medical connotation points us back in the direction of the surgical specialist. Cerreto was in fact a small town in the vicinity of Norcia, an isolated commune in the mountains of eastern Umbria, which was the centre of an important local medical tradition.[72] At least as early as the fourteenth century, Norcia and its neighbouring towns of Borgo alle Preci and Poggio alla Croce began to export large numbers of empirical surgeons. Between 1386 and 1444, for example, the Florentine Guild of Doctors, Apothecaries and Grocers enrolled an extraordinary 26 doctors from Norcia and its territories, including a number of the hernia doctors that appeared in the *catasto* of 1427. (By way of comparison, during the same period the much closer and larger medical centre of Bologna provided Florence with only two immigrant practitioners.) Although Florence may have had an unusually high number of the surgical specialists known as Norcini in the fifteenth century, it did not have a monopoly on immigrant practitioners from the area: in the sixteenth and seventeenth centuries, there were documented communities of Norcini in Urbino, Bologna and Genoa, and by the eighteenth century, they were found in all the principal Italian cities.[73]

The Norcini seem initially to have specialized in surgery for hernia and stone, although they soon became associated with operations on the eyes as well. The origins of this regional family-based tradition is obscure; the most likely explanation traces it to the practice of castration, which plays an important role in the raising of pigs and production of sausages, for which Norcia, blessed with extensive oak forests, is still renowned.[74] Whatever the roots of their practice, however, the Norcini maintained a high profile and clear identity long into the early modern period, well after Durante Scacchi (scion of one of their oldest families) committed many of their techniques to paper in 1581.[75] And they were never, to my knowledge, identified as a group with mountebanks, even in the later period, when professional lines were more clearly drawn. Thus Mercurio Scipione's discussion of charlatans in his *Popular Errors of Italy* (1645) contrasted these explicitly with 'two most honoured brothers from Norcia, who, because they are excellent in castrating and removing stones, make an impressive and honourable living'.[76]

The importance and strength of the tradition of the Norcini underlines the general point with which I began this chapter: although surgical specialists, like other empirics, appear in some medical treatises as an undesirable and undifferentiated gaggle of marginal practitioners, other documents reveal a much more complicated reality. The specialized surgeons who practised in the cities of fourteenth- and fifteenth-century Italy were an exceedingly diverse lot, ranging from part-time ringworm doctors and cataract operators through well-established and respected families expert in the demanding treatment of bones, hernia and stone. They included doctors who lived largely or entirely from private practice, and doctors who built their work around institutional clients such as hospitals and the state. Some lived and practised in the same city for their entire lives, while others were itinerants for at least part of their careers.

As I said at the beginning, I have not considered the actual operations performed by these surgical specialists, and I make no claims about their effectiveness. However, there is some evidence that in the course of their migrations, they may have been important in disseminating, if not developing, knowledge of new techniques. The eminent physician and anatomist Alessandro Benedetti claimed to have learned a superior method of hernia surgery from a Spanish itinerant.[77] A similar experience was described by the author of an anonymous fragment in a fourteenth-century Florentine manuscript, written in Latin and thus certainly the work of a university-educated physician or surgeon; the writer described what he called

> a new way of treating a rupture or intestinal hernia, ... not mentioned by the medical authors and ... better and safer than all of the other ones they mention, for it is not dangerous or uncomfort-

> able for the patient. It was invented by a certain Maestro Giovanni of Verona, who is now staying in Urbino.

After detailing this operation, the author concluded, 'I learned this operation from the said Maestro in 1373 according to the Florentine calendar'.[78]

Like this text, much of the material I have been able to put together raises as many questions as it answers. It would be useful to know, for example, how typical Florence actually was in the number and range of surgical specialists it supported and the privileges they enjoyed. Notoriously lax in its licensing procedures, was it especially hospitable to empirics, or were they equally numerous and well established in other Italian cities? How would the inclusion of women surgical specialists (presumably less mobile than the men) change the picture? Were there other regions that, like Norcia, possessed distinctive healing traditions recognized throughout large portions of northern and central Italy? Above all, in a society where bone doctors might also be physicians, where hernia doctors received lucrative state contracts, where empirically trained specialists, barbers and wise women were consulted by both rich and poor, do we need to rethink the apparently incoherent category of 'popular medicine'?

Notes

* Niccolò Falcucci, *Sermones medicinales*, 4 vols, Venice, 1490–21, vol. 4, fol. 45v; on the figure of the *vetula* as emblematic of experience-based practice in learned medical polemics, see Jole Agrimi and Chiari Crisciani, 'Medici e "vetulae" dal dugento al Quattrocento: problemi di ricerca', in Paolo Rossi, et al., *Cultura popolare e cultura dotta nel Seicento: Atti del convegno di studio di Genova (23–25 novembre, 1982)*, Milan, 1983, pp. 144–59. This chapter has benefited from the helpful suggestions of Vivian Nutton and other participants in the original conference.

1. Act of the legislative council of Florence, 24 April 1406, Archivio di stato, Florence: Provvisioni-Registri (hereafter PR) 95, fol. 3r–v. Unless otherwise indicated, all archival references are to documents in the Florentine state archives.
2. E.g., for Florence, references below and in Katharine Park, *Doctors and Medicine in Early Renaissance Florence*, Princeton, 1985, pp. 71, 88–91. For Venice, Ugo Stefanutti, *Documentazioni cronologiche per la storia della medicina, chirurgia e farmacia in Venezia dal 1258 al 1332*, Venice, 1961, pp. 67–8, 81, 85, 86, 90, 95, 99, 100, 101–2.
3. E.g. Leonardo da Bertipaglia, *Cirurgia, passim*, as cited in Lynn Thorndike, *Science and Thought in the Fifteenth Century*, New York, 1929, esp. pp. 96–7; Guido da Arezzo, *Liber Mitis*, as cited in Ugo Viviani, 'Ciarlatanismo medico', *Rivista di storia delle scienze mediche e naturali*, 10 (1919), p. 104; Dino Del Garbo, as cited in Nancy G. Siraisi, 'How to Write a Latin

Book on Surgery', in Luis García-Ballester, Roger French, Jon Arrizabalaga and Andrew Cunningham, eds, *Practical Medicine from Salerno to the Black Death*, Cambridge, 1994, pp. 108–9.

4. Cited in Michael R. McVaugh, 'Royal Surgeons in the Crown of Aragon', in García-Ballester et al., eds, *Practical Medicine*, p. 236.
5. On the dangers of taking at face value contemporary descriptions of particular groups of doctors as 'quacks', see Margaret Pelling and Charles Webster, 'Medical Practitioners', in Charles Webster, ed., *Health, Medicine and Mortality in the Sixteenth Century*, Cambridge, 1979, p. 166. For a fine overview of medical practice and practitioners in this period, see Nancy G. Siraisi, *Medieval and Early Renaissance Medicine: An Introduction to Knowledge and Practice*, Chicago, 1990, chs 2 and 6. Throughout this chapter I have used the English 'doctor' to translate the Latin *medicus* or Italian *medico*; despite the etymological incongruity – the Latin root of 'doctor' suggests a university graduate, and by no means all *medici* had academic degrees – the word as currently used has the same degree of generality as the Latin and Italian terms.
6. E.g., Tiziana Pesenti Marangon, '"Professores chirurgie", "medici ciroici" e "barbitonsores" a Padova nell' età di Leonardo Buffi da Bertipaglia (+ dopo il 1448)', *Quaderni per la storia dell' università di Padova*, 11 (1978), esp. p. 36; Cornelius O'Boyle, 'Physicians and Surgeons in Paris', in Garcìa-Ballester et al., eds, *Practical Medicine*, p. 182. (This excellent collection includes a number of important articles on surgery, with a strong emphasis on learned surgery, in the later Middle Ages.) On the increasing stratification of medical practice in sixteenth- and seventeenth-century Italy, see Gianna Pomata's remarkable study of Bologna: *La promessa di guarigione: Malati e curatori in Antico Regime*, Rome and Bari, 1994, esp. chs 3 and 6.
7. Michael R. McVaugh, *Medicine before the Plague: Practitioners and their Patients in the Crown of Aragon, 1285–1385*, Cambridge, 1993, pp. 160–61.
8. There are almost no scholarly studies of surgical specialists in the later Middle Ages and Renaissance. The rare exceptions include Giovanni Sacino's sketchy survey, 'Primi albori di specializzazione della medicina toscana nel Medioevo', in *Atti del XXI congresso internazionale di storia della medicina*, 2 vols, Siena, 1968, vol. 1, pp. 100–105; Ugo Stefanutti's narrowly focused but well-documented study, 'Sulla liceità deontologica dei patti conclusi "ante curam" fra medici chirurghi e pazienti', in his *Fatti e personaggi di storia della medicina*, Venice, 1959, pp. 21–36; and some of the suggestive, if often uncritical and severely underdocumented articles on the Norcini and Preciani (see note 72 below). On their ancient predecessors, see Gerhard Baader, 'Spezialärtzte in der Spätantike', *Medizinhistorisches Journal*, 2 (1967), pp. 231–8.
9. On the details of some of their operations, which I will not be considering, see Michael R. McVaugh's contribution to this volume (Chapter 7).
10. See in general Monica H. Green, 'Documenting Medieval Women's Medical Practice', in García-Ballester et al., eds, *Practical Medicine*, Cambridge, 1994, pp. 322–52.
11. Raffaele Calvanico, *Fonti per la storia della medicina e della chirurgia per il regno di Napoli nel periodo angioino (a. 1273–1410)*, Naples, 1962, *passim*. On this source and on women's practice and the gendering of healing

in general, see Katharine Park, 'The Healing Arts: Magic and Medicine', in Robert Davis and Judith Brown, eds, *Gender and Society in Renaissance Italy*, London, 1998; and Monica H. Green, 'Women's Medical Practice and Health Care in Medieval Europe', in Judith M. Bennett et al., eds, *Sisters and Workers in the Middle Ages*, Chicago, 1989, esp. p. 48.

12. Complete list in Park, *Doctors and Medicine*, Appendix III. In much of the discussion that follows I have collated information from the *catasto* with information from a range of other archival sources, including notarial records, other tax distributions, books of public legislation, private and institutional account books, and matriculation lists for the Guild of Doctors, Apothecaries and Grocers. On the *catasto* itself, see David Herlihy and Christiane Klapisch-Zuber, *Les toscans et leurs familles: une étude du catasto florentin de 1427*, Paris, 1978; ch. 1 describes the *catasto* records in some detail.
13. Catasto–Campioni del Monte–S. Giovanni/Drago–1427, fols 604v–5r (*campione*, or official summary); Catasto 52, fol. 267r (*portata*, or declaration).
14. Catasto 78, fol. 242r; Catasto 48, fol. 647r.
15. Catasto–Campioni del Monte–S. Giovanni/Drago–1427, fol. 605v; Catasto 52, fol. 267v.
16. Catasto 88, fol. 178r (declaration only). Maestro Piero was one of two doctors living immediately outside the city gates and hence taxed as a resident of the countryside.
17. Catasto–Campioni del Monte–S. Giovanni/Leon d'oro–1427, fols 666v–7v; Catasto 51, fol. 1091r–3v.
18. Catasto 81, fols 251v–252v; Catasto 61, fols 708r–9r.
19. Catasto 67, fol. 310v; Catasto 24, fol. 1154r.
20. I should perhaps also add to these the 'wound doctors' who commonly followed the army in times of war or treated tortured prisoners and victims of civil assault, although most of the references I have found to that specialty date from before 1350.
21. See, e.g., Stefanutti, *Documentazioni*, p. 117, concerning Maestro Domenico da Chioggia, 'chirugico et specialiter de crepatis et curatione lapidum', and the reference to the two doctors from Parma in n. 60. Stefanutti also includes documents concerning doctors identified exclusively as concerned with stone; see, e.g., pp. 83, 99.
22. Prestanze 5, fol. 64v.
23. Arte dei medici e speziali (AMS) 21, *ad annum*.
24. It is important to stress that this statement is based almost exclusively on documents concerning male doctors and heads of household. Female doctors, legally incompetent and rarely listed as heads of household, are virtually invisible in the tax records, and there is no way of knowing their numbers and specialties. In addition to Monna Neccia, the ringworm doctor (see note 22), I have found only one reference to another woman specialist, Monna Iacopa, 'chi medicava d' impiastri nel tempo della mortalità del 74'; Biblioteca Nazionale di Firenze: MS Magl. xxv, 113, cited in Giovanni Targioni-Tozzetti, *Notizie sulla storia delle scienze fisiche in Toscana*, Florence, 1952, p. 155.
25. Park, *Doctors and Medicine*, pp. 31–2, 175–6; this became increasingly rare over the course of the later fourteenth and fifteenth centuries.
26. Maestro Stefano's father, Maestro Lodovico di maestro Francesco di

maestro Bonino, matriculated in the Guild of Doctors, Apothecaries and Grocers as a poultice doctor before the Black Death, while Maestro Domenico's father, Maestro Giovanni di maestro Ciuccio da Civitavecchia, who matriculated in 1385, was a bone doctor.

27. See Aryeh Feigenbaum, 'Early History of Cataract and the Ancient Operation for Cataract', *American Journal of Ophthalmology*, 49 (1960), pp. 305–26; and Michel Feugère, Ernst Künzl and Ursula Weisser, 'Die Starnadeln von Montbellet (Saône-et-Loire): ein Beitrag zur antiken und islamischen Augenheilkunde', *Jahrbuch des römisch-germanischen Zentralmuseums (Mainz)*, 32 (1985), pp. 436–508.
28. See Margaret Pelling, 'Occupational Diversity: Barbersurgeons and the Trades of Norwich', *Bulletin of the History of Medicine*, 56 (1982), pp. 484–511.
29. Arte dei medici e speziali 9 and 21. The only exception was the tooth doctor, Maestro Simone di Pacino, who as an inhabitant of the countryside (albeit the very near countryside, since he lived just outside the city walls) was not required to matriculate in the city guild. On the process of matriculation and the nature of the guild's role in regulating medical practice, see Park, *Doctors and Medicine*, ch. 1.
30. E.g., Stefanutti, *Documentazioni*, pp. 81 (Biagio, hernia doctor); 86 (Maestro Domenico di S. Fosca, bone doctor), 99 (Maestro Gambertono da Fana, stone doctor); 101–2 (Draga the Slav, podagra and eyes). On Florence's licensing procedures, Park, *Doctors and Medicine*, pp. 25–8.
31. Records of Maestro Giovanni's employment in, e.g., Spedale di Santa Maria Nuova (hereafter SMN) 4458 (1404–06), fol. 103v; records relating to the salary of Maestro Domenico, 'nostro medico', in, e.g., SMN 4477 (1426–28), fols 103v and 113v; SMN 4479 (1428–30), fols 43v, 104v.
32. Percentile figures from Herlihy and Klapisch-Zuber, *Les toscans et leurs familles*, p. 258.
33. Estimo 306; Prestanze 156, fol. 20r. In each case their assessments were surpassed (among doctors) only by three of the most illustrious physicians in the city.
34. Mario Battistini, *I medici e la medicina in Volterra nel Medioevo*, Castelfiorentino, 1923, p. 22; PR 77, fols. 178r–9r (new numeration).
35. See McVaugh, 'Royal Surgeons', pp. 221, 233.
36. Catasto 91, fols 708r–9r.
37. Marchionne di Coppo Stefani, *Istoria fiorentina*, in Ildefonso di San Luigi, ed., *Delizie degli eruditi toscani*, 24 vols, Florence, 1770–89, vol. 17, p. 7.
38. PR 27, fol. 98r (1336). He was hired in 1326: Raffaele Ciasca, *L'arte dei medici e speziali nella storia e nel commercio fiorentino dal secolo XII al XV*, Florence, 1927, p. 299. This position and its attendant tax exemption were written into the communal statutes; see, e.g., Statuti del Commune–Statuti del Capitano–1355, IV, 74, fol. 146v. Maestro Iacopo was the father of Maestro Stefano, whose wealth I have already mentioned.
39. PR 77, fols 178v–9r.
40. PR 90, fol. 289r–91r.
41. PR 105, fols 358v–60v.
42. Ibid. The other physician was Maestro Iacopo d'Arquà, in 1382 (PR 71,

fols 51v–2v), who seems never to have taken advantage of the grant to settle in Florence.

43. PR 23, fol. 12v; PR 27, fol. 98r (quotation); PR 32, fol. 115r (new numeration); PR 36, fol. 30r; PR 52, fol. 138r. By 1344, Maestro Iacopo was receiving 10 lire a month, plus use of a horse to visit far-flung patients, a salary also enjoyed by his sons.
44. E.g., PR 38, 57r–v. By analogy with Venice and Milan, both of which had similar employees, we can conclude that another of his tasks was probably to treat suspects after torture; see B. Cecchetti, *La medicina in Venezia nel 1300*, Venice, 1883, pp. 41–4. The Florentine prison doctors in the fourteenth and early fifteenth centuries were Maestro Filippo di ser Bindo; Maestro Andrea di Bartolo (appointed 1350, PR 38, fol. 57r–v); Maestro Niccolò di Valore (appointed 1378, PR 67, fols 45v–6r); Maestro Nello di Berto (appointed 1413, PR 102, fols 80v–81v); and Maestro Piero di Feo (appointed 1416, PR 106, fol. 181r). The standard annual salary was 50 lire.
45. PR 48, fol. 42v; PR 161, entry of 19 June 1363. In 1364, the city also hired a local wound doctor, Maestro Michele di Coluccino of Barga, for the same purpose: Camerlinghi della camera del commune–Uscita 165, fol. [7r].
46. PR 48, fols 149v–50r. Maestro Gregorio received 70 lire and served for one year in 1362–63.
47. PR 47, fol. 33r. Maestro Beltrame received 100 lire a year, later raised to 50 florins, and served from 1354 to 1362.
48. Ciasca, *L' arte dei medici e speciali*, p. 296.
49. Details and literature in Vivian Nutton, 'Continuity or Rediscovery? The City Physician in Classical Antiquity and Mediaeval Italy', in Andrew W. Russell ed., *The Town and State Physician in Europe from the Middle Ages to the Enlightenment*, Wolfenbüttel, 1981, pp. 24–34.
50. Stefanutti, *Documentazioni*, pp. 90 (Latin, p. 117), 95, and 85 (quotation; Latin, p. 114). Stefanutti also includes many documents giving surgical specialists permission to practise in Venice without going through the regular licensing procedure administered by the College of Doctors.
51. Bartolomeo da Montagnana, *Consilia*, in his *Opera medica*, Venice, 1497, fols 115v–16v; cited in Marangon, '"Professores chirurgie"', p. 12. For other testimonies to the same effect, see Marangon, ibid., pp. 10–12, and G. B. Fabbri, 'Della litotomia antica e dei litotomi ed oculisti norcini o preciani', *Memorie dell'accademia delle scienze dell'istituto di Bologna*, ser. 3, 9, 1 (1870), pp. 244–6.
52. Leonardo da Bertipaglia, *Cirurgia*, Vienna MS 4751, fol. 83r, as cited in Lynn Thorndike, *Science and Thought in the Fifteenth Century*, New York, 1929, p. 100.
53. McVaugh, Chapter 7 in this volume.
54. Umberto Dallari, *I rotuli dei lettori legisti e artisti dello studio bolognese dal 1380 al 1405*, 4 vols, Bologna, 1888–1924, vol. 4, pp. 19, 53, 55, 57, 59, 63, 65.
55. Archivio di stato di Prato: Archivio Datini-Carteggio privato 1093 (24 August 1392).
56. The hernia doctor Maestro Luca di maestro Antonio da Norcia declared in 1451 a rented shop: Catasto 711, fol. 582r.
57. PR 27, fol. 98r.

58. Cataso 24, fol. 1154r. By 1430, he owned two mules for that purpose: Catasto 397, fol. 258v.
59. PR 85, fols 122v–3r.
60. Transcribed in Ugo Viviani, 'Ciarlatanismo medico', *Rivista di storia critica delle scienze mediche e naturali*, 10, 3–4, May–August (1919), p. 56.
61. PR 27, fol. 98r; PR 38, fol. 57v; PR 48, fol. 149v. Pomata notes that in seventeenth-century Bologna, the authorities tended to tolerate the practice of unofficial healers who treated the poor out of charity; *La promessa di quarigione*, p. 79.
62. Transcribed in Stefanutti, 'Sulla liceità, doc. 6 (pp. 34–5); other examples in ibid., doc. 4 (leg ulcer), and Guido Rizzi, 'Un contratto notarile quattrocentesco per operazione di cataratta', in *Atti del IIo convegno della Marca per la storia della medicina*, Fermo, 1958, 59–61 (cataract).
63. Stefanutti, 'Sulla liceità', pp. 22–3.
64. As in, for example, ibid., docs 3 and 5.
65. Pomata, *La promessa di guarigione*, ch. 2, esp. pp. 76–99.
66. For Venice, Stefanutti, *Documentazioni, passim*. Barber doctors began to matriculate in the Florentine Guild in significant numbers in the second half of the fourteenth century; see Arte dei medici e speziali (AMS) 9. Marangon places empirical surgeons below barbers in the fifteenth-century hierarchy of medical practitioners ('"Professores chirurgie"', pp. 29–36), but without convincing evidence, and she may have been misled by the polemics of academic writers, who did not see barber-doctors as a competitive threat and who therefore spared them in their polemics.
67. Barbers were made subject to the Florentine Guild of Doctors, Apothecaries, and Grocers in 1384; see Raffaele Ciasca, *Statuti dell'arte dei medici e speziali*, Florence, 1922, pp. 320–21. There are one or two Florentine instances of men matriculated as barber-doctors who appeared in later documents as 'surgeons', with the surgeon's honorific, but such cases were very rare. I know of none where a barber-doctor later developed a surgical specialty, although Niccolò di Valore, who matriculated in 1372 as 'barber or doctor' later became the official doctor to the city prison.
68. Although the word *ciarlatano* (from *ciarlare*, to prattle) is documented in late fifteenth-century Tuscan, it was rare and does not seem to have any particularly medical associations, referring more generally to travelling confidence men, notably preachers and friars. As a point of departure, see Yakov Malkiel, 'Italian *ciarlatano* and its Romance Offshoots', *Romance Philology*, 2 (1948–49), pp. 317–26, and Salvatore Battaglia, *Grande dizionario della lingua italiana*, 15 vols to date, Turin, 1961, s. v. 'ciarlatano'. The work of Malkiel and his fellow philologists is fraught with confusions growing out of their unfamiliarity with late medieval social and medical practices.
69. William Eamon vividly describes the world of the sixteenth-century *ciarlatani* in his *Science and the Secrets of Nature: Books of Secrets in Medieval and Early Modern Culture*, Princeton, 1994, pp. 236–60. See also Pomata, *La promessa di guarigione*, pp. 151–5; Alison Klairmont Lingo, 'Empirics and Charlatans in Early Modern France: The Genesis of the Classification of the "Other" in Medical Practice', *Journal of Social History*, 19 (1986), pp. 583–604; J.-P. Goubert, 'L'art de guérir: médicine savante et médicine populaire dans la France de 1790', *Annales ESC*, 32

(1977), pp. 908–26; Pietro Camporesi, 'Speziali e ciarlatani', in Giuseppe Adani and Gastone Tamagnini, eds, *Medicina, Erbe e Magia*, Milan, Silvana, 1981, 139–59.

70. Park, *Doctors and Medicine*, especially pp. 34–46.
71. Marangon, '"Professores chirurgie"', pp. 35–37.
72. The meagre historical literature on the early history of this tradition is underdocumented, uncritical and repetitious, and it should be used with extreme care. The principal studies are Cristiano Dominici, 'La scuola chirurgica preciana', *Rivista di storia della medicina*, 9 (1965), pp. 198–215; Ansano Fabbi, 'The *Norcini* and their Families', *Medicina nei secoli*, 9, 3 (1972), pp. 67–89; *idem*, 'Il lebbrosario della Valnerina e la scuola chirurgica di Preci', *Bollettino della deputazione di storia patria per l'Umbria*, 61 (1964), pp. 5–55; G. B. Fabbri, 'Della litotomia antica e dei litotomi ed oculisti norcini o preciani', *Memorie della accademia delle scienze dell'istituto di Bologna*, ser. 2, 9 (1869–70), pp. 239–66; and Pietro Pizzoni, 'La litotomia e i litotomi norcini', *Bollettino della deputazione di storia patria per l'Umbria*, 48 (1951), pp. 202–11.
73. Pizzoni, 'La litotomia', pp. 205–8; for Bologna, see Pomata, *La promessa di guarigione*, p. 155.
74. I have found no evidence to support the hypothesis of Fabbri and others that the locals initially learned their skills from the local Benedictine abbey of S. Eutizio.
75. Durante Scacchi's *Subsidium medicinae* was published in 1596. Other famous later Norcini included Orazio da Norcia, whose work with hernias was mentioned by Fabrizio, and the Benevoli family, chief lithotomists and ophthalmologists to the Florentine hospital of Santa Maria Nuova in the later seventeenth century.
76. Quoted in Andrea Corsini, *Medici ciarlatani e ciarlatani medici*, Bologna, Nicola Zanichelli, 1922, p. 55. On the 'quasi-professional' status of the *norcini* in seventeenth-century Bologna, see Pomata, *La promessa di guarigione*, p. 155.
77. Cited in Michele Jandolo, 'Storia della chirurgia dell'ernia inguinale', *Castalia*, 15 (1959), p. 61.
78. Biblioteca nazionale di Firenze: MS Palatino 811, fol. 69v.

CHAPTER SEVEN

Treatment of Hernia in the Later Middle Ages: Surgical Correction and Social Construction

Michael R. McVaugh

Practical medicine in the Middle Ages – assuming that by that we mean medical practice[1] – is not an easy thing to come to grips with. Our evidence for what we might call the practice of internal medicine, the realm of the *physicus* or physician, includes virtually nothing that might be called a case history. It comes instead mostly from textbooks embodying a physiology and a pathology that are difficult to relate to our own experience of reality, and a therapeutics that it is even more difficult to believe had any practical consequences. The apparent dependence of so many medical authors upon the written sources available to them, century after century, makes it hard to credit that their judgements were controlled by their own experience. Discoveries and innovations – *experimenta* – appear sometimes to have struck the medieval physician almost as awkwardnesses, inconvenient intrusions that had to be fitted into an already rationally finished, completed system,[2] a science that today seems to us very much a construction utterly peculiar to another society. We may well despair of understanding how internal medicine functioned 'in practice'.

Surgery, however, would seem to hold more promise for a historian of practical medicine.[3] True, medieval surgery too built up a textual tradition, and certain surgical authors could be just as imitative as medical writers: the late thirteenth-century surgeries of Bruno Longoburgo and Teodorico Borgognoni are so closely related that it is still not clear who copied from whom. But surgeons (*cirurgici*) of that period were conscious of the immaturity of their craft, of its need to establish its disciplinary dignity, and while they supposed that this required them to achieve the same sort of rational systematization of knowledge as that enjoyed by medicine, they also accepted that there were still problems and techniques remaining for them to discover. For surgeons, therefore, arguing from practical results, as opposed to reason or authority, was perhaps easier to justify intellectually than it was for physicians, and their writings do often cite their own experience with particular procedures.[4] Furthermore, the increasing prominence given to anatomy in medieval surgeries, beginning with that of Guglielmo da Saliceto (1276), means that the world described by surgical authors seems to correspond more closely to our objective reality than do the humours and medicinal degrees, say, of the medieval physicians. Finally, it is easy for us to imagine that surgical treatments must have succeeded or failed more obviously than medical cures, and that the reactions of their patients would have forced medieval surgeons to learn from their mistakes, thus ensuring the positive technical 'progress' of surgery.[5] Let us therefore examine the history of one such procedure in the fourteenth century, the correction of a type of hernia, to see if indeed surgery offers a useful index to the character and potential strengths of practical medicine in the later Middle Ages.

At the end of the thirteenth century, the Latin surgical tradition had come to believe in the technical possibility of operating to correct what today would be called indirect inguinal hernia. This condition arises when the internal inguinal ring in the abdomen (through which pass the spermatic cord and investing fascia down the inguinal canal to the testicle) 'stretches' enough to allow dilation and distention of a vestigial peritoneal sac (the processus vaginalis) by intestine or omentum; the resulting hernia may ultimately descend along the spermatic cord within its surrounding fascia and into the scrotum. In extreme cases, when the intestine passes through the ring within the peritoneal sac and is caught, the trapped intestine becomes gangrenous and the patient can die.[6]

In describing this condition, medieval surgeons spoke not of the spermatic cord but of what they called the *didymus*; perhaps confused by the investing fascia, they assumed that the spermatic cord was enveloped by a peritoneal membrane continuous with the abdominal peritoneum, in effect constituting an open tube – the *didymus* – uniting the peritoneal cavity and the cavity of the tunica vaginalis surrounding the testicle. Indeed, on physical examination it *feels* like a tube. 'The spermatic vessels', explained the famous early fourteenth-century anatomist Mondino dei Liuzzi,

> are covered by a membrane, which springs from *siphac* [the peritoneum], called *didymus*; the end is dilated to hold the testicles and here it is called *osceum* [the scrotum]. ... The special disease of the *didymus* is an unnatural expansion of its orifice, which causes the contents of the *siphac* to descend to the *osceum*; the descent is called hernia.[7]

Neither Mondino nor his contemporaries show an awareness of their debt to antiquity, but in this they were merely reasserting an anatomical model already developed by Galen. Actually, medieval and classical anatomists were all mistaken; the spermatic fascia have no structural integrity, and normally no such extended open channel exists continuous with the peritoneum.[8] Galen's account of inguinal anatomy was based on dissections of macaques, in which the processus vaginalis – the peritoneal sac that precedes the testis in its descent into the scrotum during fetal development – never atrophies and disappears (as it usually does in man) but remains open; during operations for hernia, Galen probably encountered instances of an incompletely closed human processus vaginalis that helped confirm him in his belief that the simian and human structures were identical.[9]

Today the problem is corrected by surgically excising the hernial sac and reconstructing the ligamentous sheathing around the spermatic cord and the inguinal floor, but the medieval surgeons who first conceived of the *didymus* as an open conduit through which the hernia was introduced recognized a different general solution, one that we can trace back, through the Arabic author Albucasis (translated into Latin in the twelfth century), to the classical world in the surgery of Paul of Aegina: it was somehow to sever or destroy the *didymus* high up, towards the abdomen, so that when it healed the scar would block the channel broaching the peritoneal wall.[10] As Teodorico Borgognoni explained, writing in the 1260s, the *didymus* could be severed in three ways. Two of these he described relatively briefly. In one, after reducing the hernia, the surgeon forces a heated cautery iron down through the skin at the spot where the hernia is visible until the cautery is stopped by the pubic bone; in the other, designed 'for the many who fear the knife and have no less abhorrence for the fire', he repeatedly applies what Teodorico calls the 'potential cautery', corrosive medicines (for example, quicklime), to the same spot, over and over again, which eat away the tissue until the pubic bone is reached. In both cases the expectation was that the procedure would encounter the *didymus* as it did its damage and destroy it, sealing the passage through the inguinal ring by cicatrization.[11]

Teodorico's description of a third procedure is much more circumstantial than the other two, which suggests that this was the one in commonest use in the thirteenth century: reading it in full may help us visualize a medieval operation a little better. After voiding the patient's bowels, have him

> lie down on a bench or plank prepared for the purpose ... , so that his hips are elevated and his head is low. And let him be tied to the bench or plank with three bandages, one on his legs round the ankles, the second over his thighs above the knees, and the third over his chest restraining his hands and arms. Now then bring the

> testicle up to the rupture and let the assistant place his finger upon the spot of the rupture so that the intestine cannot slip back. Then cut the skin lengthwise above the testicle and make an incision large enough that the testicle can be drawn out from it. And after the testicle has been drawn out, instruct the assistant to draw it upward while you free the *didymus* from underlying tissue back up to the groin with some instrument adapted for this purpose, not particularly sharp, or with the fingernails, which is safer. And then search about with your fingers to be sure that none of the intestine is still present in the *didymus*; and if you find any, push it back inside the abdomen. Next take a large square needle in which there is strong thread and wrap the *didymus* many times quite tightly, letting the ends of this thread hang outside. Then, having secured the bench, cut all around the *didymus* next to the tied-off portion with a broad cautery iron heated very hot, and let it be well seared with two other cauteries heated very hot; but be careful not to cut or burn any part of the stitches. Finally, make a cut in the lower part of the skin of the scrotum, so that blood and pus can escape; and pack into the wound some lint soaked in oil of roses or white of egg, and a wick into the incision that you made in the lower portion of the scrotum, and bind it all up with a suitable bandage.[12]

While surgeons recognized that these procedures were feasible, and recognized too that inguinal hernia could be fatal – 'I have already seen two men die from this [condition]', wrote Teodorico[13] – they knew quite well that such treatments were scarcely less dangerous than the hernia itself. They recommended that they be performed only after explaining the risks fully and candidly to the patient, before witnesses, and then only if the surgeon 'has performed the operation before or has assisted a knowledgeable surgeon in it or has seen such an operation performed on someone, and is able and intelligent, since it is easy to kill the patient by an incompetent and unintelligent procedure'.[14]

A terribly painful, life-threatening condition and a risky resolution of the anatomical problem producing it which by removing the testicle seemed to threaten sterility even if it were successful: these were circumstances made to order for the unsupervised, competitive, rapidly expanding craft of surgery as it existed after 1300. Established surgeons like Lanfranco of Milan, in the generation after Teodorico, complained about the greed that characterized the many, unskilled and untrained, who claimed to be able to cure inguinal hernia without using the knife and without destroying the testicle's function: 'Many people', he declared, 'rashly attempt this treatment knowing nothing of the anatomy or of the difference in the conditions, and continually go wrong in operating, but they do not learn from their mistakes; rather, the less they know, the more operations they perform.'[15] Lanfranco himself was able to distinguish between direct and indirect inguinal hernia (the former is produced by a weakness and rupture of the fascia of the inguinal floor rather than by a stretching of the inguinal ring), and he insisted that the two had to be differentiated in diagnosis since their different anatomies required different treatments.[16]

Lanfranco described summarily the variety of approaches being promoted by these self-styled surgeons:

> Some apply a corrosive medicine over the site of the *didymus* until the *didymus* has been laid bare and then corrode the *didymus* itself, after which some remove the testicle and others allow it to rot away. Others force two pointed cauteries intersecting like a cross through the *didymus*, and place wooden sticks through the resulting holes, and cauterize upon them, including part of the *didymus*, and heal it up when the eschar has fallen away. Others do not cauterize but cut the skin and expose and strip the *didymus*; then they tie it with thread, tightening the thread a little every day, until the thread has cut through the *didymus*. Others open the skin and then cauterize the *didymus* partially but not entirely, and this technique is less bad then the others. Others insert two needles into the *didymus* and external skin at right angles, each with a doubled thread; then they tie these threads tightly below the needles and twist them like a tourniquet until all the tissue included in the needles has been severed. Others have still other different techniques, and I would list them all if I were not afraid of lengthening my book.[17]

In fact, these practices were probably not entirely those of unlearned empirics, since at least two are identical with techniques described by Rolando da Parma in his *Surgery*, a hundred years before Lanfranco.[18] But Lanfranco preferred not to acknowledge this, because, his expressions of disdain notwithstanding, these men were his competitors in the search to sign up prospective patients; he himself was exploring – and publicizing – his own variants on the standard procedures.

The 'potential cautery', corrosive medicines, Lanfranco condemns outright in the harshest of terms – 'the worst of all methods' – as causing great pain and death,[19] and the knife he passes over in silence; the tool he prefers to use is the true or actual cautery. Lanfranco explains three different ways to use it, each to be employed according to the circumstances of the particular case.[20] One he describes as quick, easy and sure, if the patient is willing to lose the testicle. It is identical with Albucasis's method (though Lanfranco does not credit his source), and employs a thin, broad, blade, semi-circular in shape, which is heated white-hot and forced down to meet the pubic bone; its breadth ensures that it will encounter and destroy the *didymus* and create a strong scar. Since the testicle will lose its nutriment and die, an incision must also be made in the scrotum and a wick inserted to draw off the putrefying matter. The second approach, even quicker but uncertain in its results and suitable only when the aperture to be sealed is a small one, involves a series of needle-pointed cauteries to be inserted in a line along the spermatic cord, scarring it shut and preventing passage of the intestine.

It is Lanfranco's third technique that he praises most highly and for which he explicitly insists on his own originality: 'although I got the idea from someone else', he says, 'it was perfected by my own ingenuity'.[21] First, use a knife to expose the *didymus*; then, lifting it up with hooks and strings, place a flat piece of iron under the *didymus* for protection and cauterize *beneath* this shield, down to the pubic bone. In healing, Lanfranco says, the external flesh will weld so tightly to the pubic bone around the *didymus* that the intestine will no longer be able to slip down through, and yet the testicle will still be nourished through the conduit, which remains intact. Some practitioners of this technique, he adds, also scar the *didymus* slightly with the cautery in order to constrict the passage still further – a practice 'not altogether harmful', he concedes grudgingly, 'as long as it is done with moderation'.[22]

Teodorico and Lanfranco are describing the variety of surgeons' procedures as they stood about 1300; at the same time they allow us to make inferences about patient psychology. It is not easy now to understand why men should have been as eager as they clearly were to seek surgical correction of a hernia. Granted, a strangulated hernia could prove fatal, but such an eventuality was rare; most inguinal hernias would have been uncomfortable and bothersome but not, we might think, such a problem as to warrant an extremely painful and serious operation. Lanfranco himself was unhappy with surgical intervention for hernia, and urged conservative treatment instead, with bandages and a truss: the condition may not be cured in this way, he wrote, but it will not get any worse, and the patient will not live a day less. Yet Lanfranco's stories about his practice suggest that he had to work hard to convince his own patients that it would be better for them to endure discomfort for a lifetime than to risk everything for the chance of a permanent cure. What may have weighed heavily in their decision was an element of public humiliation associated with the condition. In some societies today men who suffer from hernia become the butts of sexual and scatological ridicule, and it seems possible that the same was true in medieval Europe, to judge from literary sources.[23] Such men would have had a strong psychological incentive to undergo the operation and to be re-constructed, as it were, as 'normal' males. The throng of empiric surgeons of whom Lanfranco complains was less scrupulous than he and gave the public what it wanted, no doubt without stressing the dangers involved. In self-defence, therefore, even a deeply sceptical practitioner like Lanfranco had to offer the operation in order not to lose patients to potential competitors.

Under these circumstances, patient preferences shaped the development of surgical technique and turned the treatment of indirect inguinal hernia into the first fourteenth-century surgical speciality. Surgeons shared an understanding of the anatomical problem and a knowledge of various approaches that could resolve it; to attract a client away from his competitors, a surgeon had to be able to offer a procedure that responded to the sufferer's particular concerns. Teodorico warns that some patients have a particular dread of the razor, others of the cautery; Lanfranco adds that many will resist any method that risks destroying virility by removing a testicle. Later fourteenth-century surgeons followed Lanfranco in exploring variations on the established procedure that would appeal to as wide a range of patients as possible.

In the great mid-century encyclopedia of surgical practice, the *Inventarium* or *Chirurgia Magna* of Guy de Chauliac, these tendencies beginning to emerge in Lanfranco's day appear fully developed. Guy's career exemplifies the permeable barrier between medicine and surgery in the fourteenth century, the tendency of many practitioners to acquire medical learning as an accompaniment to surgical training. Guy studied surgery at Bologna with Bertuccio, Mondino dei Liuzzi's student, but he also received a medical degree at Montpellier with Raymond de Moleriis, who was chancellor there in 1335. His entire life as a practitioner was spent, as far as we know, in southern France, first in Lyons and then, in the 1340s and 1350s, as physician to the popes in Avignon, where his *Chirurgia Magna* was composed in 1363, five years before he died.[24] Three other earlier compositions of his are mentioned in the *Chirurgia*, one of them a 'Libellus de ruptura'; evidently the treatment of hernia attracted special attention from the Montpellier milieu to which Guy was attached, as well as from the Parisian and north Italian worlds that Lanfranco knew. Unfortunately, Guy's 'Libellus' is lost today, but since he referred his reader to it in the chapter on hernia in the *Chirurgia*, we can imagine that the latter discussion was closely based on the former.[25]

Guy's discussion of hernia in the *Chirurgia Magna* gives a thorough and generally straightforward account of six procedures in use at mid-century.[26] The first that he describes is tying off and cutting through the *didymus* at its exit from the abdomen; the second is destroying the *didymus* by a cautery driven down through the skin to the pubic bone. Guy's habit throughout the *Chirurgia Magna* was to identify his sources, and these two long-familiar procedures he traces to the great names of surgical literature, from Albucasis to Teodorico. Almost all the other methods he describes, however, he associates not with surgical authors of the past but with specific contemporary practitioners. The next one he takes up, the use of the potential cautery, is Guy's own preferred technique, one that he says he shares with Giovanni de Crepatis of

Bologna, André of Montpellier, and Pierre d'Orlhac of Avignon.[27] The fourth is the progressive constriction and eventual severing of the exposed *didymus* with a cord, a practice mentioned in passing by Lanfranco but here attributed to Ruggiero Frugardi, the earliest of the medieval Latin surgical authors;[28] the fifth is Lanfranco's cauterization of tissue in a way that preserved the *didymus* intact, which in Guy's day was touted by one Pierre de Die; while the sixth was evidently new, the invention of a certain Béraud Metis, and involved exposing the *didymus* and wrapping it tightly with gold wire to narrow its channel mechanically and permanently prevent the entrance of the intestine.[29]

In Guy's view, only the first four of these techniques can be truly satisfactory, because they are the only ones that seal the intestines off irrevocably from the scrotum; the other two leave the *didymus* intact and so leave an opening, even though they narrow it, and therefore while they may sometimes be useful if the hernia is a small one, they cannot guarantee prevention. Guy rehearses the argument that one might use to reassure a patient who feared the loss of the testicle that the four first procedures entailed: 'I have seen plenty of fathers who had only one testicle, and the lesser of two evils is always to be preferred.' As for choosing among these four, the knife is always a dangerous instrument, while the white-hot cautery produces terror in the patient, so that his own preferred technique employs the potential cautery. By the unremitting application of quicklime and arsenic to the skin of the abdomen over the hernia, the tissues will be destroyed in two weeks, creating an eschar just above the *didymus*; when this is removed, an incision is made in the *didymus*, further corrosives are introduced, and in two weeks more the cord will be destroyed and the healing process may begin. After the wound has healed, a truss and inaction will still be needed for 30 days.

Guy had already remarked that Pierre d'Orlhac was another proponent of this procedure; now, in a remarkable aside, he comments on the minor differences between their methods and reveals something of the technical interplay that competition enforced.

> Master Pierre, whom I saw treat thirty patients suffering from hernia, never kept them inactive but allowed them to go about in town so that they might forget the pain of the corrosive medicine, something I do not recommend unless the intestine is firmly withheld. In the operation itself, although he cut around the eschar as far as he could, he never forced its removal until it fell away by itself, and he put nothing in the wound from beginning to end except cloth and bandages, feeling that the eschar protected the flesh from the corrosives; I consider this to be unsound, because as long as the eschar is there it is very difficult to know when you have reached the *didymus*, while when the eschar is gone both

touch and sight reveal the truth. It took him eight weeks to complete the operation, a period that I reduced by three weeks. ...

Then, hearing that in treating Louis de Brissac of Vienne ... I had used the curved cultellar cautery for additional certainty, once the *didymus* had been reached [this was the instrument mentioned by Lanfranco, following Albucasis], *he* began to use the cautery from the beginning of every operation ... at every stage, saying that it helped in three ways: [preventing] the flow of blood, cutting deeper without cutting the eschar (since this was destroyed by the cautery), and mitigating the pain of the corrosive medicine. I cannot really object to this, even though (as Galen says in his commentary on the first of the *Aphorisms*) to combine distinct procedures is not faithful to the art and is not honourable, for in this operation the danger is so great that the surgeon should take advantage of everything that may help and cannot hurt, especially because the eschar prevents the cautery from being felt – as long as you are careful that the patient does not see it.[30]

It has seemed worth quoting this passage in full because it shows so vividly how individual surgical practice was shaped, at the level of technical detail, not just by considerations of efficacy, safety and speed (though these considerations are all there), but also by knowledge of a competitor's practice (to criticize or to borrow from) and of patient psychology.

Guy's *Chirurgia Magna* marks the culmination of the medieval surgical tradition that had attempted with some success to make the craft into a learned, literate discipline. It soon became something of a canonical authority, not just for students of the written word but for practitioners – and, indeed, at times too for the lay public. I have already said that public authorities in western Europe were beginning to impose controls over admission to medical and surgical practice during the fourteenth century: the process has been particularly closely studied in Valencia, in eastern Spain.[31] Here licences for the practice of general medicine or surgery were being required by the city as early as 1329, at least in principle, and by 1380 the city fathers were also beginning to grant licences to perform one specific surgical procedure: the operation to correct hernia. Typically, the city would appoint skilled examiners to test the applicant's knowledge, orally or in an actual operation,[32] and then ratify the examiner's judgement; six such licences survive from the 1380s, testifying in individualized language to the recipients' skill in this narrow specialty. Their terms thus show us the elements of craft concern that were accepted by the lay public, and give us a little more insight into the social perception of the treatment of hernia – and of its dangers.

The examiners' own understanding of the problem had been shaped by the new learned surgery, and in particular by Guy de Chauliac's

Chirurgia Magna: in 1388, defining the particular condition that Andreu Martí was to be allowed to treat, his examiners used a curious mix of Catalan vernacular and Latin technical terminology quoted directly from Guy's text.[33] But the examiners did not insist on book-learning as a requirement for practice: when Johan de Sena asked them for permission to treat cataract, hernia and bladder stone, but nothing else, the examiners agreed, commenting that 'the said things pertain more to experience and manual activity than to scientific understanding'.[34] The very practical issue of patient fears was of more immediate concern to them. Patient mistrust of the knife probably helps explain the odd explicitness with which Joan de Venecia was licensed to treat hernia *with* the knife, in distinction from Francesc Assensi de Toscana (an immigrant to Valencia from Perugia), whom the examiners agreed was competent to provide such treatment '*with or without* cutting'.[35] More revealing yet of lay concerns are the conditions that the court added when ratifying the examination given to Tomás de Mestre Tone (another Italian immigrant, from Ancona): '[he must] inform patients suffering from hernia of ... the danger of death that they could run in undergoing the said operation; and [he must] forewarn patients who will have to have an affected testicle destroyed, or both if the said complaint [involves] both.'[36] However dispassionately practitioners like Guy de Chauliac may have been able to contemplate the sacrifice of a patient's testicle, their public was clearly not convinced.

The *Chirurgia Magna* may have become canonical for the later Middle Ages, but Guy's preferred method for correcting hernia did not drive out all others. This is brought out by the *Philonium* of Valesco de Taranta, a witness to late fourteenth-century medicine who is still surprisingly unexploited by historians.[37] Valesco was Portuguese in origin; he began his studies in the liberal arts at Lisbon and completed them at Paris before proceeding to study medicine at Montpellier,[38] where he studied with the university's chancellor, Jean de Tournemire. In 1387 Valesco became *licenciatus*[39] and then entered the service of the counts of Foix, remaining there until he died; but his practice was not simply a local one, since he mentions cases he has seen in Bordeaux and to medical experience *in regnis Hispanie*, from his native Portugal to Catalunya.[40]

The *Philonium* – compiled near the end of Valesco's life, in 1418 – is unusual as an encyclopedic survey by an academically-trained physician who apparently never became a master or taught in the schools. A remarkable feature of the work is the number and variety of medical authorities it cites, not just Greco-Arabic sources but recent and even contemporary Latin practitioners as well, the latter almost all figures from the Montpellier tradition in which Valesco had been trained. These citations of recent authors may partly be a consequence of the enlarged medical literature in the fourteenth century, and of the size of his patrons' library, but it may also reflect Valesco's removal from an academic community, where professional jealousies were inevitable. Valesco is not hesitant to praise the practice – as distinct from the writings – of his own masters at Montpellier; of other masters there in his time, like François Conill and Jean Jacme ('quem ego vidi');[41] or of other practitioners of his acquaintance, like Guillem sa Garriga of Girona in Catalunya, not a physician but a surgeon.[42]

For, like Guy, Valesco was a practitioner who cared little for the frontier between medicine and surgery. Book VII of the *Philonium* not only incorporates an independent treatise on surgery, it also includes separate discussion of a number of surgical topics of interest to its author, and one of these is hernia. It is typical of his approach elsewhere in the *Philonium* that Valesco's survey of treatments for hernia draws intelligently from the whole of the relevant literature – in this case the literature of the surgical tradition, dating back to Albucasis and Ruggiero Frugardi and culminating in Guy de Chauliac.[43] It generally follows the list of procedures provided by Guy in his *Chirurgia Magna*, and it conscientiously quotes almost all of Guy's account of his preferred treatment by potential cautery.

But Valesco was far from a slavish borrower, and his account of the traditional methods often incorporates new elements which seem again to represent contemporary practice and innovations in technique. Surgical severing of the *didymus*, for example, he sets into an astrological context (it should not be carried out at the full moon or when the moon is in Libra, Virgo or Scorpio) – astrology was an increasingly prominent feature of medicine and surgery after 1350 – and he adds the detail not found in either Teodorico or Guy that the *didymus* should be cut between two ligatures.[44] Of Ruggiero's progressive constriction and eventual severing of the *didymus* with a cord, Valesco reports that instead of using hemp thread to cut the *didymus*, some practitioners are using a four-fold golden wire, 'and they do this so that they can seem to be doing something with gold wire'.[45] If this is not simply Valesco's second-hand misunderstanding of the gold-wire approach invented by Béraud Metis (it was Béraud who had introduced gold wire to wrap around the *didymus*, to keep the channel narrow), it would suggest that certain surgeons were applying Béraud's new technology to an older procedure, not because it *was* more effective but because it would *seem* more effective – because more costly – to prospective patients. Describing Lanfranco's method of cauterizing beneath the *didymus*, shielded from the cautery with iron to keep it unharmed, Valesco mentions that Jean de Tournemire – yet another medical master involved in surgery – recommended the same technique.

And Valesco does not limit himself to the procedures that Guy listed. He has an entirely new one to describe, one that he tells us he has seen employed by a certain Guillaume Brito; it saves the testicle while preventing recurrence of the hernia.[46] The surgeon cuts down to expose the *didymus*; then he passes a three-inch needle and cord through the *didymus* a little way in from one edge – it has to be pulled through with pliers, Valesco explains, because the *didymus* is so tough – and back through it again a corresponding distance from the other edge; the cord, now encircling the central section of the *didymus*, is pulled tight and knotted firmly with two knots. The loop is tightened further, day after day, until it has completely cut through the tissue and come free. As the *didymus* heals and cicatrizes at its centre, it becomes so small a channel that the intestine can never enter it, yet at its intact edges the generative force and nutriment can still flow in to the testicle. With a similar rationale, Valesco adds, some surgeons cut the *didymus* halfway through and cauterize, leaving intact half the *didymus* through which nothing harmful can pass – 'and I have seen this done'.[47]

Nancy Siraisi has concluded that the Italian surgeons of the late thirteenth century were strongly attracted by the contemporary model of institutionalized academic medicine, with its promise of 'ordered wisdom', and that consequently they tended to depend heavily on authoritative sources and rational argumentation in their accounts of their craft.[48] The 'strong authorial presence' that we also find in their works she sees as ensuring self-advertisement as much as reinforcing pedagogical emphasis. As an illustration of self-promotion through ostensible instruction, Siraisi recounts a story told by Lanfranco, where he explained his own method for treating a wound while ridiculing the empiric whom he had bested; if she had chosen to, she could perfectly well have cited Lanfranco's discussion of hernia as combining the same two functions.[49] Lanfranco gave only cursory and disdainful mention to the treatments of hernia offered by others in his day, and while he conceded that one of his own procedures was adapted from somebody else's, he was conspicuously silent on the identity of the actual inventor and stressed instead his own inventiveness and superiority.

Guy de Chauliac's account of treatments for hernia, 60 years later, reveals a very different attitude towards craft experience, one that is more respectful of its collective worth. Where Lanfranco explained his own treatments carefully but dismissed his competitor's methods in very few words, Guy set out all contemporary procedures for hernia repair with almost equal seriousness, and, by ascribing many of these procedures to other contemporary surgeons as well as to classical authorities, he promoted his colleagues' practice together with his own. Valesco de Taranta's *Philonium* continues to display the same open-mindedness to contemporary practices.

For Guy and Valesco, practical observations from whatever source have their own independent worth. Observations still have to be guaranteed by personal authority, certainly; but whereas in the thirteenth century the eminence of the guarantor was critical (Galen or Avicenna, for example), and determined how much weight should be given to his observations in rational argument, the eminence of Guy's authorities – or Valesco's – is of little importance. It is not *who* vouches for the fact that matters now, but *that* it can credibly be vouched for, and in this regard even unlettered practitioners can be as credible as the great names of the past. Far from casting doubt on potential competitors, both Guy and Valesco prove eager to establish personally the credibility of these modern authorities ('I saw master Pierre treat thirty patients in this way'; 'and I have seen this done'), and they do not try to force the observations into a pre-established system; Guy, it will be remembered, was actually willing to concede that a colleague was correct to act in accordance with practical experience even though his actions contradicted a Galenic principle and, by implication, were an improvement on Guy's own methods. The contrast with Lanfranco's refusal to acknowledge the work of his competitors, even those he borrowed from, could scarcely be more direct.

How should we explain this change in attitude towards authority and experience? It may be that Guy and Valesco, both on the interface between medicine and surgery, were thereby less directly caught up in occupational competitiveness than Lanfranco and felt freer to give credit to their contemporaries. It is also possible that surgery itself had come to be governed by standards of practice, internally or externally imposed, that made competition within the recently organized craft generally less intense than it had been in Lanfranco's day. It may even prove that this increased appreciation of craft experience was not so much widespread among Western practitioners after 1350 as it was simply one aspect of a regional tradition. Ordinarily two writers would not justify us in talking of a 'tradition', but I think Guy and Valesco between them do establish the existence of a surgical tradition in southern France that drew on shared practical experience to develop and refine earlier procedures for the treatment of indirect inguinal hernia.[50]

Thus many of the expectations held out at the beginning of this chapter have apparently been confirmed: focusing on the surgical correction of hernia has allowed us to recognize that medieval surgical practice could indeed be developed and articulated in response to patient needs and desires. Even the most sympathetic accounts of medieval surgery have assumed that it was crude and barbaric in execution, however 'progressive' its direction may have been, and historians seem often to have felt that the medieval treatment of hernia shows surgeons at their most insensitive.[51] Yet in fact, as I have tried to show, medieval surgeons are better understood as having thoughtfully and purposefully explored the implications of the anatomical and physiological model that they had inherited from their classical predecessors.

But did the articulation and development of practice equate to progress? Here we may reasonably be sceptical; we may wonder dubiously whether Valesco's preferred procedure (sewing through the exposed spermatic cord) would really have treated hernias better and more effectively than Guy's (corroding the cord with caustic chemicals) or indeed Lanfranco's (opening the groin and cauterizing beneath the cord). And our scepticism is likely to be reinforced when we learn that none of the medieval techniques is likely ever to have been successful in preventing the return of the hernia. The irritation, granulation and scarring that any of them would have produced might temporarily have impeded a hernia's reappearance through the inguinal ring, but they could not have provided structural solidity, and eventually intra-abdominal pressure would probably have caused the hernia to recur.[52] By the standard of permanent repair, the medieval procedures were all failures.

Why then did medieval surgeons not learn from their failures, as an empiricist model would suggest they should? Plausibly, I would suggest, because to these surgeons and their patients the results were *not* all failures. We should not automatically assume that medieval patients expected a permanent cure and felt betrayed when one was not forthcoming; even temporary alleviation of the condition could have seemed a surgical triumph. Surgeons, for their part, could certainly find explanations for reports of post-operative recurrence of hernias: as due to accidents, to flaws inherent in the particular methods employed, or to incompetence and even fraud. Perhaps the *didymus* had not been completely destroyed? This, remember, was the reason Guy de Chauliac had advanced to explain why the methods of Lanfranco and Béraud Metis might permit hernias to return. Perhaps the surgeon had been negligent? Pierre Franco in the sixteenth century accused some dishonest practitioners of using hempen thread instead of gold wire to tie off the *didymus*; unlike the gold, the hemp would eventually disintegrate and the hernia would reappear – but *after* the surgeons had vanished.[53] Whether his accusation had any basis in fact (probably it did), it still shows how second-hand reports of failures could easily be rationalized. Such rationalizations at once presumed and reinforced the medieval surgeons' confident belief in their model of inguinal anatomy, their belief in the *didymus* as a strong conduit connecting the abdomen with the scrotum, which remained unaltered into the early modern period.[54] The surgeon Pierre Franco, just mentioned, still accepted this model unquestioningly in 1561; so did the anatomist Andreas Vesalius in 1555.[55] As long as the surgeons felt confidence in their visualization of the anatomical situation, and could explain away reports of failures, they were bound to continue making subtle changes in existing procedures rather than try to develop a totally new one.

The history of the medieval treatment of inguinal hernia may not demonstrate the inevitability of surgical progress, if by that we continue to understand a steady improvement in technique grounded in anatomical experience and achieving more or less permanent repair. Yet curiously if we recast our definition of surgical success, a different kind of progress does become apparent. Contemporary surgical literature suggests that patients were not so much preoccupied with permanence of cure as with two other features of the operation that desperately concerned them, and that surgeons exerted considerable ingenuity in trying to provide. One thing patients clearly wanted was minimization of their fear and pain, and here the variousness of patient psychology encouraged the evolution of a great many different techniques – some involving only the knife *or* the cautery *or* caustic medicines, others using these tools in various combinations, depending on what the patient might tolerate or might dread – as well as methods of distracting their patients from their pain or of shortening its duration, even though these methods might then require compromises in technique. In these innovations, unexpectedly, we are forced to recognize a kind of progress in surgical technique, for they unquestionably gave the patient increasing control over the kind of operation – and of agony – that he would have to endure.

Secondly, surgeons were being forced to respond to their patients' dread of the hemi-castration required by the operative technique that was first introduced to correct inguinal hernia. Here once again, even more forcibly, we have to acknowledge what amounts to surgical progress, rapid procedural innovation focused on a single theme: the search for a procedure that would correct the hernia but keep the affected testicle intact. First there was Lanfranco's method of cauterizing beneath the protected *didymus*; then, avoiding the cautery and appealing more directly to the anatomical model, came methods that mechanically constricted the *didymus* by wrapping it with gold wire or by excising its centre with tightened loops of thread. These new approaches that deliberately preserved the *didymus*, for the sake of testicular function, were of course those that Guy de Chauliac criticised for exactly that reason, since it was liable to allow the hernia to recur. Thus in choosing among the increasing variety of procedures, patients were able to decide what they wanted more from the operation: a greater likelihood of a lasting cure, or the safeguarding of their virility. The fact that variations on the new approaches were still being described by Valesco de Taranta in the early fifteenth century and Pierre Franco in the mid-sixteenth indicates that to many sufferers the latter outcome was more important.

It no longer seems particularly radical to interpret the success of new biomedical theories (humours and temperaments, for example) as socially constructed, and I am trying to suggest that we may be able usefully to approach 'progress' in surgical practice in the same way. In terms of fourteenth-century hopes and fears, the grisly sequence of horrors I have described, each to us seemingly more agonizing than the next, may well have appeared to be a steady advance – whether or not the operation repaired the hernia it was supposed to correct. For these procedures allowed practitioners to believe that they were devising increasingly sound procedures, physiologically, for preventing or at least minimizing the chance of a hernia's recurrence while preserving a testicle; and at the same time they provided sufferers with increasing control over pain – the power to choose the torture they feared the least. Even though we have no direct testimony from patients, it seems reasonable to conclude, from the proliferation of so many new procedures in the surgical marketplace, that the public too perceived the continuing elaboration of surgical techniques as contributing to the betterment of health – and, of course, as reason to trust a surgeon who had mastered them. If all parties concerned were gaining confidence in the operation – and I think they must have been – don't we have to acknowledge real surgical progress, even though we believe that by our standards the operation itself was a fundamentally mistaken one?

Acknowledgements

I am grateful for discussions of preliminary versions of this paper in a colloquium on 'The Doctor and Patient in Medieval and Renaissance Europe', Duke University, and at seminars in the Department of the History of Science, Medicine, and Technology, Johns Hopkins University, and the Department of History of Science, Harvard University.

Notes

1. I make this qualification since *medicina practica* and medical practice would have meant different things to, say, a serious student of Haly Abbas's *Pantegni*.

2. Chiara Crisciani, 'History, Novelty, and Progress in Scholastic Medicine', *Osiris*, 2nd series, 6 (1990), pp. 127–30.
3. Jole Agrimi and Chiara Crisciani, 'The science and practice of medicine in the thirteenth century according to Guglielmo da Saliceto, Italian surgeon', in Luis García-Ballester, Roger French, Jon Arrizabalaga and Andrew Cunningham, eds, *Practical Medicine from Salerno to the Black Death*, (Cambridge, Cambridge University Press, 1994), pp. 60–87.
4. Crisciani, 'History', pp. 131–4; Nancy G. Siraisi, 'How to Write a Latin Book on Surgery: Organizing Principles and Authorial Devices in Guglielmo da Saliceto and Dino del Garbo', in García-Ballester et al., *Practical Medicine*, pp. 88–109.
5. Robert Gottfried, *Doctors and Patients in Medieval England 1340–1530* (Princeton, Princeton University Press, 1986), presents what I believe to be a naïvely extreme and untenable version of this thesis that surgeons, by virtue of their immersion in a practical craft that forced them to learn from experience, were bound to progress towards modern medicine. The same view is expressed much more moderately by John M. Riddle, 'Theory and Practice in Medieval Medicine', *Viator*, 5 (1974), p. 182, and is implicit in the discussion of surgery in C. H. Talbot, *Medicine in Medieval England* (London, Oldbourne, 1967), pp. 88–104 ('Unlike the work of the physicians, which in the thirteenth century made no apparent progress, the work of surgery went forward at an exhilarating pace'; p. 88).
6. My account is based on Lloyd M. Nyhus and Robert E. Condon, *Hernia*, 2nd edn (Philadelphia and Toronto, Lippincott, 1978), and Leo M. Zimmerman and Barry J. Anson, *Anatomy and Surgery of Hernia*, 2nd edn (Baltimore, Williams and Wilkins, 1967). I am deeply grateful to Drs George F. Sheldon and Colin G. Thomas, Jr, of the Department of Surgery, University of North Carolina, for their advice and constructive comments.
7. 'Ista vasa ... contenta sunt et velata panniculo orto a siphac qui nominatur didimus cuius orificium est in fine illorum clausum secundum naturam ... in fine eius dilatatur ad quantitatem testiculorum et in parte illa vocatur bursa testiculorum sive oseum. ... Egritudo eius specialis ... est dillatatio orificii eius preter naturam que causa est ut illa que intra siphach continentur descendant in oseum et talis descensus dicitur hernia.' Ernest Wickersheimer, *Anatomies de Mondino dei Luzzi et de Guido de Vigevano* (rpt Geneva, Slatkine, 1977), p. 27; my translation slightly modifies that of Charles Singer, *The Fasciculo di Medicina, Venice 1493* (Florence, R. Lier, 1925), part I, p. 77. For a French perspective, cf. Henri de Mondeville, *Cyrurgia*, I.11: 'Interior pars ossei, quae ab intra osseum circumdat testiculos sicut syphac nutritivorum regionem, est de substantia dicti syphacis ... ; hujusmodi pars syphacis sic mediocriter stricta, quae est inter concavitatem syphacis et concavitatem ossei et transit inter carnem exteriorem et os pectis a duobus lateribus vergae, dicitur dindimus i. e. dubitativus quia semper debemus dubitare de relaxatione et ruptura' (Julius Leopold Pagel, 'Die Chirurgie des Heinrich von Mondeville [Hermondaville]', *Archiv für klinische Chirurgie*, 40 [1890], p. 309).

   Mondeville's derivation of *di(n)dimus* from 'doubt' had a long history, going back at least to the *Anatomia* of Ricardus Anglicus in the twelfth century: 'Est autem quidam nervus bifurcatus, utrique testiculo colligatus, superius autem collimitatur cum siphac et intestinis et uocatur didimus id est dubius, an magis ab intestinis aut magis a testiculis originem trahat' (Karl Sudhoff, 'Der "Micrologus" – Text der "Anatomia" Richards des Engländers', *Archiv für Geschichte der Medizin*, 19 [1927], p. 230). (I am grateful to Professor John Baldwin for drawing my attention to this passage.) This derivation evidently reflects a misconstruction of the gospel account of the apostle Thomas – 'unu ex duodecim, qui dicitur Didymus' (John 20.24) – for 'didymos' actually means 'twin' in Greek. Thomas's nickname is not explained in the gospel passage that follows, which describes his scepticism that Christ could really have appeared to his fellows as they had claimed; presumably some early anatomist supposed that 'Didymus' must refer to his scepticism, but it is a little surprising to find Mondeville still accepting the derivation. Guy de Chauliac, for one, was well aware that the *didymus* was so called because it was a paired or twinned structure: see Guy de Chauliac, *Inventarium sive Chirurgia Magna*, I.2.7 – 'vocatur dindimus, quia duplicatus' (ed. Michael R. McVaugh [Leiden, Brill, 1997], vol. 1, p. 53).

8. The discrepancy between the modern and medieval understandings has created great difficulties for historians, who have regularly failed to understand what *didymus* meant to a medieval or early modern surgeon. Campbell and Colton translated it as 'scrotum' in the passage from Teodorico Borgognoni (II.104) quoted below in n. 12; Leo M. Zimmerman and Ilza Veith (*Great Ideas in the History of Surgery*, 2nd edn [New York, Dover, 1967], pp. 196–200) translated it as '[hernial] sac' in their English rendering of Pierre Franco's treatise (1561) – yet Franco is clear enough about his anatomical picture, which is still the medieval one (E. Nicaise, ed., *Chirurgie de Pierre Franco de Turriers en Provence composée en 1561* [Paris, 1895], pp. 34–5).

9. Galen sets the model out perhaps most clearly in *On anatomical procedures*, XII.7 (*Galen On Anatomical Procedures: The Later Books*, tr. W. L. H. Duckworth [Cambridge, Cambridge University Press, 1962], pp. 123–9). Duckworth somewhat misleadingly equates the structure that Galen referred to there as 'the channel which many anatomists call "the conducting canal"' with the spermatic cord itself, but since Galen described this structure as lying immediately beneath the cremaster muscle he seems to have understood the investing fasciae as the outer boundary of the 'channel'. (In *On anat. proc.*, VI.5, he also refers briefly to the hernia formed when peritoneum 'breaks into the passage to the testicles'; *Galen On Anatomical Procedures*, tr. Charles Singer [London, Oxford University Press, 1956], p. 157.) A briefer acount occurs in *De usu partium*, XIV.13, where Galen refers to 'the flute-like channel from the peritoneum' as containing the constituents of the spermatic cord (*Galen on the Usefulness of the Parts of the Body*, tr. Margaret Tallmadge May [Ithaca, Cornell University Press, 1968], vol. 2, pp. 648–9); May identifies this 'channel' with the inguinal canal, which, however, is merely a space framed by a number of ligaments and muscles and is unlikely to have been thought of by Galen as a discrete 'flute-like' structure. Historians have long recognized that Galen believed in such a passageway between abdomen and scrotum, though they have not fully appreciated its consequences for surgical treatment: see John E. Raaf, 'Hernia Healers', *Annals of Medical History*, n.s. 4 (1932), p. 380, and Edmund Andrews,

'A History of the Development of the Technique of Herniotomy', *Annals of Medical History*, n.s. 7 (1935), pp. 456–7.

Medieval physicians and surgeons could not have been acquainted with any of these Galenic accounts before 1300. Books X–XV of *On Anatomical Procedures* (as well as a portion of book IX) survive only in Arabic and were unknown to the Middle Ages. The medieval abridgement of *De usu partium* called *De iuvamentis membrorum* omitted book XIV; the full text was eventually translated from Greek in the fourteenth century by Niccolo da Reggio (and is quoted, for example, in the surgery of Guy de Chauliac). Here at last Galen could be read describing 'porus ... qui a peritoneo velut fistula quadam nutrientia testiculos vasa deduxit' (MS Vatican City, Vat. Lat. 2380, f. 91va) – in Latin, *fistula* meant, not simply a passage, but a pipe or quill or catheter; that is, a tubular structure.

10. *The Seven Books of Paulus Aegineta*, tr. Francis Adams (London, 1846), vol. 2, pp. 372–7. Although Galen alludes to 'the operation for hernia' (*On Anatomical Procedures*, tr. Duckworth, p. 125), so far as I know he never describes it. Celsus appears to describe a different operation (*De medicina*, VII.19; tr. W. G. Spencer [Cambridge, MA, Harvard University Press; London, Heinemann, 1938], vol. 3, pp. 399–409), one that preserved the testicle, but it is not easy to say with any precision what the operation entailed because the physiological model that Celsus's account presupposes and the anatomical language that it employs are so vague. Interpretations by modern historians of herniotomy of its supposed details seem to me to be somewhat overconfident.
11. Teodorico, *Surgery*, III.34; *The Surgery of Theodoric*, tr. Eldridge Campbell and James Colton (New York, Appleton–Century–Crofts, 1960), vol. 2, pp. 100–102. Bruno's *Surgery* (on which Teodorico seems to have drawn heavily for most of his book) gives the first of these treatments verbatim, but omits any account of the use of the potential cautery (Susan P. Hall, 'The *Cyrurgia Magna* of Brunus Longoburgensis: A Critical Edition', Dissertation, Oxford, 1957, pp. 279–80), and in this it follows Albucasis, who discussed the actual but not the potential cautery in cases of inguinal hernia (*Albucasis on Surgery and Instruments*, ed. and tr. M. S. Spink and G. L. Lewis [Berkeley, University of California Press, 1973], pp. 134–9; ch. 45). The earliest reference I have so far seen to this application of the potential cautery is in a commentary on the *Surgery* of Guillaume de Congenis of Montpellier, in the first half of the thirteenth century: the text speaks of cutting down to the *didymus* with a knife, but his student-commentator adds that once he saw Guillaume apply a corrosive medicine instead – 'sed cum aliquantulum corrosisset in profundum, homo dolorem sustinere noluit et sic magister in cura non processit' (Karl Sudhoff, *Beiträge zur Geschichte der Chirurgie im Mittelalter* [Leipzig, Barth, 1918], vol. 2, p. 370).

Surgeons were well aware that if the potential cautery were to be used successfully, the patient would have to have continuing psychological support: 'Necessarium est cyrurgico scire, quod corrosivorum quaedam statim cum applicentur, inferunt dolorem patienti, quaedam non statim sed post aliquas horas, et hoc debet scire propter duo: 1^{m} quia aliqui patientes facilius dolorem sustinent una hora quam altera, ut post comestionem quam ante, et aliqui ex contrario, et aliqui stantes in societate aut convivio nolunt molestari in praesentia aliorum. Et quia aliquando cyrurgicus non potest continue assistere patienti, ideo scitis praedictis ipse debet applicare corrosivum, quod corrodat hora, quae est magis conveniens patienti; 2m quia si patiens sit delicatus et cyrurgicus applicat corrosivum quod statim operatur, fortasse patiens procurabit quod cyrurgicus amovebit, et si applicet corrosivum quod, postquam recesserit, operatur, patiens non audebit ipsum in absentia cyrurgici amovere et cum hoc non compatietur patienti cyrurgicus in dolore.' Henri de Mondeville, *Cyrurgia*, V.7; ed. Pagel, *Arch. klin. Chirurgie*, 42 (1891), p. 702. One fourteenth-century surgeon's technique for distracting the patient from the corrosive's pain is alluded to in n. 30, below.

12. Teodorico, *Surgery*, III.35; I have modified the translation of Campbell and Colton (vol. 2, p. 104), following the Latin edition in *Ars chirurgica* (Venice, 1546), ff. 134v–184r. The same passage appears in Bruno, *Surgery* (ed. Hall, pp. 283–4). Their common description of the operation probably goes back to Albucasis (tr. Spink and Lewis, pp. 440–44; ch. 65).
13. Bruno's *Surgery* does not include this reference, so it appears to be Teodorico's own comment.
14. For the importance of delivering a warning in front of witnesses, see Teodorico, *Surgery*, III.35 (tr. Campbell and Colton, vol. 2, p. 103). The need for experience with the procedure is emphasized by Guglielmo da Saliceto: 'si usus fuerit tali operatione vel usus fuerit cum aliquo operatore rationabili vel viderit talem operationem fieri in aliquo et fuerit boni ingenii et bone ymaginationis secure potest in tali cura procedere; et per aliam viam non in hac cura presumat se aliquo modo operari quia per malam etiam edoctam operationem de levi hominem interficere posset.' *Chirurgia*, I.44; MS Oxford, St John's College, 76, f. 23r. Guglielmo's procedure is essentially the same as Teodorico's, except that he ties the *didymus* with two ligatures a finger's-breadth apart 'et illud spacium scindatur per medium ex transverso et postea cauterizetur optime'. Also, whereas Teodorico instructed the surgeon to withdraw the testicle from the incision and then to cut the *didymus* leading to it, Guglielmo criticizes this as the act of 'medici stolidi et nichil scientes', and insists that the *didymus* is to be severed while the testicle is left to rest normally in the scrotum – a less traumatic procedure than Teodorico's, presumably, though it too would inevitably end in the loss of the testicle. Zimmerman and Veith (*Great Ideas*, p. 107) are thus perhaps literally correct to say that 'Salicet is ... the first author since Celsus to reject removal of the testicle as an essential part of the operation for hernia', but their assertion is cerainly misleading; from a prospective father's viewpoint, Guglielmo's procedure would have seemed no better than Teodorico's. (The statement by Zimmerman and Veith is repeated in Lloyd M. Nyhus and Robert E. Condon, *Hernia*, 4th edn [Philadelphia and Toronto, Lippincott, 1995], p. 6.)
15. 'Nam multi de hac cura se cum audacia intromittunt qui nec loca noverunt nec aegritudinis differentiam cognoverunt, quare quotidie cadunt in suis operationibus in errorem, nec propter hoc ab eorum insania se divertunt. Sed quanto minus sciunt, tanto magis de curis se talibus intromittunt.' Lanfranco, *Chirurgia*, III.3.7 (MS Cambridge, Gonville and Caius College [=Cgc] 159/209, 329v; Middle English translation in *Lanfrank's 'Science of cirurgie,'* ed. Robert v. Fleischhacker [London, 1894], p. 270).

16. The distinction between the two is already made by Guillaume de Congenis. However, he distinguishes between indirect (*relaxatum*) and direct (*ruptum*) hernia, not anatomically, but diagnostically: the former hernia appears when the patient is asked to cough (Sudhoff, *Beiträge*, vol. 2, p. 371). Unlike Lanfranco, who describes an operation, Guillaume prescribes only diet and a truss for direct inguinal hernia.
17. 'Utplurimum supra locum pectinis supra didymum, scilicet medicamen applicant corrosivum, donec didymus detegatur, et corrodunt postea didymum, quorum aliqui extrahunt testiculum, aliqui tamen per viam illam ad finem corrumpunt testiculum. Aliqui cum duobus cauteriis punctualibus sese ad modum crucis intersecantibus supra didymum cauteriçant, et duos ibi ponunt stilos ligneos, super quos cutem iterum cauteriçant, accipientes cum suis cauteriis didymi partem, et cum eschara ceciderit, consolidant. Alii sine cauterio superficialem cutem incidunt, et didymum scarnant; postea ligant cum spago, spagum stringendo quotidie, donec totus truncatur dydymus a spago. Alii post pellis superioris apertionem partem cauteriçatam diminuunt, partemque non cauteriçatam relinquunt, et hic modus minus aliis est malus. Alii acus duas infigunt in didymum et exteriorem pellem, et unaqueque habet filum duplicem, et acus sese cruciunt adinvicem; postea accipiunt illa fila et sub acubus nectunt fortiter, et super apponunt martentinum, donec pellis tota ab acubus comprehensa solvetur. Aliqui etiam alias diversas habent operationes, et ego iam distincte ponerem illas, et predictarum modum, si libri longitudinem non timerem.' Lanfranco, *Chirurgia*, III.3.7 (MS Cgc 159/209, 330b–331a; ed. Fleischhacker, p. 271).
18. The second of the techniques described in the quotation above is already described by Ruggiero Frugardi in the late twelfth century (Sudhoff, *Beiträge*, II.221; Salvatore de Renzi, *Collectio Salernitana* [=*CS*] [Naples, 1853], vol. 2, p. 483). Rolando passes it on and adds the third (*CS*, vol. 2, pp. 683, 685).
19. 'Super omnes modos peior est ille qui fit cum caustica medicina. Nam medicina caustica propter eius magnam venenositatem et malitiam dolores multos facit, qui sunt causa attrahendi apostema, et raro fit quin per eam apostema maximum generetur. Et quod peius est, adeo per eam inflatur didymus, et contrahitur, quod aliquando vulnus exit et per eius contractionem cum eo patitur diaphragma cerebrum quod est fons omnium membrorum nervosorum ut scivisti, et sic multi spasmantur ... et spasmati subito moriuntur' (MS Cgc 159/209, 334a; ed. Fleischhacker, p. 271).
20. The passage describing these techniques is omitted in Fleischhacker's Middle English text.
21. 'Quamvis ab alio sumpserim principium, tamen est a meo ingenio completa et inventa' (MS Cgc 159/209, 332a).
22. 'Sunt enim quidam qui partem aliquam tangunt de didymo cum cauterio, ut magis constringatur; nec est illud multum malum, dummodo factum fuerit cum mensura' (MS Cgc 159/209, 334a).
23. I have come upon a few scattered indicators of such an attitude. Cf. the pejorative contexts in which the word 'potra' (hernia) is used in medieval Castilian, as far back as 1251; Joan Corominas and José A. Pascual, *Diccionario crítico etimológico castellano e hispánico* (Madrid, Gredos, 1981), vol. 4, p. 623; or the ridicule expressed in a thirteenth-century

story, 'A tant li vileniax chaï/La teste à val, les piez à mont:/Bien voient tuit cil qui i sont/Que hergneus estoit li vilains' (Barbazan, *Fabliaux et contes des poètes françois* [Paris, 1808], vol. 2, p. 77). Claudine Fabre-Vassas, 'La cure de la hernie', in *Le corps humain: nature, culture, surnaturel*, Actes du 110e Congrès National des Sociétés Savantes, (Paris, CTHS, 1985), pp. 277–88, also bears on popular attitudes towards the condition; and cf. the miracle of Saint-Foy, in L. Saltet, 'Miracle prétendu et magie: le "martelage du ventre" du VII° au XIV° siécle', *Bull. Litt. Ecclés.*, Toulouse, 1933, pp. 97–119. But much more research would have to be done to confirm this suggestion.

24. *La Grand Chirurgie de Guy de Chauliac*, ed. E. Nicaise (Paris, 1890), pp. lxxvii–lxxxviii.
25. Ibid., pp. ciii, 525.
26. Guy de Chauliac, *Inventarium*, VI.2.7; ed. McVaugh, vol. 1, pp. 372–6. Or the edition of Laurent Joubert: *Chirurgia Magna Guidonis de Cauliaco* (Lyons, 1585; rpt. Darmstadt, Wissenschaftliche Buchgesellschaft, 1976), pp. 339–43.
27. As we have seen, the procedure was described before him by Teodorico Borgognoni and had been attempted by Guillaume de Congenis; Mondino dei Liuzzi (1316) listed it – along with cutting through or simply tying off the spermatic cord – as one of the three ways to treat hernia surgically (Wickersheimer, *Anatomies*, pp. 27–8). In the sixteenth century, Ambroise Paré still endorsed the use of this technique under certain circumstances, attributing its invention jointly to Guy and Teodorico: *The Apologie and Treatise of Ambroise Paré*, ed. Geoffrey Keynes (London, Falcon, 1951), pp. 112–13.
28. I do not find this treatment described in Ruggiero's *Surgery* (Sudhoff, *Beiträge*, vol. 2, pp. 221–2).
29. The printed edition reads 'Bernardus' but the manuscripts 'Beraudus' or 'Berandus'; see also Nicaise, ed. Franco, p. 49, n. 2. Paré, *Apologie and Treatise*, p. 109, describes a version of this *punctus aureus* still in use in the sixteenth century. I am unsure why Pierre Huard and Mirko Drazen Grmek, *Mille ans de chirurgie en occident* (Paris, Dacosta, 1966), pp. 48–9, believe that Guy himself espoused this method.
30. 'Magister autem Petrus, qui in mei presentia curavit 30, nullum faciebat quiescere sed ire per villam continue ut obliviscerentur molestiam corrosivi – quod non laudo nisi intestinum penitus esset retentum. Et in operando, licet incideret in circuitu escarram quantum sibi erat possibile, nullo modo procurabat casum ipsius usque in finem que cadebat per se, nichil ponendo in foramine a principio usque ad finem nisi carpiam cum pannis et ligamine. Erat enim intencio sua quod escarra defendebat carnem a corrosivo – quod non reputo securum, quia stante escarra satis est difficile scire quando erit realiter operacio in dindimo; quando autem est remota escarra, tactus et oculus testificantur veritatem. Tempus vero tocius sue operacionis erat octo septimanarum. Ego vero sibi abbreviavi eam de tribus septimanis, salvo pluri si semper remanet escarra carnis.

    Verum post ipse audiens quod ego ad maiorem certitudinem in cura domini Ludewici de Brissiaco, dalphinatus Viennensis, post primam dindimi aperturam posueram cauterium curvum cultellare, ipse usus fuit a principio totalis operacionis in qualibet remutacione (vel de tercia in terciam) cum cauterio. Et dicebat quod iuvabat ad tria, ad fluxum sanguinis et ad profundandum magis sine abscisione escarre (quia cauterium consumebat eam), et cum hoc dicebat quod dolorem corrosivi mitigabat; quod non multum inprobo nisi quantum ad hoc quod non est artificiale neque honorabile operaciones perfectas commiscere (in commento primi Amphorismorum). Nichilominus tantum est periculum in opere quod de omnibus se debet homo iuvare de hiis que iuvare et nocere non possunt, presertim quia escarra defendit quod cauterium non sentitur, dumtaxat quod fiat caute quod patiens non videat.' *Inventarium*, ed. McVaugh, vol. 1, pp. 375–6. Franco quotes the same passage in French and renders 'vel de tertia in tertiam' as 'au moins trois en trois jours' (ed. Nicaise, p. 52).

Pierre d'Orlhac (for whom the *Inventarium* is our only historical source) apparently made something of a speciality of the use of the potential cautery, corrosive medicines, in treating hernias of all kinds, including also hydrocele (*Inventarium*, vol. 1, p. 117) and varicocele (ibid., p. 178).

31. Luis García-Ballester, Michael R. McVaugh and Agustín Rubio-Vela, *Medical Licensing and Learning in Fourteenth-Century Valencia; Transactions of the American Philosophical Society*, 79, part 6, (1989).
32. See, e.g., the text published in ibid., pp. 115–17 (doc. 27).
33. Guy had defined *ruptura dindimali* as follows: 'inflatio hernialis in qua intestinum aut zirbus dislocatur et egreditur ab interioribus ad carnem miracis, proprie in dindimo et ossio seu testiculorum bursa', ibid., pp. 18, 103 (doc. 15). The *mirach* is the omentum.
34. Ibid., p. 114 (doc. 25).
35. Ibid., pp. 112, 97 (docs 23, 12).
36. Ibid., p. 92 (doc. 10).
37. 'Surprisingly', because the text is so readily available: at least eleven editions were printed before 1600. My references below are to *Philonium ... Valesci de Tharanta* (Venice, 1521). The only study of any aspect of his work of which I am aware concerns his dentistry: Meinolf Ebbers, *Zahnheilkundliches bei Valesco de Taranta* (inaugural dissertation, Leipzig, Bielefeld, 1922), which has little to contribute.
38. For Lisbon, *Philonium*, VI.15 (f. 174vb); for Paris, I.12 (f. 11vb) and V.24 (f. 158va).
39. For Colba, *Philonium*, VI.35, f. 209vb; for Forester, 'magister noster', VII.24 (f. 183ra); for Tournemire as 'my master', III.5 (f. 69va) and IV.12 (f. 98va) as *cancellarius tempore meo*. The granting of his licence in 1387 is mentioned at II.60, though he must have begun to practise five years before since at f. 1rb he says he has practised for 36 years.
40. Bordeaux, *Philonium*, I.21 (f. 24rb); partibus Gasconie', VII.[56] (f. 207ra); 'in regnis Hispanie', VII.6 (f. 188ra); 'in regno Portugalie', VII.9 (f. 192vb); 'iste est modus dominarum de Cathalonia quando sunt puerpere etc.', V.8 (f. 136rb).
41. For Cunill, *Philonium*, III.7 (f. 72ra); for Jean Jacme, VII.[26] (f. 202rb).
42. 'Hanc curam [scrophularum] fecit magister Guil. sagarriga in Gerunda cuidam pulchre mulieri me presente'; *Philonium*, VII.[57] (f. 207va); 'et secundum istum modum operabatur magister Guilelmus de Garriga', II.62 (f. 53ra).
43. *Philonium*, VI.8 (ff. 166v–167v).
44. The detail is, however, to be found in Albucasis (tr. Spink and Lewis, p. 442) and in Guglielmo da Saliceto (above, n. 14).
45. 'Istum eundem modum operantur aliqui, sed loco fili canabis vel chorde

ponunt filum aureum quadruplicatum et ligant donec filum per se exit; stare dimittunt aliqualiter stringendo et hoc faciunt ut videantur aliquid fecisse cum filo auri. Isti enim prius scindunt pellem et carnem et accipiunt solum dydymum et curant vulnus preter foramen fili. Dicunt enim quod cum longitudine temporis dydymus stringitur et confortatur quamvis totus non abscindatur'; *Philonium*, VI.8, f. 167rb.

46. Brito is otherwise unknown. Sudhoff, *Beiträge*, vol. 2, pp. 301–2, quotes the entire passage while arguing that Guillaume Brito and Guillaume de Congenis were different people.
47. This last is a practice alluded to by Lanfranco (above, n. 17) as adopted by some of his contemporaries – one 'less bad than the others' – but not described in detail by him, nor does Valesco attribute it to Lanfranco.
48. Nancy G. Siraisi, 'How to Write', in García-Ballester et al., *Practical Medicine*, pp. 88–109.
49. Ibid., p. 101.
50. And of course it may reflect not just changing attitudes towards experience within surgery, but within all areas of medical practice. Jole Agrimi and Chiara Crisciani (*Edocere medicos* [Naples, Guerini, 1988], p. 103), see the control of textual tradition by appeals to particular experience as a more or less timeless feature of medical scholasticism, and illustrate their contention by pointing to the *Nonum Almansoris*, whose succinctness yet great utility ensured that its commentators 'ricorrono più frequentemente alle lezioni e testimonianze di docenti e professionisti più o meno contemporanei [ed] a integrazioni e confronti tratti dalla propria esperienza'. However, they draw their examples exclusively from relatively late – fifteenth-century – commentaries (by Ferrari da Grado and Arcolano). It would be interesting to compare the commentary on this work by Gerard de Solo (Montpellier, *c.*1335), to see whether Gerard too was already appealing to contemporaries' practice and to his own personal experience in order to help fill out Rhazes's text.
51. Raaf, 'Hernia Healers', pp. 382–4; Andrews, 'History', p. 462; Leo M. Zimmerman and Judith E. Zimmerman, 'The History of Hernia Treatment', in Nyhus and Condon, *Hernia*, 2nd edn, pp. 4–6. The historical introduction in the fourth edition of Nyhus and Condon's textbook (by José Felix Patiño) sharply reduces its account of medieval treatments of hernia, a different indicator of how slightingly medieval surgery tends to be considered.
52. E. J. Gurlt's assessment of the effectiveness of Valesco de Taranta's preferred treatment – 'es muss in hohem Grade bezweifelt werden' (*Geschichte der Chirurgie und ihrer Ausübung* [Berlin, 1898], vol. 2, p. 116) – could be extended to every medieval procedure for the correction of hernia. At the end of the nineteenth century, before Edoardo Bassini introduced what is essentially the modern procedure for hernia repair (1888–90), the four year recurrence rate using the best previous methods still approached 100% (Zimmerman and Zimmerman, 'History', p. 9).
53. Franco, *Chirurgie*, ed. Nicaise, pp. 45–6.
54. I have found no historical account of these developments, but an account of a concomitant historical problem, the development of an understanding of muscular and ligamentous structure in the inguinal region, is Chester B. McVay, 'The Anatomic Basis for Inguinal and Femoral

Hernioplasty', *Surgery, Gynecology and Obstetrics*, 139 (1974), pp. 931–45.

55. For Franco, see above, n. 4. For Vesalius, *Fabrica*, V.13; 2nd edn, Basel, 1555, pp. 640, 642; Nancy Siraisi has generously shared her translation of these passages with me. See too Vesalius's figure 22 to Book V, reprinted with caption translated (from the Basel, 1543, edition) by J. B. de C. M. Saunders and Charles D. O'Malley, *Vesalius: The Illustrations from his Works* (Cleveland, World Publishing, 1950), p. 168, which purports to represent 'the covering extended from [the peritoneum] to enfold the testis and seminal vessel of its side'). The authors were probably unaware that Vesalius's anatomy was here squarely in the medieval tradition, for they found it necessary to explain away his acceptance here of a conduit continuous with the peritoneum: 'The peritoneal process mentioned and seen on the right side of the illustration suggests the finding of a congenital hernial sac in the specimen.'

CHAPTER EIGHT

Thomas Fayreford: An English Fifteenth-Century Medical Practitioner

Peter Murray Jones

Evidence for the nature of medical practice in the fifteenth century is hard to come by, for England no less than for other parts of Europe. A great number of medical manuscripts written in England in this period survive, preserving texts in Latin, Middle English and Anglo-Norman, or a mixture of the three.[1] Many of these texts deal with practical medicine, the application of medical theory to diagnosis, prognosis and treatment, or simply preserve collections of remedies. But these, even the most informal and personal collections of recipes, are prescriptive in character and do not tell us which remedies were used, on which patients, for which complaints, by which practitioner. The sources of the recipes collected can usually be identified, because so often they were copied from standard academic or encyclopedic texts, such as Book 7 on illnesses and poisons in the *De proprietatibus rerum* of Bartholomaeus Anglicus, the *Thesaurus pauperum* of Petrus Hispanus, the *Lilium medicinae* of Bernard Gordon, or the *Compendium medicinae* of Gilbertus Anglicus. In other words even the most practical-looking text can often be shown to derive from academic authorities.

Of course there is also evidence which brings us closer to the biographies of medical men, preserved in academic or ecclesiastical records (since so many were clerics), evidence which shows up their preferments and property, their ownership of books, medical and otherwise, and their testamentary intentions.[2] From a less flattering perspective, there are occasional cases brought by patients to secure redress after treatment or lack of it, or by doctors to obtain fees withheld by their patients.[3] The glimpses these give of the realities of medical life in the fifteenth century are invaluable, though they often tantalize by what they fail to tell as much as they inform. But they are in the end just glimpses, and do not allow us to see the interactions of practitioner and patients over time. Only the extraordinary case histories written by the English surgeon John of Arderne in the 1370s preserve a picture of the treatment meted out to a small band of his patients, most of them unnamed.[4]

For the fifteenth century we have the commonplace book of John Argentine, royal doctor and later Provost of King's College, Cambridge. This book preserves a number of *experimenta*, the cases which he treated or observed near Cambridge or in Hertfordshire, amongst remedies copied from various academic sources.[5] At the other end of the scale of medical practice we have the book of John Crophill, bailiff of a house of Benedictine nuns at Wix in Essex, who earned some extra income by treating patients on his travels about the estates of the priory. We learn something about who his patients were, some of them with little money to spend on medicines, but there is not much that can be said about how Crophill treated them. His list of patients is more of an accounting device than a record of medical practice.[6]

But the medical practitioner about whom we can learn the most in fifteenth-century England is without doubt Thomas Fayreford, despite the fact that our only real information about him comes from his own writings. British Library Harley MS 2558 preserves a list of the cures he claims to have made, his commonplace book on medicine and surgery, and other medical texts he copied.[7] The list of cures is a record of patients treated by Fayreford, an otherwise obscure practitioner in Somerset and Devon in the first half of the fifteenth century. As well as the evidence of Fayreford's scribal hand, we have internal evidence for Fayreford's writing his text in the fifteenth rather than fourteenth century – he mentions at one point a case of the Oxford physician Nicholas Colnet, who did not proceed BA until 1395, and probably was not licensed to practise physic until after 1400.[8]

Fayreford's list of cures, which occupies two sides of paper manuscript made up in booklets, gives details of the patients' names, sometimes their occupations and places of residence, the ailments from which they suffered in more or less detail, with the prognosis before treatment and Fayreford's remedies in some instances. For once, we are taken outside the enclosed and self-referential world of medical texts which tell us only what it is recommended should be done, and have some access to the character of medical practice itself.[9] Although in places the tiny writing is hard to read, and sometimes even harder to interpret, this list is thus a unique document for our understanding of the nature of medical practice at this time, and all the more interesting for being concerned not with a prestigious university or court doctor, but a provincial practitioner with no university qualification or status as a retainer.

The document on folio 9 of Harley MS 2558 is entitled (in Latin, as is the rest of the list) 'the list of cures performed by Thomas Fayreford in different places'. It is a list compiled and written by Fayreford himself. There are 103 entries in the list, though it is not easy to calculate a

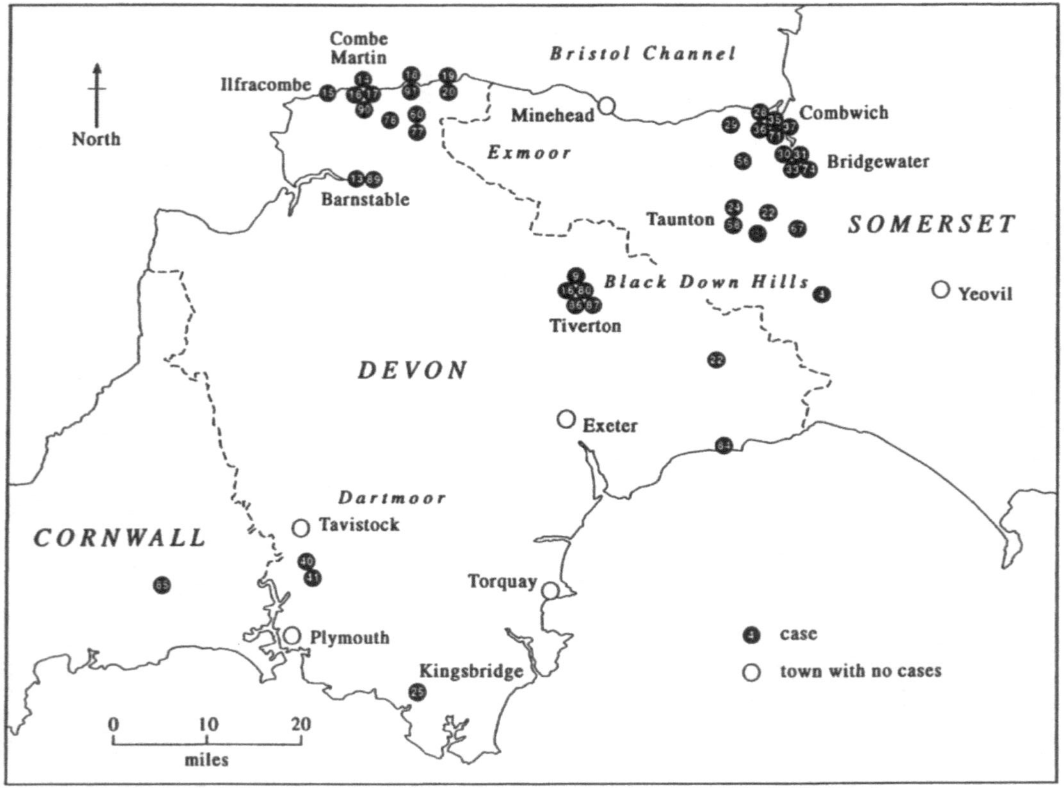

8.1 Forty-two cases plotted by number

number of patients treated, as some of the entries are very abbreviated, and may refer to more than one person treated. Unfortunately Fayreford gives no dates for the cures, but it is clear that the bulk of them were performed in Somerset and Devon, and since most places he names can be identified, it is possible to plot them on a map (see Figure 8.1). One of his patients is named as being from Fairford in Gloucestershire, so it is likely that this was Thomas Fayreford's own place of origin and the source of his name. There is no record of a person of this name attending university at the right date (nor indeed any independent evidence for the existence of our Thomas Fayreford, other than this manuscript). However, given the nearness of Fairford to Oxford as well as the mention of Nicholas Colnet of Oxford – a well-known doctor, later in royal service – it may be that Fayreford learnt some or all of his medicine there.

In assessing the list of cures we do have to bear in mind that it is not simply a series of day-to-day memoranda. Looking at it closely we can see that it was not created out of journal entries made every time Fayreford treated a patient. It seems to have been written in two campaigns, corresponding to the recto and verso of leaf 9 of the manuscript. The first 43 cases on the recto side are written in a darker ink than the remainder on the verso, and the recto is written as one text block, whereas the verso is in two columns. Generally speaking the list is fuller in the information it provides at the beginning than it is at the end. The first two entries in particular are very detailed, the rest of the list of cures is progressively less so, and after item 28 on the list the entries are sometimes very abbreviated (the last just reads 'Item Iohannes peterton'). It may be that this reflects a process of recollection, so that Fayreford begins with cases he has reason to remember best, and after the first quarter of the list or so has come to those cases for which he remembers the barest details.

(Harley MS 2558, ff. 9–9v)
De curis factis per T Fayreford in diversis locis[10]

1. In primis in dominam de ponynges / que habuit frenesim & sincopacionem & squinanciam & suffocacionem matricis simul & semel & in iii ebdomadis fuit perfecte sanitatis domino dante
2. Item in Johannem Wyse qui habuit yctericiam manifestam & fagina super regionem epatis fere usque ad mortem & constipacionem per vi dies & corupcionem appetitus cum siti vehementi
3. Item in Johannem Cloode / qui fuit in ethica & alienacione mentis & ebullicione epatis & c
4. Item mulier de Northover[11] eius lingua fuit sequestrata cum cephalargica & tremore in stomacho & c

5. Item mulier de sydyntonne[12]/ que fuit in suffocacione matricis fere ad mortem & indignitate stomachi
6. Item in filia. W. poulet / que habuit lumbricos & in epilentica passione quatuor in una nocte
7. Item T. parmyter de kyngeston[13] qui in colica tribus vicibus fuit ad mortem / cum pillule dissolute & c.
8. Item Ricardus Webber / qui bis fuit ita constipatus quod disperavit de vita / cum pillule & clistere /
9. Item iuvenis de tyvertone[14]/ qui perdidit visum unius oculi & recuperavit cum sanguine yrundinis & betonica
10. Item Ricardus de combe[15]/ qui fuit ptisicus per iii annos cum rascatione sanguinis & saniei / quod omnes disperaverunt
11. Item lytul boy de choldecombe[16]/ qui habuit ictericiam manifestam & inclinacionem corporis super terram continue
12. Item henricus cros <*superscript:* gedlye> de devon / qui fuit in ethica febre & peracute de quo omnes disperaverunt
13. Item mulier de barstaple[17] / que habuit oculos reumatizantes per teren[18] in tribus noctis fuit finaliter sanata
14. Item pope de cowmartyn[19] / qui habuit tibiam fractum quod plicata fuit quod talus fuit in popplice
15. Item quidam in ylfyrcombe[20] / qui habuit crus fractum cum malo de puppa <?> in mari
16. Item mulier in cowmartyn[21] / de continue motu in stomacho suo
17. Item quidam homo de eodem / de fluxu / continenter per multos annos
18. Item mulier de martyngho mylle[22] / de tussi inveterata & ptysi <*illegible word*> vetula
19. Item quidam homo de lynton[23] / de ptisi quod perdidit vocem & fortitudinem & laborem / & fuit sanatus
20. Item Thomas dene / ibidem de lesione mirabili quod omnes disperaverunt de vita eius
21. Item ii homines & mulier quaedam / que habuerunt sciatitam passionem / quod non potuerunt movere
22. Item quidam homo de monektone[24] / qui habuit manum secundum omnes deperditum / & recuperavit
23. Item alius de porloyiston[25] / cum pollice //
24. Item alius de stapulgrene[26] cum tibia lesa
25. Item alius de kyng bryt[27] / cum apostemate dure melancolice in fauce / quod disperavit de vita & ego similiter
26. Item egritudinem per lumbricos vidi / quam plures liberatos per pulverem nostrum
27. Item mulier quedam de crisu menstruorum in villa de kyngestone alicuius parochia <*last three words uncertain*>[28]

28. Item gelamtonem iuxta cowmyche[29] / qui fuit constipatus & in stomacho aggravatus & appetitum deperdit desperaverunt omnes de vita sua
29. Item homo ad mortem de stokinsy[30] //
30. Item sacerdos de bruggewater[31] cum ictericia & c //
31. Item uxor garstunis ibidem
32. Item Thomas digon de scalpatione & pruritu //
33. Item celerarius de bruggewater[32] //
34. Item filius gelantone in febre
35. Item uxor gardyner de cowmyche[33] //
36. Item duo filii eiusdem unus de ptisi alter de febre //
37. Item carnifex[34] ibidem in febre//
38. Item knyt de yldebare[35] //
39. Item uxor Iohannes cade //
40. Item frater Iohannes <*superscript:* bis> de boklond[36] ad mortem //
41. Item frater Iohannes moles ibidem ad mortis portam //
42. Item puer cum <*dirup?*> cifac[37] //
43. Item homo de noaton[38] cum pede piccridis

(f. 9v)

<an interpolated note on where to find a medicinal simple> Gracia dei . ut dicitur est ut lilium sed eius flos est inter album & rubium & folia duriora ut gladius & valde virida & habet una stipes ubi unicum florem erectum & concavum ut campana & habetur iuxta holdych[39] & Robertus taylor de holdysch scit ubi

44. Item uxor roberti yerd in dolore capitis ad alienationem mentis
45. Item uxor Jo Walals de adustione ignis ad disperationem
46. Item puer goode de combustione ignis
47. Item puer ad pewenam[40] de combustione ignis
48. Item puer knygt de tussi vehementi
49. Item Johannes Fowl de pede lesa & dispareta
50. Item uxor .t. delme de apostemate super epar
51. Femines plures curavi in domo parsone
52. Item puer de stapulgrene[41] cum tibia astremata
53. Item iuvenis super contak <?> de dolore currenti de loco ad locum
54. mulier de brenfeld cum emigranea
55. Item gale de petertonne[42] in colica magna
56. Item rector de spaxton[43] de indignitate stomachi & goute[44]
57. Item dominus ponynges de goute & dolore renum
58. Item mulier in london de suffocacione matricis
59. Item mulier de borialibus de dolore circa iunccuras

60. Item uxor de percumbia[45] de spina in pede
61. Item. tom. mot de fayreford[46] de spina in manu
62. Item Iohannes smyth de morsu cati
63. Item uxor gerneys de morsu canis
64. Item Ricardus smyth de heele[47] de tumescente ventris
65. Item due mulieres de continua motu cordis ibidem
66. Item Iohannes Inyl <?> de consolidatione nervorum & spina & fluxu
67. Item mulier de northcory[48] de ydropici //
68. Item iii mulieres de inflacione mamillarum
69. Item mulier de havyngdone de inflacione tibie mirabile
70. Item unus ad eton stunlantus[49] cum daggare punctu
71. Item uxor Roger mors de cowmysche[50] de suffocacione matricis
72. Item filia bone <?> de febre & lesione manus
73. Item mas <?> de lye[51] de stomacho infrigidato & c.
74. Item uxor danser de bruggwater[52]
75. Item Robertus lucas mylle <?> de conquassacione per causam <*two indistinct words*: pepla instro?>
76. Item Iohanes Ick de tiverton[53] de iecur <?>
77. Item uxor .Io. baal de percombe[54] de suffocacione matricis
78. Item mulier de kyntisbury[55] de suffocacione matricis
79. Item uxor pym de merrywede[56] stomacho infrigidato
80. Item molendinarius de tivertone[57] de colice ad mortem
81. Item tyfane de conquassione corporis & disperans
82. Item puer in ydropico in domo freind //
83. Item filia tyfane
84. Item Iohannes foyes in pestilencie //
85. Item mulier de likiard[58] in epilentica
86. Item puer tyverton[59] in pestilencie //
87. Item mulier ibidem in dolore brachii
88. Item mulier de brancome[60] de albaras <?>
89. Item quidam homo de barstaple[61] de cardiaca & sincopacione
90. Item filius cuiusdam de cowmartin[62] cum tibia lesa in mari
91. Item uxor ambrosye de matynho[63] cum suffocacione matricis
92. Item puer transfixus in medio manus in axiam <?>
93. Item quidem frythhay de ptisi ad portam mortis
94. Item uxor Willelmi pethulle de rampcom[64] de suffocacione matricis
95. Item filia cok geffrey de yliaca gravi & colice
96. Item uxor cowmysch <?>[65] de suffocacione matricis
97. Item Thomas dene cum felone in pollice gravi
98. Item Willelmus squier de nopton[66] de siti & calore <*illegible word*> & calcium
99. De dolore dentium quamplures liberavi

100. de emorowdes similiter diversis per operam dedi & curavi
101. Item mulier de taunton in poulstret de suffocacione
102. Robertus benet de northunton[67] de apostemate
103. Item Iohannes peterton

Fayreford's patients

The list of cures shows that Fayreford treated men, women, and children – 63 definitely male, and 42 female, and amongst them 17 children. The men are commonly named, although some appear as, for instance, 'quidam homo de monektone', perhaps because Fayreford simply could not recall the name. The women appear simply as 'mulier', or 'uxor' or 'filia' in relation to named men; none of them are named personally, not even Fayreford's most important patient, Lady Ponynges (we cannot be sure whether he means the first or second wife of Robert de Poynings, 4th Baron Poynings – the first Eleanor died by 1434, the second Margaret died in 1448).[68] The children appears as 'puer', 'iuvenis', or 'filia', and are similarly only identified by association with adult males. This practice in recording names is what we might expect if we look at the identification of individuals in other comparable records, for instance those of miracles at the tombs of particular saints. A number of entries on the list identify individuals only as a man or a woman from a certain named place, as with the case of the man from Monkton. In the last resort even this rudimentary identification might fail, as in one entry simply referring to 'iii mulieres de inflacione mamillarum'.

The list is rather tantalizing on the subject of the patients' class and social occupation. At the top end we have Lord and Lady Ponynges, both treated by Fayreford, for gout and suffocation of the womb respectively. We can suspect from the amount of space devoted to the symptoms of Lady Ponynges in particular that Fayreford devoted more time to their cases than to others of lower rank. They had estates in Somerset which must have brought them at times within the geographical range of Fayreford's practice, though they were likely to have spent much more of their lives on other properties, outside that range. There are at least three ecclesiastics on the list. One of them was the rector of Spaxton in Somerset, another a priest (sacerdos) from Bridgwater. A brother John Moles of Buckland in Devon appears twice on the list. Clergy are always well represented amongst patients of physicians named in contemporary records, and in case histories like those of John of Arderne – as we might expect from the social standing of the higher clergy, and their willingness and ability to travel to seek medical treatment. Together with the Ponynges family their appearance as patients suggests that Fayreford knew how to behave at the tables of gentlemen – as John of Arderne suggested was essential for the good surgeon. Otherwise Fayreford tells us only about a miller from Tiverton in Devon, a cellarer from Bridgwater, and one 'cook Geffrey', whose daughter he treated. There is certainly not enough here to generalize about the social makeup of Fayreford's patients as a group. Presumably like Arderne he charged a sliding scale of fees, adjusted not only to the patient's prognosis and the cost of medicaments, but also to the ability of the patient to pay. There is no information in the list about his fees.

Places of residence of the patients

What can we learn about Thomas Fayreford's practice from the places that the patients come from? The list is headed 'cures made by Thomas Fayreford in different places', which suggests that he travelled about to see his patients rather than that they came to him.[69] In fact as many as 61 of 103 entries on the list indicate place names, many of which can be identified with reasonable confidence. When no place name is mentioned, the use of a personal name may well signify that Fayreford was actually resident in the same place as the patient. Case 82 refers to a boy with dropsy 'in domo frend'. This *domus* must have been known to Fayreford, though he does not say where it is. The exceptions to the general pattern – a pattern suggesting Fayreford visiting his patients or being visited locally – are two cases of women mentioned, one as being 'in London', the other as being 'from the north'. Fayreford might exceptionally have treated the first woman in London, though the other obviously came to him.

As for the rest of the places named, they enable us to divide up Fayreford's practice into different sectors, corresponding presumably to different places in which he was based at different times. Two of the cases would seem to have been treated in Gloucestershire – case 61 is that of Tom Mot of Fayrford, cured of a thorn in the hand. This Fayrford or Fairford is surely Thomas's birthplace, about 25 miles to the west of Oxford. Another case was treated in Siddington, just south of Cirencester, and a further 7 or 8 miles west of Fairford. There cannot be much doubt that these were cases treated by Fayreford while he was resident in his home town, perhaps early in his career.

But these cases are a long way from the others mentioned in the list, which are all in Devon and Somerset. Bridgwater in Somerset seems to have been the epicentre for a cluster of cases, which all belong to the Somerset levels. Presumably Fayreford lived there, or in the vicinity, for a period – unfortunately since he does not give dates we cannot have an idea how long this period was. Case 101 refers to a woman living in 'poulstret' in Taunton, so it must have been a town which Fayreford knew well. Secondly, as many as six cases are reported for the town of Tiverton in Devon, which certainly lies outside a day's travel from Bridgwater. We can pencil it in as a second base – or rather third, counting Fairford – from which Fayreford conducted his practice.

Three more cases lie in south Devon, and it is difficult to see how Fayreford could have travelled easily to these from either Tiverton or Bridgwater. It is unlikely that he would have travelled so far specially to treat these patients, who are not mentioned as of high social status; perhaps he made visits to the area on an occasional basis, rather like the steward of far-flung estates (Crophill had to do this, but over a smaller area) or a travelling senior ecclesiastic. Or perhaps these patients travelled some distance before coming to see Fayreford in his base in Tiverton. The final large group of cases lies to the far north of Devon, well to the west of Bridgwater, along the north Devon coast from Porlock in the east to Barnstaple in the west. It is not so clear here where Fayreford's base would have been – perhaps Ilfracombe or Combe Martin. But again we are talking of a group of places which could be visited within a day's ride, and which imply residence by Fayreford in this area over a period of time.

The picture which we can piece together from all these suggests that Fayreford was not one of those practitioners who stayed in a particular town throughout his career, and expected to make his living by seeing patients there. Instead he must have had at least three bases in Somerset and Devon, together with one in Gloucestershire, and travelled out from them. He may even have made longer journeys not so much to visit particular patients as to drum up business for himself in new areas where itinerant doctors were infrequent visitors. Even when resident in a particular town for a longer period Fayreford must have expected to have to visit patients up to a day's ride away, presumably on summons from the patient, or his or her relatives or friends. Presumably the fees charged would also have reflected the expense and time he incurred on these visits, as well as the cost of medicaments and the notional value of his opinion on the case.[70] Except in the case of Lady Ponynges, who took three weeks to cure, Fayreford does not mention the length of time his cures took, but we can suppose that her case was indeed exceptional because of her status, and the complications of the symptoms presented. Many of Fayreford's poorer patients would have had to come to him, rather than summon his assistance and pay his travelling costs. Nor could they have afforded medicines over a long period of time.

What can be said about the diseases from which the patients on Fayreford's list suffered? Can this evidence be used to give us information on the kind of practice Fayreford was engaged in, and some sort of mapping of the world of illness as actually encountered by one practitioner? Here the problems involved in expanding Fayreford's abbreviations, and the distinctly gnomic character of most of the entries, pose considerable difficulties of interpretation. On the other hand we can for the first time bring in evidence from outside the list itself, namely the other writings in the same manuscript by Fayreford – what he terms his *Practica*, his surgery, and a herbal called, deceptively 'Circa instans' (it is *not* the well-known herbal of that name but something put together by Fayreford himself). It will prove easier to interpret Fayreford's recording of diseases in the list of cures once we understand better its relation to the rest of the material he compiled.

Description of the manuscript

There are three items before the list of cures in the Fayreford manuscript written by earlier scribes, and these can be left out of consideration. The part of the manuscript written by Fayreford himself contains the following:[71]

4. ff.9r–v	*De curis factis per T. Ffayreford in diversis locis*
5. ff.10r–11v	A list of ailments with the name of the relevant remedial herb, beginning *Pro dolore capitis capitulo absinthium*, forming an index to the 'chapters' of item 9
6. f.12r	*Tabula super practicam scriptam post 'Circa instans' in hoc volumine per Thomam Ffayreford collectam et plurimum expertam etiam experiendam Deo concedente.* This table is a guide (with medieval folio references) to item 11
7. f.12v	*De cirurgia collecta secundum Ffayrford.* Gives medieval folio references to cures contained in item 12
8. f.12v	A short text *De saporibus et gradibus*, beginning *Novem sunt species saporum* ... (ThK 955)
9. ff.13r–64v	An alphabetical herbal, beginning *Absinthium est calidum et siccum in tertio gradu* ... (ThK 11). This is *not* the *Circa instans* herbal, despite the title given to it in item 6.
10. ff.65r–72r	The *Modus medendi* of Pontius de Sancto Egidio (s.xiii) (ThK 37; this MS only)
11.ff.72v–124v	*Ffayreford* (written in gold). A medical commonplace book in Latin, with passages of Middle English, which

begins deceptively with the opening lines of Roger Baron's *Practica*, beginning *Sicut ab antiquis habemus auctoribus* ... (ThK 1479). See item 6.

12.ff.125r–151r A surgical commonplace book with the rubric *Incipit Cirurgia secundum Ffayreforde*. See item 7.

The remaining items in the manuscript are earlier in date, and can be ignored here in relation to the list of cures.

Both items 11 and 12 are compiled on what I have called the commonplace book principle – that is to say that Fayreford has allotted each heading its own share of blank paper or parchment, and then added to each section beneath its own heading at different times, as can be seen from changes in the colour of the ink, and from the occasional spaces left unfilled in the text at the end of each section. It may be that a good number of medical texts were compiled originally in this way, particularly recipe books where recipes are grouped under disease headings – but of course except in the case of the autograph manuscript itself – the Fayreford part of Harley MS 2558 – the signs of this method of compilation disappear once the exemplar has been copied. As a result very few medical manuscripts with texts compiled on this principle are known to us. But we can be sure that texts 11 and 12 in our manuscript were not copied by a scribe from an exemplar but written by the author. The tables of contents to items 11 and 12 are found as items 6 and 7. Tables 6 and 7 both state that the texts were 'collected' by Thomas Fayreford, who is therefore both author and scribe. No copies of these texts in any other manuscript have as yet been identified.

It is clear nevertheless that Fayreford's manuscript as a whole was compiled with an audience in mind, and not just for his own use. This can be seen from the decoration of the manuscript. The *Practica* is headed at the top of the first folio by the word 'Ffayreford', written in large textura hand in gold within a cartouche. The beginning of the herbal (item 9) is given an elaborate illuminated bar border on the top and gutter edges of the written space, and a decorated three line initial. In all three of the main texts compiled by Fayreford himself we find rubricated initials for major sections, painted in red and blue. Fayreford himself has supplied the tiny guide letters for the rubricator to follow. Professional illuminators and rubricators must have been employed at Fayreford's expense to provide this decoration.

Fayreford has also supplied his own foliation so that users of the manuscript can consult the tables and find the information they want in the texts he compiled. He also makes use of handy cross-references from one section in the text to another – to relate for instance the occurrence of syncope to suffocation of the womb, as in the case of

Lady Ponynges, or sometimes to save repeating recipes. At several points in his texts Fayreford has supplied pen drawings in his own hand. Though these are informal and usually have been added outside the text block, they serve to illustrate the shape of a plaster, the appearance of an ailment or the description of a plant. His models may well have been other contemporary English medical and surgical manuscripts, particularly those written in the vernacular, which employed decoration and marginal illustrations to enhance the texts of well-known authors like Guy de Chauliac and John of Arderne (Fayreford's drawing of a patient in spasm is clearly copied from an Arderne manuscript[72]). But the decorated title to Fayreford's *Practica* (item 11) proclaims clearly that Fayreford intended his book to redound to his own fame.

Diagnosis and prognosis: the case histories

In items 11 and 12, the *Practica* and surgery, we find not only headings which correspond to diseases mentioned in the list of cures, but also case histories, some of which are based on Fayreford's own practice, and indeed can be identified in four instances with individuals entered in the list of cures. With the help of these other pieces of evidence we can arrive at a better understanding of some entries on the list of cures, and even speculate further about the nature of courses of treatment when these are not specified in the list.

One of the cases mentioned in the list of cures, and described in more detail in the *Practica*, is that of John Cloode, who suffered from ethica fever, delirium (*alienacio mentis*), and 'boiling up' (*ebullicio*) of the liver (case 3). We learn from the case history on f. 75 that:

> one (identified as 'Cloode' by Fayreford's hand in the margin) often had headache to the point of delirium. I had his head shaved and with plantain juice, mixed with houseleek and verbena, I washed his head using sharp wine. Then I anointed him with an ointment made of poplar buds, rose and camomile oil mixed up together. Immediately he said that his head was healed, although for a long time he had suffered from hectic fever.[73]

It seems that Fayreford's remedy was to soothe the patient with herbal remedies applied externally to a shaven head. It is worth noting that the patient declares himself cured in the head, rather than freed from the hectic fever. The case history occurs under the heading '*dolor capitis*' rather than that of '*De febribus*' (f. 124v). Fayreford's treatment is much more down to earth than the rather high-flown passages on hectic fever he copied into his book would suggest. Nor does Fayreford tell us whether the liver complaint was treated separately, or regarded as associated with the fever. There is a heading 'De epate' in the commonplace book, where diagnosis of heating of the liver is discussed, and most of the material copied is quoted from Avicenna or other authorities. There is no discussion of *ebullicio*, though at the end comes a recipe for an electuary 'For the fever and het of the lyver and the jandys'.

These commonplace book entries bear out the diagnostic features of the list of cures. While Fayreford obviously read and copied into his book procedures for arriving at a differential diagnosis of, for instance, fevers or liver complaints, neither his case histories nor his list of cures indicate how he arrived at a diagnosis in specific cases. As in the case of John Cloode the diagnosis is stated as if established for certain, and consists of a statement of several conditions from which the patient is suffering. Sometimes these conditions can be related to each other in terms of Galenic humoral medicine, as signs and causes, but at other times it seems that in Galenic terms the conditions are unrelated – as with the *frenesis* and *squinancia* of Lady Ponynges (case 1).

When Fayreford wanted to do more than indicate the conditions afflicting his patients, he sometimes characterized them as putting the patient in danger of death. So Thomas Parmynter of Kingston was troubled by colic, on three occasions to the point of death, yet was cured by Fayreford with the use of pills in solution, while Richard Webber, who was similarly twice endangered by constipation, was cured by pills and clysters (cases 7 and 8). We might not immediately think of colic or constipation as life-threatening ailments, but of course we are not dealing here with modern clinical conditions. Saying that the patient is on the point of death also serves to dramatize the success of the practitioner who effects the cure, and there may be a degree of exaggeration here for rhetorical effect. The most elaborately described such case is that of John Wyse, who suffered from manifest jaundice (*ictericia manifesta*), and a deep ulcer (*fagina*) over the area of the liver, which threatened his life. Fayreford adds that he was constipated for six days and additionally suffered from corruption of his appetite and a vehement thirst (case 2). The *fagina* or ulcer over the liver is an intriguing diagnostic detail, not so far as I know brought out in connection with jaundice in any of the academic treatises. But the subtleties of diagnosis should not blind us to the fact that one of the principal aims may have been to establish a prognosis, determining simply whether a patient was likely to die if left untreated. Case 25 describes a patient whose life was despaired of by the patient, but also by Fayreford himself (*quod disperavit de vita et ego similiter*). On the basis of a prognosis of life or death a medical practitioner might negotiate with the patient, or his family and friends, a contract stipulating that the practitioner was not liable for the death of his patient as a result of his treatment.

Suffocation of the womb

The case of Lady Ponynges, the first on the list, is the most detailed in terms of the listing of ailments – probably as much because of the importance of the patient, and the amount of time and effort devoted by Fayreford to the case, as because of its intrinsic complexity. She is described as suffering from frenzy (*frenesis*), and sincope (*sincopacio*), and suffocation of the womb (*suffocacio matricis*), and quinsy (*squinancia*), all at the same time – yet she is described as having been cured within three weeks, as if the ailments were closely related and met with one course of treatment. Sincope is often represented as a sign of suffocation of the womb, and indeed is specifically mentioned as such within Fayreford's *Practica* under the heading of suffocation of the womb.[74] Frenzy is not mentioned in this way within the text on *suffocacio matris*, though is it given a separate heading in the commonplace book, and in the frenzy section suffocation of the womb receives no mention. Frenzy would normally have a chapter devoted to it within the standard *practica* text of the period. Bartholomaeus Anglicus describes frenzy as arising in two manners – the first from overheated choler, the second from fumes arising to the brain. In this second way, Fayreford is likely to have associated frenzy with the symptoms of the underlying complaint in Lady Ponynges's case, suffocation of the womb. Gilbertus Anglicus, and following him the so-called Trotula texts in Middle English translation, describe how corrupt fumes ascend from the womb to the brain in cases of suffocation of the womb.[75] It is probable then that Fayreford saw frenzy as being closely related to suffocation of the womb. With quinsy on the other hand there is no obvious connection with suffocation of the womb, and quinsy is allocated a heading of its own in Fayreford's *Practica*. So we have at least two distinct ailments which Fayreford thought he was treating in the case of Lady Ponynges, although he may have identified suffocation of the womb as the most important underlying malady that had to be tackled.

My reason for attaching such significance to suffocation of the womb relative to other ailments in this case is that this ailment is not only the commonest listed for Fayreford's female patients, but the commonest ailment mentioned in the entire list. For the other female patients Fayreford does not go into the same amount of detail about related ailments as in the case of Lady Ponynges. Amongst the 103 entries on the list are ten cases of suffocation of the womb successfully treated by Fayreford. It is well known that this ailment is one of the most problematic and intriguing of all the categories of ailment described in medical literature, one whose diagnosis and nosological identity have been much debated, and not only for the Middle Ages. It is of exceptional interest that this ailment should have assumed such a prominent part in Fayreford's list of cures, and the strongest possible evidence that gynaecological problems were not regarded as the province of women healers alone. Fayreford seems to have prided himself on his ability to deal with suffocation of the womb, and to have related it to a variety of conditions he found amongst his patients (male and female, for he finds that remedies for suffocation of the womb are also useful for those suffering from *tussis*, cough).[76]

Lady Ponynges's case of suffocation of the womb may also be referred to by Fayreford in one of the case histories in the *Practica*. Under *Suffocacio matricis* he describes the conventional approach in treating suffocation of the womb, by subfumigating with sweet-smelling substances heated over coals and applied to the woman's vagina, while foul-smelling substances are applied to the nostrils (thus driving the womb, which is attracted to sweet smells and repelled by foul, back towards its rightful place). It is necessary to bind the limbs of the woman, and rub her extremities with oil of camomile. If necessary the womb must be pressed down by hand or by a cord tied to her left side

> since by this treatment I kept a woman from sincope for three days nearly, until she began to mend, and I kept her awake since I observed that her pulse rate determined when she would be likely to pass out. In this way she was relieved of her illness and cured, and when her fainting fits were over I then permitted her to sleep sweetly for a time.[77]

The coincidence of suffocation of the womb and sincope, and the title of lady granted to the patient, suggest that this case may be that of Lady Ponynges. Whereas the list of cures says that it took three weeks for Lady Ponynges to recover, this case history speaks of only three days. It is possible of course that Lady Ponynges's other ailments took longer to cure, or that the three *days* are a slip for three *weeks*. But, whether the case is that of Lady Ponynges or not, for our purposes the entries in the *Practica* for suffocation of the womb with sincope are a good basis for assessing the way in which Fayreford cured his most prestigious patient.

In treating suffocation of the womb Fayreford would have been able to take guidance from Gilbertus, Roger or the so-called Trotula texts. In fact his entries in the *Practica* suggest that he did not draw on them to any great extent. Gilbertus and the others follow the standard course of fumigating and odorous treatments, and indeed Gilbertus mentions the use of binding the legs at the onset of suffocation, though he goes on to recommend scarification of the skin of the feet. But the detail of the remedies prescribed by Fayreford does not tally with that of the Gilbertus-derived texts, except for one recipe using lovage, hyssop, wormwood and fern-leaves boiled together for a plaster to be applied to the woman's lower belly.[78] Fayreford does cite two other sources for recipes, Johannes de Sancto Paulo and Gualterus Agilon, but it is clear that he also relied on his own trial of remedies. He talks of a powder given in drink which is of wonderful efficacy (*mirabile efficacie*), 'as I have often proved in various sicknesses'. For another remedy against suffocation of the womb, he recommends the plant called *palma christi*, with leaves similar to that of southernwood, over each of which the practitioner should say five pater nosters and five ave marias, etc. Fayreford's own plant lore thus finds its place amongst his *experimenta*,[79] as does his monitoring of the patient's pulse when she is in danger of sincope.

There were other female ailments treated by Fayreford. The list of cures includes a crisis of menstrual blood (*crisus menstruorum*), and swelling of the breasts – mentioned once each. There are sections on provoking and restraining menstrual fluxes in the *Practica*, and another on disorders of womens' breasts. The *Practica* also has extensive sections on a variety of complaints associated with the womb, under the standard headings for gynaecological texts of *pro matrice, pro precipitacione matricis, pro mola matricis*, and *de compressione specialium*. There is also a section on the delivery of women in labour, although Fayreford never mentions any cases to do with childbirth in his list of cures. But the evidence of the list makes it quite clear that we are not dealing here with a purely academic or theoretical acquaintance with gynaecological disorders on Fayreford's part. We must conclude that treating women for specifically gynaecological conditions was an integral, indeed one of the most important parts of Fayreford's practice – there was no sense in which women's complaints were off limits to Fayreford's as a male medical practitioner.[80] On the contrary, Fayreford's successes in this area are the most prominent amongst his cures.

Other kinds of ailment

Interestingly Fayreford's list deals both with categories of ailment which we may think of as peculiar to the academic physician, since their nature as disease gives rise to intellectual debate, and with those others that tend to get left out of the textbooks, even the surgeries, because of their straightforward character (like thorns in the hand, burns or simple fractures). Thus on the one hand, under the academic rubric, a number of fevers are differentiated, most frequently hectic and acute. *Alienacio mentis* is mentioned, as well as frenzy, amongst disorders which are the subject of careful distinctions by the medical authorities. As in all the *practica* literature, headaches of various kinds are prominent amongst disease categories. Simple *dolor capitis* is distinguished from *cephalargica* and *emigranea*. Case 4 is that of a woman from Northover, Somerset, suffering from *cephalargica* and a tremor in the stomach. Her treatment is described under *dolor capitis* in the *Practica*, but what Fayreford treats sounds almost like the results of a stroke. The old woman had her mouth twisted upwards, and her tongue was extruded so that she could hardly swallow or speak. She was in great pain, and her stomach was also trembling or vibrating with a continuous action. One of the two causes of *cephalargica*, according to Bartholomaeus Anglicus following Constantine, is sharp humours in the stomach, so it is likely that Fayreford would have linked his diagnosis of *cephalargica* to the stomach problems of the woman from Northover. Fayreford's treatment, which was spread over three weeks, involved gargling, injection through the nostrils, anointing the head, bloodletting beneath the tongue, Jerusalem pills, purging and a theriac – an impressive demonstration of the range of therapeutic agents at his disposal, and their deployment to meet the requirements of a very precise diagnosis.[81]

Eye ailments are similarly carefully differentiated, and here there is another case (case 9) where the list and a case history in the *Practica* evidently correspond. Fayreford refers in the list of cures to a youth of Tiverton who lost the sight of his eye and recovered it with swallow's blood and betony. In the section headed *de oculis* in the *Practica* we find the following:

> there was a boy from Tiverton in Devon about twelve years of age who lost the sight of one eye after a blow to it, so that he could not see at all with the other eye closed. Twice daily I put in the affected eye swallow's blood and daily he drank betony mashed up with ale, and within fifteen days he recovered his sight by the grace of God. And certainly in many cases I have discovered betony to be effective in getting rid of all fleshy growths in eyes when drunk in this fashion, and after bathing with rosewater as mentioned elsewhere.[82]

The use of swallow's blood for eye problems is mentioned in a number of academic authorities, and probably achieved widest currency through the chapter on the swallow in the well-known encyclopedia of Bartholomaeus Anglicus, *De proprietatibus rerum* (which itself follows Constantinus Africanus), where blood from the right wing of the swallow is said to have the power of healing eyes.[83] Fayreford's remedies for the Tiverton boy, despite the exotic impression they make at first sight, are not his own invention but derive from standard academic sources (most obviously Macer's herbal for the use of betony, which is copied in an earlier hand in Harley MS 2558, ff. 197r–233v)). Another case, that of a woman of Barnstaple with eyes troubled by rheum, is cured within three nights with another medicine compounded by Fayreford.[84]

At the other end of the scale to such relatively sophisticated diagnostic judgements as those in the case of Lady Ponynges or the old woman from Northover, are the simple surgical categories of ailment – broken bones, bites of animals, burns by fire or water, thorns or injuries from sharp implements. These obviously fall within the surgical rather than medical areas of Fayreford's practice, though he thinks them just as worthy of record as the more complex internal ailments. John Smith bitten by a dog is not overlooked, though we learn little about the treatment of such cases. There are sections on thorns, on dog-bites, and on wounds in the head of Fayreford's surgery, though there are no suggestions for operative techniques in these sections, just medicines. The most important sources for these recipes were Gilbertus Anglicus and the writings of the English fourteenth-century surgeon, John of Arderne. But it is clear that Fayreford would set a broken bone or extract a thorn, as well as prescribe remedies. However, the strictly manual side of his practice probably did not need *aides-mémoire* or written recommendations – the techniques used must have been learnt from copying the example of others, not from books.

Looking at the list of cures in the light of the headings which occur in the *Practica* and surgery in Fayreford's manuscript, it becomes apparent that the list of cures does not include diseases associated with the kidney and bladder, and such typical textbook ailments as paralysis or spasm, and pneumonia. While he thought it worth while to record remedies separately under such common headings in the *Practica* and surgery, none of the patients on his list was treated for these diseases. Of course it would be too simplistic to suppose that just because Fayreford's list of cures does not include them, that he did not treat such ailments – indeed his gathering remedies for them under the appropriate headings in the *Practica* or surgery rather suggests the opposite. Since these ailments are neither more nor less difficult to cure than many which do appear on the list, perhaps we can assume that he did not come across many cases. But these gaps in the picture of disease incidence provided by the list are no reason for supposing Fayreford was a specialist medical practitioner. It looks as if he would attempt to treat any medical or surgical condition that he came across in the course of his practice.

Two cases are mentioned in the list of patients with *pestilentia* – which of course may or may not be a visitation of the plague. We are probably safe in assuming that *pestilentia* does signify an epidemic disease, and these two cases are the only such in the list. There are no remedies for plague or other epidemic disease to be found in Fayreford's *Practica*, and no indication in the list itself of the methods by which he decided to treat *pestilentia*. If indeed the cases of John Foyes and the boy in Tiverton (cases 84 and 86) were those of plague, in one of its periodic visitations on Devon, then it would have been fascinating to have known Fayreford's successful method of cure.

Charms and remedies

One dimension of Fayreford's practice is not brought out by the list of cures, and only becomes apparent in looking at the commonplace book. Many of the remedies described in the commonplace book are attributed to information and experience gathered from other practitioners, are validated by 'probatum est', or based on Fayreford's own experience ('*probavi in puero epilentico cui dedi* ... '). Whereas the list of cures may give the impression that Fayreford's diagnostic techniques and the rationale of treatment were founded on his understanding of causes and signs, and of the theory of treatment by opposites – both based in scholastic medical knowledge – study of his commonplace book shows that many of the remedies he collected were grounded only in the outcome of experience. This does not mean that Fayreford was unusually credulous or empirical in his therapeutics. Distinguished academics like John Argentine allowed considerable space to empirical therapeutics in his commonplace book too. It is of the nature of such collections of remedies that many or most of them should come with no scholastic apparatus, and scholastic medical authorities included many such *experimenta* in their *practica* or surgery. The Fayreford commonplace book takes an inclusive and pragmatic view of the value of recipes handed on by word of mouth or by personal observation. Thus Fayreford is able to say: 'again I heard of a wonderful *experimentum*, but one that lacks any rational explanation. The patient urinates over the greater seed-bearing nettle whenever he needs to in the course of three days. When the nettle dries then the patient will be cured ...'.[85]

The extent to which Fayreford himself relied on local knowledge of the whereabouts of particular samples of medicinal value is shown by the appearance of the note on where to find *gracia dei* in the midst of the list of cures (see p. 161 above). He describes it as being like the lily, except that the colour of its flower is between white and red, it has harder sword-shaped green leaves, and each stem holds a single erect bell-shaped flower. This plant is found near Holditch, Devon, and a man named Robert Taylor there knows how to find it. This is just the sort of information that we do not find in academic medical sources or even recipe-books, although common sense tells us that medical practitioners using simples must either know themselves where to find them growing wild, or who to ask. As well as Robert Taylor he had no doubt others whom he could ask about plants, or from whom he could obtain recipes, like Lady Ponynges and the friar John of London, who both gave him recipes for *demigreyne*.[86]

One particular kind of empirical remedy, which plays a large part in the commonplace book of Thomas Fayreford, is the charm. There are at least twenty of these scattered through the text, but not randomly. Some ailments more than others seem to invite treatment by the use of charms. One concentration occurs in the section on tooth problems, where St Appollonia and St Nichasius are much invoked, and there are instructions for writing characters on the patient's cheek. Another concentration relates to childbirth, where charms are invoked in difficult labours. A third concentration occurs in the section on epilepsy, where charms are deployed to forestall fits or recover patients from them. One remedy to prevent epileptic seizures requires writing a word of power, *ananizapta*, on to a parchment. This, together with a bit of mistletoe taken from an oak, is for the patient to wear around the neck. The patient must say three masses of the Trinity and eat root of peony daily. A second charm to revive someone fallen in a seizure requires, besides smoke made from burning a goat's hoof, and sharp wine in the nose, that *ananizapta* be said three times in the ears of the patient. A third remedy 'Contra epilenticam passionem' contains the directions for ritually assembling herbs, psalms and gospels at the most propitious times to make an amulet to be used with daily pater nosters and ave marias. Every seventh day *ananizapta* must be ingested – 'eat this name written *ananizapta* three times' (et omni ebdomada commede hoc nomen scriptum ananizapta ter).[87]

The amulets to ward off epileptic seizures and the directions for speaking and ingesting the word *ananizapta* are typical of the medical functions of such cryptic words and signs as we find on medieval rings, brooches and pendants. Fayreford's fondness for suspensions and ligatures of all kinds, from coral round the neck, to silken threads tied round the arm, do not mark him out as an eccentric, or unusually credulous. Moreover, the uses of *ananizapta* suggested by Fayreford – in ingested prophylactic treatments, spoken charms and amulets – are consistent with the similar uses of the divine name *tetragramaton* and other words of power in medical charms found elsewhere. There is nothing extraordinary in Fayreford's use of charms for these three kinds of ailment; together with the flow of blood or other bodily fluids, they are traditionally the areas of therapeutics where charms are most frequently deployed. Nor are such charms only to be found in verbal 'folk' traditions – standard academic texts like the *Lilium medicine* of Bernard Gordon support the use of similar charms against epilepsy.[88]

What the prevalence of charms in Fayreford's commonplace book should do is remind us that the practice of medicine in the fifteenth century, even in the hands of learned academic physicians, did not spurn empirical remedies or charms. In certain kinds of ailment charms played a crucial role The daughter of W. Poulet, whom Fayreford treated successfully after she had three epileptic fits in one night (case 6), was very probably cured by the use of one or more charms.

Conclusion

Thomas Fayreford blurs some of the boundaries historians have found convenient to set up in describing fifteenth-century medicine. He attended the University of Oxford, and probably picked up a great deal of knowledge of medical texts there, as well as observing Nicholas Colnet and others in their medical practice. But he never seems to have matriculated or taken a medical degree at Oxford or elsewhere. His own medical practice was concentrated in areas of the West Country with no major towns or cities, whereas most learned university doctors gravitated to London, or to courts and universities. He does not seem to have been retained by any particular noble or clerical household over long periods of time, thus was not able to draw a regular income from fees and annuities. There is no indication in his manuscript that he made his bread from clerical or administrative duties, to which medicine was a sideline, as in the case of John Crophill, bailiff of Wix. We do not know his scale of charges, nor how many patients he treated in a given period. Fayreford does not seem to have a single geographical base – instead he may have moved several times within the West Country at different stages of his life.

Fayreford's patients, to judge from his list of cures, were not predominantly from any one social class or grouping. There were noble patients (Lord and Lady Ponynges), millers and cooks. He probably travelled to attend some patients, no doubt residing in the household of Lady Ponynges. Others came to him, like the old lady of Northover, who asked him for permission to return to her home once treatment was completed. His patients were men, women and children, with no obvious bias in gender or age. The ailments from which they suffered ranged from those which could only be identified by a sophisticated academic diagnosis, to cases of thorns in the hand or burns. Fayreford's practice was both medical and surgical, whether judged by the standards of the fifteenth century or our own. Many of the cures of which he was so proud were of patients whose life was despaired of by themselves, or by others.

There is only one striking feature of Fayreford's practice, as witnessed by his list of cures. Cases of suffocation of the womb make up about 10 per cent of the cures he mentions. This is extraordinary not because Fayreford was a male practitioner treating female patients for a gynaecological complaint, but because there are no other sources indicating such a high profile for this ailment. Fayreford seems to have regarded this ailment as a common and fundamental condition amongst women, linked causally to other ailments like frenzy and sincope. It is probable that he saw suffocation of the womb almost in terms of defining the nature of gynaecological disease.

Fayreford's methods of treatment, on the other hand, were by no means exceptional. Whether he relied on the treatments suggested by the standard academic texts of practical medicine, or on secrets he obtained from barbers or his patients, the sorts of remedies collected in his commonplace book would have been recognizable to another commonplace-book maker from a very different milieu, John Argentine, the royal doctor. A great many of these remedies were warranted only by the proof of experience, Fayreford's own or others, and not accounted for by rational medicine. Fayreford placed significant reliance on charms, inscribed on suspensions worn by the patient, or said ritually by the patient. Certain kinds of illness, tooth problems, childbirth, epilepsy, required the use of charms more than others. It does not seem that Fayreford thought of charms as a last desperate resort, but as a legitimate part of the armamentarium of the medical practitioner.

Notes

1. See Linda Ehrsam Voigts, 'Scientific and Medical Books', in Jeremy Griffiths and Derek Pearsall (eds), *Book Production and Publishing in Britain 1375–1475* (Cambridge, Cambridge University Press, 1989), pp. 345–402, esp. pp. 380–84.
2. C. H. Talbot and E. A. Hammond, *The Medical Practitioners of Medieval England: A Biographical Register* (London, Wellcome Historical Medical Library, 1965); supplemented by Faye Getz, 'Medical Practitioners in Medieval England', *Social History of Medicine*, 3 (1990), pp. 245–83; and Stuart Jenks, 'Medizinische Fachkrafte in England zur Zeit Heinrichs VI (1428/29–1460/61)', *Sudhoffs Archiv*, 69 (1985), pp. 214–27.
3. Madeleine Pelner Cosman, 'Medieval Medicine Malpractice: The Dicta and the Dockets', *Bulletin of the New York Academy of Medicine*, 49 (1973), pp. 22–47; Michael T. Walton, 'The Advisory Jury and Malpractice in 15th Century London: The Case of William Forest', *Journal of the History of Medicine*, 40 (1985), pp. 78–82; index references to malpractice in Carole Rawcliffe, *Medicine and Society in Later Medieval England* (Stroud, Alan Sutton, 1995); on difficulties in claiming fees, see Carole Rawcliffe, 'The Profits of Practice: The Wealth and Status of Medical Men in Later Medieval England', *Social History of Medicine*, 1 (1988), pp. 61–78.

4. P. M. Jones, 'John of Arderne and the Mediterranean Tradition of Scholastic Surgery', in L. García-Ballester, R. French, J. Arrizabalaga and A. Cunningham (eds), *Practical Medicine from Salerno to the Black Death* (Cambridge, Cambridge University Press, 1994), pp. 289–321; some of the case histories may be found in D'Arcy Power, 'The Lesser Writings of John Arderne', *XVIIth International Congress of Medicine*, London, 1913, Section XXIII History of Medicine (1914), pp. 107–33.
5. For Argentine, see D. E. Rhodes, *John Argentine. Provost of King's: His Life and his Library* (Amsterdam, Hertzberger, 1967); D. R. Leader, 'John Argentine and Learning in Medieval Cambridge', *Humanistica Lovaniensia*, 33 (1984), pp. 71–85; and for his *experimenta*, P. M. Jones, 'Information and Science', in R. Horrox (ed.), *Fifteenth Century Attitudes: Perceptions of Society in Late Medieval England* (Cambridge, Cambridge University Press, 1994), pp. 107–8.
6. On Crophill, see Lois Gean Ayoub, 'John Crophill's Books: An Edition of British Library MS Harley 1735', D.Phil thesis, Centre for Medieval Studies, University of Toronto, 1994; E. W. Talbert, 'The Notebook of a Fifteenth-Century Practicing Physician', *Texas Studies in English*, 22 (1942), pp. 5–30; and J. K. Mustain, 'A Rural Medical Practitioner in Fifteenth-Century England', *Bulletin of the History of Medicine*, 46 (1972), pp. 469–76.
7. P. M. Jones, 'Harley MS 2558: A Fifteenth-Century Medical Commonplace Book', in M. M. Schleissner (ed.), *Manuscript Sources of Medieval Medicine: A Book of Essays* (New York and London, Garland, 1995), pp. 35–54. This essay deals principally with the method of compilation and information sources used by Fayreford. It contains a full description of the manuscript on pp. 37–40.
8. On Colnet, discussed on f. 122v of Harley MS 2558, see C. H. Talbot and E. A. Hammond, *The Medical Practitioners of Medieval England: A Biographical Register* (London, Wellcome Historical Medical Library, 1965), pp. 220–22. Fayreford the medical practitioner is not the same man as the Dominican who was ordained priest in 1364 (see Alfred B. Emden, *A Biographical Register of the University of Oxford to A.D. 1500*, 3 vols (Oxford, Clarendon Press, 1957–59), vol. 2, p. 664). It is implausible that the Dominican would have started medical practice in the fifteenth century, and there is no sign in Harley MS 2558 of the interests of a priest or friar.
9. Though Jones, 'Harley', cautions against reading the document as if it was a window on the practice of fifteenth-century medicine, pointing out that the manuscript was compiled with a readership in mind, employing various rhetorical devices. Nevertheless the evidence it supplies for Fayreford's practice is invaluable, if read with this caution in mind.
10. I have expanded abbreviations throughout. Editorial interpolations are included in pointed brackets. Underlinings follow those of the manuscript.
11. Northover, Somerset. This place-name, and those following, have been established with the help of J. Bartholomew, *Survey Gazetteer of the British Isles*, 8th edn (Edinburgh, John Bartholomew, 1932) and the English Place Name Society volumes.
12. Siddington, Gloucs.?
13. Many Kingstons in Somerset and Devon.

14. Tiverton, Devon.
15. Combe Royal under Churchstow, Devon?
16. Chilcombe, Devon?
17. Barnstaple, Devon.
18. Middle English Dictionary: tere(n) = tear(s).
19. Combe Martin, Devon.
20. Ilfracombe, Devon.
21. Combe Martin, Devon.
22. Martinhoe, Devon.
23. Linton, Devon.
24. Monkton, Devon.
25. Porlock, Somerset.
26. Staplegrove, Somerset.
27. Kingsbridge, Devon.
28. Possibly a Kingstone in Devon or Somerset.
29. Combwich, Somerset.
30. Stogursey, Devon.
31. Bridgwater, Somerset.
32. Bridgwater, Somerset.
33. Combwich, Somerset.
34. This reading, based on an expansion, presumably means a butcher.
35. Ide, Devon?
36. Buckland Abbey, Devon.
37. Both words referring to the complaint are uncertain.
38. North Newton, near Bridgwater, Somerset.
39. Holditch, Devon.
40. Possibly Paignton, Devon?
41. Staplegrove, Somerset.
42. North or South Petherton, Somerset.
43. Spaxton, Somerset.
44. This reading, and that in case 57, is based on Fayreford using both Latin *gutta* and Middle English *goute* on f. 143v.
45. Parracombe, Devon.
46. Fairford, Gloucs.
47. Heele, Devon.
48. North Curry, Devon
49. Stone Easton, Somerset?
50. Combwich, Somerset.
51. Lye, Devon.
52. Bridgwater, Somerset.
53. Tiverton, Devon.
54. Parracombe, Devon.
55. Kentisbury, Devon.
56. Merrivale, nr Tavistock, Devon?
57. Tiverton, Devon.
58. Lykeard St Lawrence.
59. Tiverton, Devon.
60. Branscombe, Devon.
61. Barnstaple, Devon.
62. Combe Martin, Devon.
63. Martinhoe, Devon.

64. Ranscombe in Martinhoe, Devon?
65. Combwich, Somerset?
66. Northtowne in Milton Damarel, Devon?
67. Northam, Devon?
68. G. E. C. [George Edward Cokayne], *The Complete Peerage*, (London, The St Catherine's Press, 1945), vol. 10 pp. 663–4; *Dictionary of National Biography*, s.v. Robert Poynings (1380–1446). See further Thomas Agar Holland, 'Poynings', *Sussex Archaeological Collections*, 15, pp. 1–56, and *Victoria County History*, ed. William Page, Somerset, vol. 3, pp. 97, 170. I have retained Fayreford's spelling, Ponynges, when referring to the names given in his manuscript.
69. Although case 4, an elderly woman from Northover, Somerset, is described as seeking licence after her cure to return home ('peciit licenciam redeundi ad propria sua', f. 73r) in the case history which appears under the heading 'dolor capitis' in Fayreford's *Practica*.
70. Compare the astrologer and doctor Richard Trewythian, based in London, who treated a patient W. Boterows in April 1447, charging 7 shillings for his own travel, horse feed at 2 pence per diem for four weeks, stabling at 4 pence per diem for six weeks – a total of 30 shillings and 8 pence in addition to the cost of medicines (British Library, Sloane MS 428, f. 34v).
71. Description taken from Jones, 'Harley', see above, note 7.
72. Harley MS 2558, f. 139v. For an illustration of the spasm patient in Arderne, see *Arnaldi de Villanova Opera Medica Omnia. XVI. Translatio Libri Galieni De Rigore et Tremore et Iectigatione et Spasmo*, ed. M. R. McVaugh (Barcelona, Seminarum Historiae Medicae Gianatense, 1981), p. 19, taken from British Library Add. MS 29301, f. 5.
73. Quidam habuit dolorem capitis ut ad alienacionem mentis sepe pervenit / feci capud radi & cum succo plantaginis & semperviva & vervena mixtis cum vino acro lavari et post inungi cum popilione et oleo rosato et oleo camomile simul mixtis & et statim dixit se esse sanum in capite qui diu iacuit in ethica passione (f. 75).
74. Harley MS 2558, f. 114. There is also a cross-reference from sincope to suffocation of the womb on f. 91. Whereas Roger Baron, *Practica*, cap. 63 *De suffocatione matricis*, distinguishes between *suffocatio matricis* and sincope, despite their similar symptoms. The *Practica* is printed in *Cyrurgia Guidonis de Cauliaco. et Cyrurgia Bruni. Teodorici. Rolandi. Lanfranci. Rogerii. Bertapalie* (Venice, 1519), f. 221. Fayreford's knowledge of Roger can be assumed from his use of the incipit (see description above of item 11 in Harley MS 2558).
75. *On the Properties of Things: John Trevisa's Translation of Bartholomaeus Anglicus De Proprietatibus Rerum*, vol. 1, ed. M. C. Seymour (Oxford, Clarendon Press, 1975), book 7, cap. 5 (p. 348); *Medieval Woman's Guide to Health*, ed. and trans. Beryl Rowland (London, Croom Helm, 1981), pp. 86–7. See also Roger Bacon, *Practica*, cap. 2 *De frenesi*, f. 211 verso. The relationship of Gilbertus, Roger Baron and the so-called Trotula texts is established by Monica H. Green, 'Obstetrical and Gynecological Texts in Middle English', *Studies in the Age of Chaucer*, 14 (1992), pp. 53–88.
76. Monica Green, 'Women's Medical Practice and Health Care in Medieval Europe', *Signs: Journal of Women in Culture and Society*, 14 (1989), pp.

434–73, has exposed the fallacy of supposing that women's ailments were reserved for female practitioners, or that patients were always treated by members of the same sex. The complicated textual history of the diagnosis of *suffocatio matricis* or suffocation of the womb (less confusingly called suffocation *by* the womb, or uterine displacement) is surveyed by Ann Ellis Hanson, 'Continuity and Change: Three Case Studies in Hippocratic Gynecological Therapy and Theory', in *Women's History and Ancient History*, ed. Sarah B. Pomeroy (Chapel Hill, University of North Carolina Press, 1991), pp. 81–7; the story is taken forward with bravura to modern times by Helen King, 'Once upon a Text: Hysteria from Hippocrates', in Sander L. Gilman, Helen King, Roy Porter, G. S. Rousseau and Elaine Showalter, *Hysteria Beyond Freud* (Berkeley, University of California Press, 1993), pp. 3–90.

77. Quia per hoc custodium dominam unam a sincopi usque ad emendacionem per iii dies fere et in huiusmodo semper eam evigilavi quod cognovi per festinanciam pulsus eius in sompnolencia et sic fuit relevata et sanata et quando illa sompnolencia fuit preterita permisi eam dormire suaviter per tempus (f. 114).
78. Compare Harley MS 2558, f. 114 with *Compendium medicine Gilberti Anglici* (Lyons, 1510) f. 296v, *Cyrurgia Guidonis* (Venice, 1519) Roger, op. cit.. f. 221.
79. On Fayreford's use of *experimenta*, see Jones, 'Harley', p. 49.
80. Helen Rodnite Lemay, 'Anthonius Guainerius and Medieval Gynecology', in *Women of the Medieval World: Essays in Honour of John H. Mundy*, eds Julius Kirshner and Suzanne F. Wemple (Oxford, Basil Blackwell, 1985), pp. 317–36, suggests that Guainerius made use of a female assistant, an obstetrix, in treating women patients for *suffocatio matricis* (p. 323). Fayreford does not, it seems, require an intermediary of this sort.
81. Case 4 and f. 73 of the *Practica*. On *cephalargica*, see Bartholomaeus, *On the Properties of Things*, vol. 1, p. 343.
82. F. 78v: Erat quidam puer in etate circa xii annorum et ex percussione amisit visum unius oculi ita quod nihil potuit videre clauso alio apud tyverton in devone et inposui cotidie bis in oculo predicto sanguinem de yrundine et bibebat cotidie betonicam tritam cum servisie et infra xvnam recuperabat visum deo gracias Et certe in multis probavi betonicam esse valde evacuantem omnes ranculas sive radunculas oculorum sic potatam et lavacione aque rosarum vel aliis.
83. Bartholomaeus Anglicus, *On the Properties of Things*, vol. 1, p. 632.
84. Case 13 and f. 78v in the *Practica*.
85. Harley MS 2558, f. 121v. Item audivi mirabile experimentum sed carens rationem manifestam / mingat paciens semper quando voluerit mingere tribus diebus super urticas maiores quae semen ferunt urtica siccabitur & paciens liberabitur.
86. Harley MS 2558, f. 77v.
87. Harley MS 2558, f. 119.
88. The various use of *ananizapta* and other words of power on suspensions of all kinds will be dealt in a study of the Middleham Jewel by Lea Olsan and P. M. Jones (forthcoming). Epilepsy charms occur in Bernard Gordon's *Lilium medicinae* (Lyons, 1550), p. 226. Luke E. Demaitre, *Doctor Bernard de Gordon: Professor and Practitioner* (Toronto, Pontifical Institute of Mediaeval Studies, 1980), pp. 157–9, attributes Bernard's use of charms

for epilepsy to desperation in the face of failure of scholastic practical medicine. I suspect that Fayreford's attitude to charms was much less grudging.

CHAPTER NINE

The Death of a Medieval Text: The *Articella* and the Early Press

Jon Arrizabalaga

Introduction

Midway between the Black Death and the French Disease was an event of great historical significance in European culture, the invention of the printing press. Also between the two *termini* of this book there were changes that were to have profound effects on medicine, particularly the cultural movements of Latin humanism and Hellenism. All three interacted in many ways and it is the purpose of this chapter to look at a particular focus of the three, the medieval teaching textbook of medicine, the *Articella*.

All doctors trained within a university, and many who were not, would have been familiar with the *Articella*. It was put together as a collection of medical tracts from diverse sources in the twelfth century before the universities existed. Its career saw the introduction of medicine and its professional faculties into the universities and encompassed the Black Death, the Council of Florence and subsequent Platonism and Hellenism, the press, the English Sweats, the French Disease and the *editio princeps* of Galen. It was successfully modified to meet the changes in the needs and expectations of teacher and pupil. Yet the sequence of printed editions came to a sudden end in the 1530s: it did not die a lingering death. It was killed.

To try to find why will be the purpose of this chapter.[1] We shall look at the printed versions only, from the first edition of about 1476 to the eighteenth and last in 1534.[2] We shall examine the nature of the early press and how its products changed with the society of the time. The contents and the format of the *Articella* will pose a central question in these terms. In such a complex question some of the answers will be provisional; but, then, this is the first time the question has been asked.

From manuscript to machine: the *Articella* and practical medicine

Gutenberg's machine of the 1440s was a device to hold together separately cast type letters to produce pages of text. Although it probably took longer for the printer to set up a page in type than for a scribe to write out the same number of words, once set up the press could produce some hundreds of pages in a short time. The machine was seen at the time as a device to reduplicate the texts of manuscripts quicker and more cheaply. The earliest printers indeed confined themselves to reproducing works that had for centuries previously circulated as manuscript codices, the details of presentation of which they tried to copy. Like many machine-made things, the new texts were ugly, if undeniably cheap, and on one or the other count were sometimes seen as not being real books.

Nevertheless, from its original home in the Rhine valley the press quickly spread in the 1460s and particularly the 1470s to Italy, Paris, the Low Countries, central and northern Germany, eastern Europe, the Iberian kingdoms, the rest of France, England and the remainder of Europe. This argues that indeed the commercial possibilities of cheap texts were being realized in big print-runs and a buying market. It need not now be emphasized how important such a change was for the spread of knowledge in all fields; but we should avoid giving the press a unique responsibility for everything that happened in European intellectual history in the fifteenth and sixteenth centuries.[3]

So what was the *Articella*, which was caught up in these changes? It was a collection of short medical treatises already fixed by the beginning of the twelfth century.[4] Its core was a terse introduction to Greek medicine, the *Isagoge* of Johannitius,[5] to which were added the *Aphorisms* and *Prognostics* of Hippocrates and two short diagnostic tracts, *On Urines*, by the Byzantine Theophilus,[6] and *On Pulses* attributed to a Philaretus about whom little is known.[7] In the mid-twelfth century the collection was expanded by the addition of the text of Galen known at the time as the *Tegni*: it is his 'small art' of medicine, otherwise called the *Ars Parva* or *Microtegni*. In the thirteenth century was added the Hippocratic *Regimen for Acute Diseases (De Regimine Acutorum Morborum)*. Galen's commentaries on the above mentioned Hippocratic works, and 'Ali Ibn-Ridwan's commentary on Galen's *Tegni* already appeared to be included in one-third of the *Articella* manuscripts by the second half of the thirteenth century, but it is clear that they were not a part of this medical collection at the beginning.[8] At later periods a number of other small works of various origin were incorporated into this medical collection. Although widely known as such, its title of *Articella* or *Articella Hippocratis* was not widespread until the printed editions of the 1480s.[9] It was an essential tool for medical teaching and showed a remarkable capacity to survive: we shall look at how editorial strategies were related to this.

It is notable that of this original collection of works only the *Isagoge* deals with theoretical medicine (and in a very terse fashion). The others are practical in different ways. The *Aphorisms* is a collection of wise if cryptic pieces of advice to the practising doctor over a wide range of situations, and the *Regimen for Acute Diseases* deals with the practical aspects of dealing with, most notably, fevers. The tracts on pulses and urines describe the tactile and visual perceptions of the practising doctor. The practical doctor would expect to come upon situations met in the various aphorisms, would certainly have to deal with fever and derived much professional benefit from the practical business of taking the pulse and inspecting the urine. All of this is very relevant to a volume that deals, as this one does, with practical medicine. Every university-trained physician who later practised would have been brought up on the *Articella*. Many who practised without having been to a university, and those who were educated before the universities admitted medicine as a discipline, would also have been familiar with its practical contents. Its precepts would have had direct effect on the regimen prescribed by most doctors in feverish diseases. However much knowledge of urines and pulses became refined, it was based on the two tracts of the *Articella* and made a characteristic piece of the practice of the medieval doctor. None of the practical and often specializing medical persons discussed in the other chapters of this book would have been unaware of the significance of pulses, urine and regimen for the acutely ill.

Taking the pulse and examining the urine were also something of a ritual for the medieval doctor. We know from professional and ethical advice given at the time that the medieval doctor was quite aware of the possibilities for self-advertisement in the display of learning and skill in the examination of the patient in these two ways. If the doctor could pronounce a diagnosis and point to a prognosis from a sample of urine even when the patient was distant, it did a great deal of good for his reputation. The colourful charts that he carried with him were symbols of his mastery of a technical craft. The rationale behind the two techniques was that they supplied information about what was happening at two very important centres of the body: the vital faculty of the heart, which made vital spirit and arterial blood, and the natural faculty of the liver, which generated blood, the food of the body. To hint at such profundities may well have been part of the doctor's patter; the ethics of the time suggest that it was.

The 'early press'

Although bibliophiles commonly make the year 1500 the major chronological watershed in early printed books (separating *incunabula* from later books) this has little meaning in historical terms. What is important is the period of transition from manuscript to print. For our purposes this period was approximately between 1470 and 1530. It is not until the 1470s that university medicine and natural philosophy become visible products of the European presses and an active part of the university book market. At the other end of the period, it was only by 1530 that the bulk of the ancient and medieval intellectual heritage (ancient and Byzantine Greek, Latin and Arabic) had been published in Latin at least once. By then, too, Greek versions were becoming more frequent as the Hellenists pursued their ideals, and a great range of vernacular texts were printed. Important landmarks in this process were Pliny's *Historia Naturalis* (Latin edition of 1469) the Latin version of the *Canon* of Avicenna (1473), the *Materia Medica* of Dioscorides (1478; Greek edition 1499), the works of Plato (1484/85; Greek, 1513), those of Galen (1490; Greek, 1525), of Aristotle (1482; Greek, 1495–97) and the *Corpus Hippocraticum* (1525, and in Greek in 1526).[10]

Clearly the intellectual orientation of the scholars of the period was towards ancient and medieval authority, which was increasingly seen as Greek. Within medicine the number of books published during the lifetimes of their authors was accordingly very small until the 1490s, when it rose suddenly.[11] After this date living authors seem to have gradually realized the huge opportunities which presses offered for diffusion of their studies, and found publishers ready to finance their printing, although they do not seem to have surpassed the number of dead authors until the second half of the sixteenth century.

The printed *Articella*

The *Articella* was printed with surprising regularity over this period. Its eighteen editions average out over its publishing history at about one edition every three years. No two editions were, in the event, more than eight years apart before its sudden demise. But the geographical spread was far less even than the chronological. The presses of only four cities printed all the *Articella* editions: Padua, Venice, Pavia and Lyons. Here again the distribution was uneven, for there was only one Paduan edition and two Pavian. Half the entire number of editions were printed in Venice (nine) and a third of them in Lyons (six editions). The differences are even more marked when we realize that the press was a latecomer to Lyons and that its earliest *Articella* was not printed until 1505; thereafter it produced comfortably more editions than Venice. An equally dramatic change is in format, for all the fifteenth-century editions were in folio, but most sixteenth-century editions were octavos. (This was accompanied by a general move away from the two-column format, less convenient on the smaller page.)

In other words, well over 80 per cent of the editions of the *Articella*, a text designed for university teaching, were produced by non-university towns, rather than by the presses of the towns that housed the prestigious medical schools. Why should this have been so? The answer seems to lie in the nature of the printing and publishing business. The universities must have represented a major market, but Padua, Ferrara or Bologna were not far from Venice, and most of the journey from Lyons to Montpellier would have been down the Rhône, so we can guess that transport costs were not prohibitive. What was important was the nature of book production. On the one hand the early press was marked by changes in technology and scholarship to supply an increasingly demanding market. On the other, printing and publishing was a savagely competitive business and often unscrupulous. The early printing houses on average enjoyed only a brief life. Some such reason might be thought to lie behind the fact that most of the printers of the *Articella* did not go on to print a second edition,[12] but in fact only the printer of the first edition went out of business soon after. He is thought to have been Nicolaus Petri of Haarlem, and he printed the *Articella* in about 1476. Records are found of his activities in Padua in 1476 and in Vicenza between 1475 and 1477, but nothing thereafter. However, his business partner in the Vicenza period, Hermann Liechtenstein of Cologne, was the printer of the second edition of the *Articella* in Venice in 1483. We can guess that Liechtenstein had gained some experience of the market for the textbook and saw that a better edition would be a viable business proposition.[13]

Certainly from a scholar's viewpoint a corrected edition was badly needed. The edition of 1476 is eccentric when compared to the standard text adopted by later editions and seems to have been based on a corrupt manuscript. University doctors would have been able to compare Petri's edition with manuscript versions of the *Articella*, many of which were very carefully written. The second edition had an editor, Francesc Argilagues, and it is more than convention when he tells the reader that the first edition was full of mistakes and misprints, so that 'most passages remained corrupted and spoiled rather than corrected' and 'neither sense nor opinion could be obtained from them'.[14] Argilagues condemned Petri's carelessness as a printer as energetically as he praised Liechtenstein as 'a great lover of the art of books (*librarie artis*) practised by him in such an exquisite way that he is undoubtedly superior to the other printers'.[15] It seems reasonable to guess that in the competitive world of fifteenth-century printing Liechtenstein had learned from the mistakes as well as from the business opportunities of Petri.

It was not only the nature of the printing and publishing trade that determined who operated the presses and where. The university in the manuscript age had its own ways of supplying itself with texts. The university stationer, the *pecia* system of copying texts, the extraordinary lectures of the bachelors all in different ways were connected to the slow business of generating and correcting texts. Correcting was routine, for there would always be a certain if small percentage of errors. In the case of the parallel textbook of natural philosophy, the teacher took the class through Aristotle's text so that they could gloss the scribal errors. Indeed, the scribe had anticipated this and other kinds of gloss by leaving extra space between the lines of text. With these systems in place it is not surprising that the universities did not seek to compete in printing. The arrival of invariant printed texts, cheaply produced at competing commercial centres must have soon destroyed the old systems, but that was not perhaps at first apparent.[16]

The nature of the printed book also meant changes in the way in which text was produced. We saw that the first printed works were seen simply as replicated manuscripts. But manuscripts were often produced on commission, in religious houses or in universities, in other words in some regulated system. But the printer worked in an open market. He was first a technical expert, able to cast type and handle the press. He needed funds to set up and, perhaps, took a partner for this purpose. He needed to sell his wares, which was a different business from making them. Two-thirds of the printers of the *Articella* also acted as their own publisher. People in this position needed to advertise, sell and distribute. One way to advertise was to print something eye-catching at the front of the text, and many an early book begins with a direct address to a potential customer: 'READER, you have here ... '. Title-pages and addresses to the reader served the same function, as we saw when Argilagues drew attention to the superiority of his own edition of the *Articella*. But to sell to a specialist market, like the medical, meant having specialist skills. There was no author available to provide material useful for selling texts like the *Articella* and the printer himself was unlikely to know much medicine.

The editor

In a competitive situation these circumstances led to the birth of two new occupations, that of editor and of proofreader. The proofreader was needed because the text was invariant. The printer did not make allowances for glosses to be inserted between the lines and the printed book did not get the same treatment in the university as manuscripts. Any changes had to be made before the print-run began. It was an opportunity to put the work into a final form consistent with the textual and philological accuracy sought after by the humanist movement for as much as a century. The editor played a related role. He had to have specialist knowledge of the subject area of the text and to be responsible for the contents and style. He had to secure and compare manuscripts, and in a humanist way seek the intention of the author within the changes imposed by time. The text had to be true to the original as far as possible, but also attractive to the reader. The two aims were not always strictly compatible and editorial components of printed books were additions and explanations not in the original text. Chapters, sub-chapters, headings, marginal summaries, full references for authorial quotations, tables, contents, indices, variant readings, corrigenda and addenda all helped to guide the reader but were all imposed on the text.

The editor could also address the reader or a patron at the beginning of the work and explain its significance or superiority or something else that would help to sell it or add to his own reputation. He could also advise the publisher on what would be publishable, advice which ultimately led to the publication of new materials. Here the editor was the agent who expanded the intellectual horizons of the reading public. He could also point the publisher towards new translations of well-known (and publishable) works. Some of these possibilities are demonstrated in the *Articella*. Works added to the printed collection in fact fall into two different categories: those that were incorporated for the first time into a printed edition of the *Articella* and those that were now first printed at all. In brief, to the seven texts that were canonical by the thirteenth century, more than twenty new works were added in the different printed editions of the *Articella*. Likewise some editors added as many as three new translations to the one or more already traditional in the medieval collection.

Clearly, many things were needed by the man who was going to fill the new occupation of editor successfully. He would need to like the job and to be able to learn from experience. He needed previous training in the subject area of the books involved and a great deal of skill and patience for rigorous textual work. Such qualifications might well have been obtained in a university. So while, as we have seen, there was some separation of the universities and the publishers, yet there were two important connections, first that the universities were a sizeable market for the books, and second that university men made good editors. With the authority with which his training invested him the editor endorsed the quality of the final product: university qualifications, previous editing experience and prestige as a university teacher or medical practitioner all increasingly combined to promote the value of the book. The editor must be an important focus when we follow the story of how the *Articella* reacted to external forces and finally became extinct.

These general points are illustrated by the known editors of the *Articella*. The first edition, to the best of our knowledge, did not have an editor: another of its medieval features. Of the remaining seventeen editions only two (Venice, 1502 and Lyons, 1505) do not have editors' names. In fifteen editions, then, the names of the editors are given, often in eye-catching places, such as the title-page (in six editions). Undoubtedly the name of the editor helped to sell the book. Their reputations or qualifications were valuable in this. There were five of them, and we know a little about them. They were Francesc Argilagues, Gregorio della Volpe (*Gregorius a Vulpe*), Pietro Antonio Rustico (*Rusticus Placentinus*), Pere Pomar (*Petrus Pomarius*) and Girolamo Salio (*Hieronymus de Saliis*). Argilagues and Pomar were Spaniards, both of them from Valencia; the other three came from the north Italian cities of Vicenza, Piacenza and Faenza, respectively.[17] Among their qualifications for editing the *Articella* was the fact that all of them were doctors of arts and medicine. In addition Rustico was a principal teacher – *lector ordinarius* – of theoretical medicine at the University of Pavia. Moreover, three of them were also involved in other editorial activities and thus were adding to their reputations and authority. In particular Argilagues prepared three editions of Pietro d'Abano's *Conciliator* (Venice, 1483 and 1496; Pavia, 1490): a book that centres on the actual or potential differences between medical men and philosophers, and which had been famous since it was finished in the early fourteenth century. It was a model of high scholastic technique and did not always meet with the approval of the Hellenists and humanists of the late fifteenth and early sixteenth centuries. Their preferred authorities were the whole texts and arguments of the ancients, not broken up for analysis and commentary in the scholastic manner. The editions of Galen's works were therefore important, and the reputation of Rustico, the professor of Pavia, must have been enhanced by his position of editor of the fourth edition of the *Galeni Opera*, published in his university town in 1515–16 in three volumes (Girolamo Salio also edited other texts, notably some works of Ptolemy and Filippo Beroaldo.)

Medicine, humanism and Hellenism

The conceptual framework of physicians trained in the universities of northern Italy in the second half of the fifteenth century may be described as late medieval Galenism, sometimes also called Avicennan Galenism. Its doctrines rested on the supposed harmony of classical – Greek and Roman – medicine and the Arabic re-creation of it. In particular Avicenna, as the foremost Arabic author, was held to agree with Galen, the great interpreter of Hippocrates. This did not prevent future doctors coming out of university lecture rooms imbued with the concepts and values of the humanist movement. They could not be called humanists, for humanism was a style of teaching rather than a body of doctrine, and one which suited the literary subjects best, but by the middle of the fifteenth century, as Kristeller observes, the influence of the humanist movement had gone beyond the limits of the *studia humanitatis* and to a greater or lesser extent affected every intellectual sphere. Medicine and natural philosophy, as technical subjects, had been humanized as much as their nature would allow by the period of the printed *Articella*.[18]

A 'humanized' medical man might well share with the literary humanists a desire to restore what the ancient authors had truly said. He would be prepared to use or accept textual criticism of the major medical sources and strove to recognize that the historical circumstances in which the authors had written had a bearing on what they wrote. The medical 'establishment' was also a profession and it taught structured courses within universities governed by statutes. These are not circumstances that promote change, and however 'humanized' he was the doctors did not want to abandon their authoritative Avicenna, who was neither ancient nor Greek nor Roman. Nor did they agree with the new fashion of medical Hellenism of the 1480s. This movement, with origins in the Council of Ferrara–Florence (1438–39) and the collapse of Constantinople in 1453, sought to radicalize the humanist programme, advocating a return to the *prisca medicina* of the ancient Greeks, which they claimed was the true source of medicine.[19]

The medical Hellenists were not an intellectually homogeneous group. Some of them followed the natural philosophy of Aristotle, as taught in the schools of western Europe since the thirteenth century, which they read now in Greek. Others identified themselves with the Platonic philosophy then being revitalized in Florence by Marsilio Ficino and his circle, and studied the Greek Plato and Greek neo-Platonists. But all of them agreed, in the face of the academic medical 'establishment', that a return to the Greek *prisca medicina* was the best, if indeed not the only, way of achieving the reform of medicine which, they maintained, could no longer be postponed. They sought a 'rebirth' of Greek medicine, which they maintained had spent centuries in the dark.

Many in the medical 'establishment' did not agree. Theirs was a professional and practical business. It had been taught in Latin for centuries, and these doctors read their Greeks and Arabs in Latin, beginning with the *Articella*. Latin was more than the language of mere commentators, whom the Hellenists decried, and was part of their culture, which they called, in reaction to the Hellenists, the *res Latina*. While they did not deny the importance of the Greek authors they thought that to limit medicine to ancient texts was to ignore the additions made to medicine by the commentators, who 'aggregated' new knowledge to the old, or made refinements within the broad principles of the ancients. Some even felt that in restricting themselves to Greek sources the Hellenists were avoiding the technical difficulties of medicine (and natural philosophy) or were discussing words rather than things.

This was the context in which the *Articella* was printed. There were many things about it that did not appeal to the medical Hellenists. It was in Latin. It had technical terms that could look barbaric. Some of the component tracts were of late origin, and all were small. It was full of commentaries, often with more than one for an individual work. Its editors introduced additional works composed in Arabic or Latin long after the end of the classical period. Ultimately, the medical Hellenists won their battle. New translations from the Greek replaced those medieval ones from Arabic and Greek, and among the texts used for teaching those that allowed the Greek authors to 'speak for themselves' were preferred to the analysis and commentary of the Latin tradition. The medical Hellenists killed the *Articella* by destroying the market for it.

The Hellenist medical movement, the earliest nuclei of which crystallized round physicians like Nicolò Leoniceno (1428–1524) at the university of Ferrara and Giorgio Valla (1447–1500), quickly spread through the medical faculties of Italy and then the rest of Europe, coming into full flower in the sixteenth century. Among its leaders were Lorenzo Lorenzano (1450–*c.*1502), Giovanni Manardi (1462–1536), Jean de la Ruelle (*c.*1479–1537), Wilhelm Kop (1460–*c.*1532), Johan Guinther von Andernacht (1505–74), and Thomas Linacre (*c.* 1460–1524). Their most characteristic activity of course was the translation and editing of ancient and Byzantine Greek works. Works of Galen, Hippocrates and others began to circulate, first in manuscript, from about 1480, although most of them were not printed until well after 1500.[20]

Changes in the *Articella*

The changes made by their editors in the different editions of the *Articella* are of two major kinds. The first kind involves those made in reaction to medical humanism both Latin and Greek; and the second relates to the changing nature and function of the printed book. We shall look at the different editions on a broadly chronological basis.

The first edition, of about 1476, remained close to manuscript conventions. It seems to have had no editor other than the printer, who probably worked from a single manuscript exemplar and as we have seen, not a very good one. Like a manuscript, it has no page or folio numbers, no title page, list of contents or colophon; its beginning and end are marked only by an *incipit* and *explicit*. The edition consists of the seven works that were canonical in the thirteenth century: the initial trio of *Isagoge, Urines* and *Pulses* is followed by the Hippocratic *Aphorisms* together with the commentary on them by Galen, in the Arabic/Latin translation by Constantine the African (died before 1098–99);[21] this is followed in turn by the Hippocratic *Prognostics* in two versions, again with Galen's commentary in one single version.[22] Then comes the Hippocratic *Regimen in Acute Diseases*, also in two versions, once more with Galen's commentary in one single version.[23] Finally comes Galen's *Tegni* in two translations, the *translatio antiqua*, completed but not begun by Burgundio of Pisa (1110–93) and the *translatio ex Arabico* by Gerard of Cremona, accompanied by a Latin version of its standard commentary by 'Ali Ibn-Ridwan (Haly Rodoan).[24]

This is the *Articella* at its most basic and medieval. The translations are mostly from the Arabic; Galen is better represented as a commentator than author; and the number of medieval or Byzantine works matches the number of Hippocratic. These features were changed by later editors in a number of ways that relate to the context of late fifteenth-century medicine as seen by the editors.

The Articellae *of Argilagues*

The first editor was Argilagues, who produced the Venice editions of 1483 and 1487. He had been trained in the medical faculties of Siena and Pisa during the 1470s and was a typical member of the Italian medical 'establishment' that we have characterized as being Avicennan–Galenist.[25] He resented the claims of the medical Hellenists and took a belligerent attitude to them. Undoubtedly this affected what he chose to include in the *Articella*, that is, what he took a proper medical education to be. First, in an introductory note to the tracts in the *Articella* he took pains to resolve an academic question posed by apparent contradictions in Hippocrates, Galen and Avicenna. It was a question of how to calculate the critical days in post-partum fever, and it arose as part of the subject matter of the Hippocratic *Prognostics*. Galen's commentary on the point seemed to differ from Avicenna's explanation of it, and it is clearly the action of an 'establishment' figure to try to reconcile Avicenna with the Greek sources.[26] Leoniceno, the arch-Hellenist, would have delighted in showing that Avicenna was in error.

Second, Argilagues has a word of advice for the reader in connection with the Hippocratic *Regimen in Acute Diseases*. Only the first three sections of the work, he says, have previously been printed, and not the last, of which only a single translation existed, containing some difficulties. Humanist, physician and Hellenist alike would agree that it was good now to publish the remaining part of the text, but in doing so in a less than perfect translation Argilagues knew that he would run the gauntlet of criticism from the Hellenists.

> If in this fourth section there are some Greek words wrongly written in our Latin letters, which might make any expert in Greek letters laugh, there is no reason at all for criticism, since the translation of these words is faithful and true. None of the codices of which I made use in my editing differs on these words, in spite of the fact that they often appear written in different ways in the commentary and in the text. When one knows the essence of something, one must not worry about the words; it was Galen's wish to learn and teach without using words. Thus it is found, in contradiction to many, in the second particle of the *Aphorisms*, commentary 22, that [Galen] says, 'I want to avoid the views of the new physicians who always chatter about names, believing that they are talking about the things they are the names of'. And in the third book of the *Tegni*, near its end, he says that 'it is possible not to give names of causes at all, like the sophists who neglect theory in the investigation of the great diversity of things and reduce their lives to a matter of names'. Averroes for his part says that Aristotle had little concern with names. The Latin translations should be enough for you, reader, since the Latin language is not to be considered inferior to Greek in dignity and excellence. In the foreword to his *Tusculan Questions* Cicero says 'I have always thought that our forefathers were in themselves wiser than the Greeks in all things, or that they improved all that they took from them'. Let Priscianus and many others think the opposite.[27]

This passage has been given at length because it shows so clearly Argilagues as a careful editor, working from a range of manuscripts and clearly within the late medieval medical tradition. He stoutly defends the sense of the Latin translation (despite some infelicities of Greek transcription) and in arguing strongly for the importance of thing over name he has eloquently chosen a medical model, Galen, and a Latin hero, Cicero, significantly where Cicero is challenging Greek cultural superiority. The argument about things and names might have been sharpened by the medieval dispute between the nominalists and realists, but it found forceful application in the hands of another group of 'establishment' medical figures, the anatomists, who often thought that in concentrating on Greekifying the terminology the Hellenists had forgotten the real business of anatomy.[28] In just the same way Argilagues argues that the philological concern of the Hellenists was in some sense an evasion of the technical and difficult issues of real things in the business of the natural philosopher and physician. Argilagues questioned the value of Hellenistic translations that were in circulation in manuscript (we should remember that Aldo Manuzio did not start publishing medical works in Greek and Latin until 1497).

In short, as an opponent of the Hellenists, we see Argilagues as a businesslike medical man, with humanistic textual and historical skills that served him in his editing and without the Hellenists' aversion to the Arabic and medieval sources of medicine. He was full of praise for Gerard of Cremona's translations from the Arabic in the technical fields of medicine, natural philosophy and mathematics: 'a very illustrious man who translated from Arabic into our Latin 75 works of dialectics and philosophy as well as of mathematics, not to mention 21 medical works. If this place were more appropriate I would enumerate all of them here in his honour'.[29] Certainly, Gerard of Cremona (1114–87) was not someone whose memory the Hellenists would be inclined to celebrate. He not only was the leader of the Toledo school of translators (1130/40–1284), but also symbolized the kind of approach to medical and natural philosophical sources that shaped the university pattern of learning in the late Middle Ages – a pattern that Argilagues, like most members of the medical 'establishment', feared was to be displaced and substituted by the new, still evanescent one, that the Hellenists were intending to introduce.

The Hellenists' programme threw some aspects of late medieval Galenism into a new relief. Argilagues energetically attacked the carelessness of some works of the ancients then circulating and we have seen that he was scathing about the first edition of the *Articella*. The point was that such things were soft targets for the Hellenists, and threatened the repute of good Latin scholarship. Argilagues was pungent in his attack on careless editors and especially printers, who 'almost always alter and change everything they receive already corrected'. Such tension between editor and printer must have been a common feature of the early press.

In the light of all this we can understand a little better the changes that Argilagues introduced into the *Articella*. First, he brought into the collection a little work by Gentile da Foligno on arranging the books of

Galen.[30] For the Hellenist Leoniceno, Gentile was 'the old commentator' on Avicenna, because he had lived before the plague. Leoniceno did not like commentators or Avicenna, but to Argilagues both had much to offer. Gentile's advice in this text on how to divide up the books of Galen and in what order to read them began life as a commentary on Galen's *Tegni* and so was a by-product of teaching the *Articella*. In bringing it into the collection Argilagues was asserting the continuity and utility of the medical Latin tradition.

It was not necessary to be a Hellenist to see the virtues of good translations of Greek works, and Argilagues introduced into the *Articella* no less than four Hippocratic works that had not been previously published. The first was the *Epidemics* – or at least its sixth book – together with the commentary by John of Alexandria in an Arabic–Latin translation.[31] Another was, in Greek–Latin translation, *The Nature of the Foetus*, which is a tract on the development and therefore the anatomy of the unborn body.[32] The other two, also in Greek–Latin translations are concerned with legal and ethical parts of medicine and are sometimes confused, so here are their Latin titles: *De Lege*[33] and *Iusiurandum*, the latter translated by Nicolò Perotti.[34]

With his *Articella* in this new form, Argilagues exercised (or even indeed initiated) another editorial function by introducing three tables of contents. These seem to have been intended as a guide to the most important works, for they cover the *Tegni*, the *Aphorisms* and three more Hippocratic texts taken together, the *Prognostics, Epidemics* and *Regimen in Acute Diseases*. Argilagues did not think it worthwhile or important, then, to provide a guide to the first three works of the collection, Johannitius's introduction and the texts on urines and pulses. There is evidence that although they were among the oldest members of the *Articella*, these texts were regarded simply as introductory – a sort of medical *trivium* to the Hippocratic/Galenic *quadrivium* that followed – and were sometimes omitted.[35] Argilagues's treatment would be consistent with such an attitude.

Other editors followed Argilagues's lead in supplying tables of contents, but only in the folio and quarto editions (Della Volpe and Salio). No doubt it was necessary to omit as much as possible in squeezing the component tracts of the *Articella* into an octavo volume. Possibly too if the pocket-sized octavos were intended as constant companions (rather than reference or library folios) familiarity would render such guides unnecessary.

The octavo Articellae

The first octavo *Articella* was the edition of Venice, 1502. We do not know who its editor was, and so we do not have any external means of judging his cultural alignment. But there are signs of the cultural changes we have been discussing. This edition includes the first of a new series of translations made by Hellenists from the Greek: the Hippocratic *Aphorisms* in a translation by Theodore Gaza, who died in 1478. In comparison to the age of the collection as a whole, this is a fairly rapid adoption of novelty. But then the formation of the collection itself had much to do with the comparatively sudden appearance of the Arabic–Latin translations in the twelfth century, and we should not be surprised at its modification at a time of a new round of translations beginning in the late fifteenth century. The new translation made the old one a *translatio antiqua*; but it did not make it redundant. The editor retained it in his volume, despite the pressure on space in a small book.[36] One reason for this may be that the old translation was commonly taught by means of commentary, and scholastic commentary commonly proceeded by examining small sections of the text in turn. Each section was identified by a phrase – a *lemma* – taken from the text, which had to remain constant if the commentary was to work. The old commentary could not work with a new translation. To a certain extent the same thing was true of Galen's commentaries traditionally presented with the Hippocratic texts of the *Articella* (although not of the *Aphorisms* in this case): a new translation of the Hippocratic text would ideally require a new translation of Galen's commentary.

Not only did the editor retain the old translation of the *Aphorisms*, he used it a second time in presenting a *Collection of Aphorisms relating to Every Disease*, in which the aphorisms were reorganized to follow a head-to-toe sequence. The point of doing this was to add an organizing principle to the collection to make for easier learning and reference. Doubtless the old translation was retained for this purpose because it was still the most familiar (and fitted the commentaries). The editor said the arrangement was 'to ease the labour of the students' (*ad tollendum studentium laborem*), which reflects the central part played in medical education by the *Aphorisms*.[37] Indeed, it is worth pausing just a moment to reflect on the nature of medical aphorisms. The Hippocratic forms of the genre are conspicuously without theory and look like pieces of advice distilled from the lengthy and authoritative experience of the father of medicine. They were in a sense practical, for they told the doctor what to expect or do in a variety of situations. Practical, based on experience and without theory, they might have been thought to be empirical; but the university-trained, rational and learned doctor had the most pressing need never to appear to be empirical, for this was a label that had come to be applied to his rivals, the unlicensed practitioners. Although it was not explicit, in this situation one advantage of reading Galen's commentaries on the Hippocratic texts was that Galen supplied the theory that Hippocrates had chosen not to express. Indeed, to explain the *Aphorisms, Prognostics* and *Regimen in Acute Diseases* (all frequently accompanied by Galen's commentaries in the *Articella*) was to assign causes and to introduce principles. The *Aphorisms* were thus rescued from empiricism and retained their authority and practicality.

Others, too, saw the advantage of aphorisms. The editor of this *Articella* made a second change to the collection by adding a collection of aphoristic extracts made from the first five books of the *De Medicina* of Cornelius Celsus.[38] These 'flowers' (*Flosculi in Medicina ex Cornelio Celso extracti*) could be picked with profit from Celsus not only to be presented as aphorisms, but as pieces of elegant, ancient and confident *Latin* medical literature, from the '*Cicero medicorum*', at a time when the Hellenists were getting into their stride. Both humanist and Hellenist medical men thought that the new appearance of old texts was a good thing, and there is no conflict in our editor publishing Celsus and Theodore Gaza's translation of Hippocrates.

Yet another collection of aphorisms enters the story, for our editor reintroduced the collection of Yûhannâ Mâsawayh, known to the West as Mesue. This had been an infrequent member of the *Articella* in the manuscript period of its history, when it was known as the *Aphorismi Johannis Damasceni*. Like most other of the member tracts of the *Articella* this text had an independent manuscript history and was first printed in Milan in 1481; it was part of just half of the printed *Articellae* and was included also in some other printed collections.[39]

The third alteration made by the anonymous editor of the 1502 edition was more drastic. He decided not to include four of the Hippocratic works, one of which, *Regimen in Acute Diseases*, had been canonical for a long time. Of the Hippocratic texts introduced by Argilagues our editor kept only the *Iusiurandum*. Perhaps he saw Argilagues' inclusion of *De Lege* and the texts on epidemics and the nature of the foetus as unnecessary innovations. But the omission of the book on acute diseases alone is a serious loss to the Greek side of the balance, as is the absence of Galen's commentary on the surviving Hippocratic prognostics and aphorisms. The introduction of Mesue might seem to further shift the balance away from a Greek *prisca medicina*; but then Galen's *Tegni* is also without its commentary, which was originally Arabic.

We cannot be sure of all the factors influencing the decision of an editor on what to include, but it is fairly clear that the needs of the traditional medical faculties, and their statutes, formed a market that competed with another partly shaped by Hellenism. The later editions of the *Articella* show this clearly. First, there is the group of editions put out by Rustico (Pavia, 1506, 1510; Venice, 1507) and Pomar (Lyons, 1515, 1519, 1525, 1534). These were presumably targeted at the medical schools of Pavia and Montpellier.

Rustico, the *ordinarius* at Pavia, seems to have been concerned with bringing the *Articella* up to date for use in his own university. Bringing up to date meant adding rather than omitting, and Rustico accepted that the aphorisms of Mesue and the extracts from Celsus that had appeared in the 1502 edition were proper parts of the *Articella*. He also included material that was distinctly medieval rather than ancient and which was specified by the medical syllabus at Pavia, as at most late medieval faculties. This consisted of, firstly, large excerpts of Avicenna's *Canon* in its Latin translation from the Arabic by Gerard of Cremona. Systematic and comprehensive, the *Canon* was an ideal textbook, except for its size. This prevented a complete commentary being finished much before the Black Death, when Gentile da Foligno had finished all but a few sections. The text and the commentaries by Gentile, Jacques Despars (*Jacobus de Partibus*) and Gianmatteo Ferrari da Gradi (*Matthaeus de Gradibus*) were the centre of a huge publishing enterprise in the late fifteenth and early sixteenth centuries, while *Articellae* were still being printed: clearly the publisher anticipated a steady market of a traditional sort in which to recoup his investment. Rustico extracted from the *Canon* fen 1 and 2 from the first book, which were used to introduce medical theory, and book I, fen 4, and book IV, fen 1, which were used to teach practice. Avicenna's account of anatomy in *Canon* I, fen 1 was traditionally omitted.[40] Gentile thought this was wrong, believing that anatomy was the alphabet of medicine, but nevertheless followed the custom. This meant that the *Articella* was without anatomy in an age when anatomy was becoming important as Galen's anatomical works became better known and vindicated Gentile's opinion (implicit in his tract, sometimes in the *Articella*, on how to read Galen's books). By 1502 Gabriel de Zerbi had made Paduan anatomy conspicuous with his huge book, which took Galen's *On the Use of the Parts* as its guide. When Berengario da Carpi did the same to Bolognese anatomy in 1521 it became increasingly clear that the rationality and learning on which the physician had depended for so long for his professional standing, was anatomical. Both Zerbi and Berengario were 'establishment' figures: proud to call themselves 'scholastics' they saw the Hellenists as a distinct group and, while admiring their philological skill, distrusted their anatomical competence. Both had a humanistic interest in restoring Galen's anatomy in a Latin form.[41] To the extent that anatomical rationality prospered, the *Articella* was marginalized.

The *Canon* remained an important text in medical teaching throughout the sixteenth century, and the ultimate victory of the Hellenists, who disliked it, was in this respect incomplete. Rustico himself brought out a revised edition of it in Lyons in 1522, in collaboration with Symphorien Champier.[42] Moreover the 'establishment' medical men looked with favour at another of Avicenna's writings and Rustico included in his editions of the *Articella* Avicenna's *Cantica*, a medical compendium that again shows the attractions of the aphoristic form for medical teachers.[43] The authority that the Arabic authors continued to have in medicine is indicated too by Rustico's third additional text included in the *Articella*, book nine of Rhazes's work addressed to the king, Almansor, *Liber ad Almansorem Regem*. This was a text of special therapeutics, arranged in the medieval fashion from head to toe. This was popular and had a separate publishing history, first appearing in Milan or Pavia in 1472 as part of the *Practica* of Gianmatteo Ferrari da Gradi, the *Canon* commentator we met above. The whole of the *Ad Almansorem* was printed as early as 1481 and continued to appear in new editions throughout the sixteenth century;[44] it clearly formed a staple in the diet of surviving 'establishment' physicians.

Rustico's fourth addition to the *Articella* was yet another aphoristic work, the alphabetical list of remedies taken by Jacques Despars (the commentator on the *Canon*, who died in 1458) from Mesue: *Summula per Alphabetum super Plurimis Remediis ex ipsius Mesue Libris Excerptis*. This too was often printed during the fifteenth century and after Rustico's editions of the *Articella* was included also by Pomar.[45] These four additions to the collection clearly had an authority and answered a need that was not at all derived from the Hellenizing physicians. There is a fifth addition of Rustico's of which the same can be said, two brief descriptions of weights, and measures, for pharmaceutical purposes taken 'from the breviary of Aiseir' and from the breviary 'of the son of Serapion' respectively.

Lastly, Rustico added a group of short treatises on prognosis thought to be Hippocratic and called collectively the *Capsula Eburnea*,[46] the 'ivory chest'. These mostly spurious texts were probably derived from the canonical Hippocratic work on prognosis and dealt with the signs of life and death. Rustico's text was the Latin version by Gerard of Cremona of an Arabic translation or adaptation. Rustico established it as a proper part of the *Articella* and it remained in subsequent editions by Pomar and Salio.[47]

The 'establishment' physicians, like the Hellenists, saw value in the ancient Greek works in good translations directly from the Greek. The Hellenists differed in seeing value *only* in such things and in actively opposing the use of Arabic sources and Latin commentators. So it need not surprise us that Rustico took advantage of the new Greek–Latin translation of Galen's *Tegni* by the Hellenist Lorenzo Lorenzano (who had completed it in early 1500) and added it to his edition of the *Articella*. However, this was an addition, rather than a replacement of the old translation, which he retained. We can only speculate about why two translations of the same text were included in an octavo volume where space was at a premium. Possibly it was intended to make a comparison possible, in which a humanist physician could exercise his philological and historical skills in deciding which was the better key to Galen's thought. Perhaps the older translation was retained (it was in the first place) because it was still taught in the schools or taught by means of the traditional commentary by Ibn-Ridwan, which would not have fitted the new translation. (Ibn-Ridwan's commentary is not included by Rustico, either because it did not fit the new translation or for reasons of space.)

It is tempting to see the increasing number of new translations included in the *Articella* as a sign of the penetration of Hellenism. They are present to greater or lesser extent in the editions of Venice (1502), Lyons (1505) and in Rustico's editions. Rustico was followed closely by Pomar in his Lyons editions of 1515, 1519, 1525 and 1534: the *Aphorisms* and *Tegni* were present in both old, and new translations by Gaza and Lorenzano, and none had Galen's commentary; the *Capsula Eburnea* appears again, so does the *Iusiurandum* and the extracts from Celsus. In following Rustico, Pomar also included the medieval works that we noted above, but in addition he restored the traditional Hippocratic text on regimen in acute diseases. He also put back into the collection the Hippocratic works included by Argilagues and Della Volpe, but omitted from the editions of 1502 and 1505 and from Rustico's, that is, those on epidemics, the nature of the foetus and *De Lege*.

Pomar also inserted six more Hippocratic works into the collection, including *Airs, Waters and Places*.[48] The others are short and do not have traditional English titles: that on secrets, *Liber secretorum* was a member of the sub-group *Capsula Eburnea*;[49] on prognostication according to the moon, *De esse egrorum secundum lune existentiam*;[50] on the nature of the body and the elements, *De humana natura vel de elementis*;[51] on remedies, *De pharmaciis*,[52] and *De insomnis*.[53] All these had become available in printed editions in the 1480s either on their own or in collections. *De insomniis* and the texts on human nature and remedies were in Greek–Latin translations, the former by the Hellenist editor Andrea Brenta (*fl.c.*1460–85), while the latter two probably by Bartholomaeus da Messina (thirteenth century) and by Nicolò da Reggio (fourteenth century), respectively.

Tempting though it is to see this text-count as evidence of the increasing penetration of Hellenist influence in the *Articella*, we should remember that the aims of the Hellenists largely coincided with those of humanist doctors in seeking out good translations of the ancient texts. In the nature of things most ancient medical texts were Greek, so again humanist and Hellenist would have been looking for the same thing. Celsus was an exception, since he wrote in Latin, and this made him an important figure for those who saw themselves as champions of Latin culture. 'Establishment' medical men varied in their attitude to humanistic principles and to the *res Latina*, but few of them were Hellenists. Pomar, for all the Greek material he introduced to the *Articella*, also increased the number of excerpts from Avicenna's *Canon*, that is, sections of book IV dealing with surgery, presumably related to the teaching of surgery in the medical syllabus in Montpellier. That all of Pomar's editions were published in Lyons seems to indicate that they were targeted at Montpellier and designed to supply a need that the particular form of medical education took there. This is suggested too by Pomar's inclusion of still more aphorisms, those of the Montpellier teacher Arnau de Vilanova. He had died in 1311, but his two sets of aphorisms ('universal' and 'particular') remained popular works.[54] Pomar's inclusion of Arnau and Avicenna make it clear that he was no determined Hellenist.

The Hellenist Articella

We see a rather different picture when we look at the editions of Girolamo Salio. Here the comparison of different translations is carried to new lengths. The Hippocratic *Aphorisms* for example are given in three different versions in three parallel columns, strongly suggesting that the point was a textual comparison. The 'first' place – the left-hand column – is occupied by the translation from the Arabic by Constantine the African, the *translatio antiqua*, then in the middle column is the *traductio Laurentiana*, that is, of Lorenzano, and to the right is the *versio* of Leoniceno. (All include Galen's commentary.) Moreover, in the margins and in smaller type (and without Galen's commentary) Salio has provided a fourth version, the translation by Theodore Gaza. The *Laurentiana* had been first printed in Florence in 1494 and Leoniceno's version in Ferrara in 1509,[55] so Salio was bringing the collection up to date, and with the addition of the work of two notable Hellenists.

The striking thing is Salio's presentation of as many as four versions of the same work. The same is true of Galen's *Tegni*, of which we have – *lemmata* by *lemmata*, consecutively printed – the translation by Leoniceno (first edition 1506), that by Lorenzano (1506), the *translatio antiqua*, made from the Greek by Burgundio of Pisa, and the *traductio ex Arabico* by Gerard of Cremona. (All four translations were followed by the standard commentary of Ibn-Ridwan in a single version.) Something similar happens in the case of the Hippocratic *Prognostics*, of which the same two translations included as *antiqua* and *nova* in the fifteenth-century printed *Articellae* are printed consecutively *lemmata* by *lemmata* along with Galen's commentary in one single version), and followed by another from the Greek by Lorenzano.[56] Finally, the edition of Lyons 1527 added a Greek–Latin version of the Hippocratic *Epidemics* (first edition 1525) by Marco Fabio Calvi (*fl.* 1520) to the standard one,[57] not to mention its restoring the Arabic–Latin version of the Hippocratic *De regimine acutorum morborum* with some fragments lacking in earlier *Articella* editions. (The Lyonese publisher advertised these two new features on the title-page of the volume, and made it clear that the editor Michel de La Chapelle, very active in Lyons in that time, had been in charge of incorporating both of them into it.[58]

A number of things are implied by Salio's editorial methods here, although we cannot be certain of his intentions. Four versions of a single text, three of them in parallel columns clearly invite textual comparison. A humanist and Hellenist philology would be served in such a way. That the texts are displayed in certain chronological order of their translation (from the *traductio ex Arabico* to Leoniceno's or vice versa) would also serve the humanists' sense of history; but it also implies an evolution of expertise, culminating with the version of the arch-Hellenist Leoniceno, the enemy of Avicenna and the commentators, and to that extent the arrangement carries a Hellenist message. But it is a message to non-Hellenists, if only because it is in Latin. Doctors who could read Greek would not need parallel or consecutive Latin versions to help them decide what Galen meant – which must be one of the purposes of the technique. It is a message to the 'establishment' doctors, for whom it would be an unreasonable expectation that they would learn Greek. Not even Hellenists would need a Latin text; when a Greek edition of the works of Hippocrates and Galen became available such an apparatus as found in these *Articellae* became less necessary and no doubt helped to end their publishing history.

Salio's quarto editions are essentially books in three parts with independent foliation (albeit without new title-pages). Most of the traditional component texts of the *Articella* are given in the first (*Isagoge – De pulsibus – De urinis*) and second (*Aphorisms, Prognostics*, and the Hippocratic works incorporated by Pomar into the collection) part, while the third part contains (in addition to the Hippocratic *Regimen in Acute Diseases, Epidemics*, and *De natura fetus*) non-traditional matter, including Leoniceno's general introduction to his own translations of Galen from the Greek (first printed in 1508). The volume ends with

Leoniceno's discussion of the 'three doctrines' with which Galen opened the *Tegni* (also 1508).[59] This had caused great difficulty for the earlier medieval commentators, and some high scholastic commentaries on it were still printed in the sixteenth century. The problem was what kind of doctrine Galen meant: how did one use them in terms of logic? Leoniceno cut through the commentaries by radically asserting that Galen was simply discussing methods of *teaching*.[60]

In short, these two editions of Salio's can be called Hellenist *Articellae*. Over and above the permanent and original first three works of the collection, there were in these editions of 1523 and 1527, twenty works of a kind that the Hellenists perceived as their tradition. The single exception was Gentile's text on how to arrange Galen's work. Of the remaining nineteen most (thirteen) were 'Hippocratic' (since we do not know what Hippocrates wrote we have to accept a range of pseudoness). We have noted Salio's wide use of Hellenist translations. The arrangement of the entire volume implies a progression of medical knowledge, from the traditional introduction of Joannitius, up through the chronological and increasingly humanist/Hellenist range of translations and ending with a Hellenist programmatic promotion of Leoniceno's translations from the Greek and his dismissal of a question that had bothered the scholastics. It was Salio, the editor, who chose to introduce his works into an *Articella*, but it was the Greek-language activities of Leoniceno and other Hellenists that finally killed the collection.

Finally, we can look in a little more detail at Leoniceno's Hellenist programme, which is important in the third part of the Hellenist *Articella*. Whatever the reasons for his conviction of the superiority of Greek culture, one of the reasons why Leoniceno wanted to recover Greek medicine was that he believed it to be more effective at the practical level. It was simply better medicine than that of the medieval Latins and the Arabs. He had been concerned about the dangers of using the wrong things as medicines (because of poor texts) when attacking Pliny and Avicenna, and he now extended his attack to all recent medical writers, in whose books the good old medicine lay hidden in shadows.[61] The Hellenists still felt themselves to be in a minority, which lent urgency to the exhortations to battle with which they addressed each other in their books. In addressing Leoniceno another Hellenist physician, Luigi Bonacciuoli (*Ludovicus Bonaciolus*), poured scorn on the enemy, the great number of medical men who reproduced old errors and filled their books with an ignorance that went unpunished. He was angry with them too and thought that their contagion of deceit was worse than the treachery of Nero in forcing his teacher Seneca and his fellow Lucano to kill themselves, and in ordering the death of his mother Agrippina. He thought that their language (because it bristled with technical terms and neologisms taken from the Arabic) was 'stammering', a term used by the Hellenists for those who did not know or write the 'eloquence' of Greek. It was parrot-talk, he said; but at least parrots are innocent, and one can remove their tongues. He cheered what he saw as Leoniceno's attempt to destroy the medicine of these people by cutting out what was profane and polluted, and cultivating 'good arts' in place of 'bad' (that is, in translating Galen well from the Greek, rather than undertaking commentary).[62]

In a minority, the medical Hellenists sought not only to reassure each other of their superiority, but needed the help of the powerful. Before prefacing his translations from Galen, Leoniceno addressed Alfonso d'Este, duke of Ferrara (1505–34), dedicating the translations to him. He reminded Alfonso of his power (and dropped a gentle comparison with the ancient Caesars), of his wisdom in choosing good letters (of Leoniceno's kind) and of his *studium* in Ferrara, where the good letters should be cultivated. (Like many reformers, the Hellenists wanted to change the names of the things they wanted to reform, and the medieval *studia* became *gymnasia* – Leoniceno's word – or the more Platonic *academiae*.) Leoniceno also reminded him that true immortality lay in the cultivation of good letters, not in stone walls; part and parcel of the whole was Leoniceno's battle against the forces of reaction, the 'neoteric' medicine, a battle in which Leoniceno called on the help of his *humanissimus princeps*.[63] It was for related reasons that Leoniceno also addressed Francesco Castelli (*Franciscus Castellus*), the duke's physician. He too was congratulated on his association with the 'good arts'. But there was a particular reason for writing to Castelli. Leoniceno refers to the recent floods and dreadful pestilence that had recently affected Ferrara so severely that the philosophers and physicians of the *gymnasium* had left their posts. It was a critical moment – as Leoniceno says, time is the enemy of the good arts, particularly those of letters, and brings disasters like this, just as (he implies) the splendour of Greek medicine was eclipsed. Bringing in new teachers might well have brought in new doctrines; but Castelli seems to have guided Alfonso in restoring a suitably Hellenistic *gymnasium* which Leoniceno thought could make use of his new work on Galen's three doctrines.[64]

It is clear that the Hellenist part of this *Articella* offers an alternative rather than a complement to the traditional texts that precede it. It was not that the Hellenists wanted to get rid of the traditional Hippocratic and Galenic texts, but rather of their unsatisfactory translations and mode of expounding them. Leoniceno's treatment of the three doctrines with which Galen opens the *Tegni* is a paradigm. It is indeed not now the medieval *Tegni*, or even the humanist equivalent, the *Ars parva*, which had already become too common a title for the Hellenists, but the *Ars medicinalis*. Leoniceno's entire treatment of this traditional member of the *Articella* was designed to replace the traditional commentaries upon it. That by 'Ali Ibn-Ridwan was doubly barbaric to Leoniceno. First where Ibn-Ridwan thought the text to be defective, he supplied words to complete what he thought was Galen's sense. They were of course Arabic words, now rendered into medieval Latin. They were accordingly ugly and in being alien almost without meaning. Secondly, Leoniceno thought that Ibn-Ridwan had been 'violent' with his textual emendation in that the result did not in fact agree with a Galenic position. The medieval Latin writer Pietro Torrigiano (*Turisanus*, *c.*1270–*c.*1350), whose nickname *Plusquam Commentator* spoke for itself to a Hellenist, had also commented on this part of the text, and although reaching a satisfactorily Galen restoration, was still barbaric to Leoniceno because he stuttered along in a parroty Latin. Leoniceno's exercise here is to go back through Ammonius and Porphyry to Aristotle and Plato and start all over again with a Greek, not medieval or Arabic discussion.[65]

If we can assume that the Hellenist *Articella* containing these texts of Leoniceno had a fairly wide circulation, then it seems likely that the Hellenist programme expressed in them had a hand in the death of the traditional collection. Leoniceno knew what kind of objections would be offered to his programme. He knew that many traditional medical men and philosophers made Avicenna and Averroes 'into gods'. He knew that 'establishment' physicians, proud of their businesslike profession, resented being sneered at by Greekifying Hellenists who appeared to avoid getting tangled in the technicalities of medicine and philosophy in their search for the 'eloquence' of Greek. In doing so, Leoniceno recognized, the Hellenists could be grouped with those who were concerned with grammar and rhetoric and teaching in the early part of the arts course, and who only dabbled in philosophy. But in writing on the three doctrines he had taken the technical side of the theory of medicine head on and shown that Hellenism could tackle it. His linguistic skills in fact deal with technical medical problems with important practical results, not only in his famous attack on Pliny, but in the introduction to the translations of Galen.

The *Articella* and the press

Let us finally look at how the men who edited and published the *Articella* reacted to the new possibilities of a growing technology. As we saw above, seven of the eighteen volumes of the *Articella* were folios – more strictly, *in secundo* – two were quartos and the remaining nine were octavos. We must assume that these changes in format were significant, and the most ready explanation is that the format was governed by the use that the publisher or editor thought that the book would be put to. The format would also encourage or defer other potential readers.

The six *secundo* volumes of the fifteenth century and that of Venice of 1513 can be considered as direct descendants of the kind of book that Petrucci has defined as the *libro da banco*, that is, manuscript texts produced at or for the universities, designed for use in conjunction with lectures and with the largest format, two columns of text and big margins for the reception of glosses and postils.[66] We have seen that this was particularly striking in the case of the Paduan *editio princeps* of the *Articella*, where the printer seems to have limited himself to reproducing a manuscript, format and all. But we see from the details of the later editions of Argilagues and Della Volpe that publishers and editors soon came to see the huge potentialities in reaching new markets and spreading knowledge. As the editor Argilagus noted:

> Undoubtedly mankind owes the highest praise to the father of such an industry [printing] as well as to those who have day by day developed, cultivated and improved it. By their work all these people have offered such a service to mankind as was never seen by our forefathers. Future generations will accordingly bestow on them immortal glory in addition to praise.
>
> In fact people of the present can rejoice exceedingly in making use of a huge amount of books which our predecessors and fathers lacked. We see that the number of printed books has increased so much that they fill not only libraries but whole houses.[67]

Salio's two quarto editions (Venice, 1523 and Lyons, 1527) are those described above as the Hellenist *Articella*. Because of their format they fit into Petrucci's category of the humanist book, which he defined as a book 'written at or for humanist circles and destined for the libraries of learned people or of those protecting them'.[68] But it is not yet clear whether these editions of the *Articella* were meant for the libraries of Hellenist physicians or perhaps reflected the medical teaching at some northern Italian universities (it is worthy of note that Leoniceno was closely linked to that of Ferrara until his death in 1524).

The nine octavo editions wholly fit the category of handbooks, that is, *enchiridia* or Petrucci's *libretti da mano*. These were intended for more personal and continuous use by their readers;[69] implicit in these terms too is the use of the octavo as a reference work. Apart from religious and devotional books, where constant use and reference was natural, Aldo Manuzio was the first to produce octavos on any scale, from 1501.[70] The innovation was soon picked up by the De Gregori brothers and their *Articella* was one of the first titles in this format: while their edition of 1500 was a folio, by June 1502 they had re-thought their publishing strategies and printed in octavo. It must have been designed for different use. It seems to have been, as Pesenti suggests, to allow students and lecturers to have this basic text always to hand.[71] This must have had a radical effect on the nature of university teaching. As Walter Rüegg has expressively remarked,

> Teaching in the Middle Ages was dominated by the spoken word in lectures and in disputations, as well as by the ideas which were presented and elaborated in those oral forms. When the ordinary student began to buy books, the written word became dominant in university teaching. Not only were their sources made more immediately and more comprehensibly accessible, but commentaries, textbooks and polemics ceased to be monopolised by teachers and could be purchased in the market.[72]

Several other features of the octavo editions of the *Articella* suggest the same thing. Rustico and Pomar expanded the contents of the collection to cover the whole medical syllabus. In doing so they were undoubtedly aiming for a market success for an *Articella* that was now to be sold to large sections of the population of medical students. Even the second edition (Lyons, 1527) of the quarto *Articella* of Salio was addressed on the title-page 'for the sake of readers and students' (although the term was wider than simply university students).[73] So much is clear from the postface that Rustico addressed to *magister* Ambrosius Varisius Rosatus, for his appeal to this potential new market could not be more explicit. Rustico asserted that having seen the Lyons edition of 1505 and having shared with the publisher the wish to find the way 'to make the book much more worthy and valuable for all the people', he did his best,

> To publish, in a new printing and like a sort of very brief compendium, all the parts of medicine which are the topic of the ordinary lectures both theoretical and practical every year in our university [Pavia] so that the whole art of medicine may be had in a sort of handbook (*enchiridion*).[74]

This consideration about the press and the market for its productions might also explain why in these editions the commentaries have been suppressed – not only the Galenic commentaries on the Hippocratic works, but that of 'Ali Ibn-Ridwan on the *Tegni*. It might also explain why these editors included as new components of the *Articella* so many of the collections of aphorisms that we have noted in passing (those of Mesue, Arnau, the *Flosculi* of Celsus, the *Cantica* of Avicenna and others) for brief aphorisms are eminently memorable.[75] That is, not only did omitting these commentaries save space in the small octavos (and diminish their price), but it was consistent with the purposes of the student, who did not need all the scholarly apparatus of the folio editions. They simply needed a single compendium with the outline of their syllabus. Precisely the same thing happened with the parallel textbooks of natural philosophy in the arts course: many of them advertised themselves with the declaration that they contained all that was needed to proceed to the arts degrees.[76]

Apart from this there was another potential use for the octavo format. Every university physician could carry it with him in his practice as a manual or *vademecum*: a reference work, as suggested above. The presence of so many series of aphorisms also supports this hypothesis. Certainly, aphorisms were wise, terse and memorable. When they were arranged for diseases from head to toe, or alphabetically, they were capable of quick recall from the pocket-book. Such a thing was not new to the sixteenth century, and Arnau of Vilanova, in his *Repetitio super Vita Brevis* (a title reflecting the first Hippocratic aphorism) said that the medical practitioner had always to carry the general precepts [*canones universales*] of his profession in a written, aphoristic form 'in his pocket (if he is unable to carry them in his mind [*corde*] for human memory is very weak)'.[77] The 'reading' part of this equation was enormously multiplied in the sixteenth century with these octavo pocket-books.

Conclusion

No less than eighteen editions of the *Articella* issued from European presses between about 1476 and 1534. During almost 60 years the *Articella* publishers managed to sell this product at the university medical market. So, why did the printed *Articella* suddenly collapse in the mid-1530s? An immediate explanation might be that by then the printing of this medical collection stopped being a profitable business for publishers, for it did no more fill up the medical readers' expectations (despite the publishers' continuous attempts to adapt its contents and format to the market's changing demands) whereas other editorial products were better covering physicians' intellectual demands either traditional or new. At least three major features contributed to the sudden death of this medieval textbook.

First, by the mid-1530s European printers had already published Latin and vernacular versions of all the works by medieval and ancient authorities (Arab, Latin and Greek) which had been essential for the training and practice of university medical practitioners during the previous 250 years or so. Additionally, from the 1490s original Greek editions of ancient and Byzantine medical works, both those previously known in other versions and those just rescued from oblivion, and from the 1510s Hellenist translations into Latin, were increasingly issuing from the presses.

Secondly, during the first third of the sixteenth century Hellenists managed to gradually introduce substantial parts of their reformist programmes in many European medical faculties inside and outside Italy. To a greater or lesser extent this brought about changes in the medical syllabus at them including the introduction of new subjects (*materia medica*, anatomy, surgery and clinical teaching, among others) as well as of new ways of teaching the traditional ones. Medical Hellenists' Latin translations eventually replaced the older ones, and their new commentaries to these texts gradually took the place of the scholastic ones. Additionally, original works, both Latin and vernacular, dealing with medical teaching, theory and practice were increasingly printed all over Europe.

Last but not least, the widest availability (in terms of numbers and prices) of medical works at the book market promoted by the printing press made a collection of works like the *Articella* eventually become an old-fashioned textbook without any role to play at the medical book market.

Acknowledgements

This study has been partly funded by the research fellowships PB92–0910–C03–03 and PB95–0001–C03–03 of the Spanish government (Ministry of Education). My special thanks are due to Roger French who in editing the original English draft to make it more readable substantially improved the contents of this chapter. I am also grateful for their valuable remarks to Andrew Cunningham, Luis García-Ballester, Pedro Gil-Sotres, Vivian Nutton, Juan Antonio Paniagua, José Pardo-Tomás, and Fernando Salmón; to the participants at the original Cambridge–Barcelona II Joint Conference where a first version of this chapter was presented; and to those present at the First and Second Meetings of the *Articella* Steering Committee. Finally, I am also indebted to Klaus-Dietrich Fischer, Monica H. Green, Josep Perarnau, Tiziana Pesenti, Maurizio Rippa Bonatti and Thomas Rütten for the pieces of information they have provided me with.

Notes

1. For an expanded version of this article including tables and appendices see Jon Arrizabalaga, *The Articella in the Early Press, c.1476–1534*, Cambridge and Barcelona, Articella Studies: Texts and Interpretations in Medieval and Renaissance Medical Teaching, 1998.
2. For the printed editions of the *Articella*, see *Gesamtkatalog der Wiegendrucke*, 2nd edn, Stuttgart and New York, 1968–, vol. 2, cols 751–6 (nos 2678–830 [hereforth, *GW*]; *Index Aureliensis. Catalogus librorum sedecimo saeculo impressorum*, Aureliae Aquensis. 1962–, vol. 2, pp. 299–300 (nos 109.132–109.140) [henceforth, *IA*]. The *IA* omitted three editions, namely those of 1502, 1505, and 1506. For that of 1502, see Richard J. Durling, *A Catalogue of Sixteenth Century Printed Books in the National Library of Medicine*, Bethesda, MD, US Department of Health, Education, and Welfare, 1967, pp. 40–41 (no. 325). For the edition of 1506, see *A Catalogue of Printed Books in the Wellcome Historical Medical Library. I. Books Printed before 1641*, London, The Wellcome Historical Medical Library, 1962, p. 26 (no. 495). For the edition of 1505, see Ludwig Choulant, *Handbuch der Bückerkunde für die ältere Medizin ...* , Leipzig, L. Voss, 1841, p. 400. I have directly seen copies of all the eighteen editions except that of 1505 of which there is no available copy to the best of my knowledge. In this Chapter I am not concerned with a later English free adaption of the *Articella* published in London in 1612 under the title *Enchiridion medicum, containing an epitome of the whole course of physicke, with the examination of a chyrurgian ...* . See Peter Krivatsy, *A Catalogue of Seventeenth-Century Printed Books in the National Library of Medicine*, Bethesda, US Department of Health and Human Services, 1989, no. 12113 (p. 1212).
3. On the world of the printed book in late fifteenth- and early sixteenth-century Europe, see among others, Rudolph Hirsch, *Printing, Selling and Reading, 1450–1550*, 2nd edn, Wiesbaden, Otto Harrassowitz, 1974; Armando Petrucci, *Libri, editori e pubblico nell'Europa moderna. Guida storica e critica*, Rome and Bari, Laterza, 1977; Elisabeth L. Eisenstein, *The Printing Press as an Agent of Change. Communications and Cultural Transformations in Early-Modern Europe*, 2 vols, Cambridge, Cambridge University Press, 1979; Sandra L. Hindman, ed., *Printing the Written World. The Social History of Books circa 1450–1520*, Ithaca and London, Cornell University Press, 1991; Roger Chartier, *Libros, lecturas y lectores en la Edad Moderna*, Madrid, Alianza, 1993; as well as the bibliography quoted in these works. On the vigorous debate promoted by Eisenstein's work, see Robert S. Westmann, 'On communication and cultural change', *Isis*, 71(3), (1980), pp. 474–7; Peter F. McNally, ed., *The Advent of Printing: Historians of Science Respond to Elisabeth Eisenstein's 'The printing press as an agent of change'*, Montreal, McGill University, 1987, among others. Limited to particular topics but still very useful are José M. Madurell and Jorge Rubió y Balaguer, *Documentos para la historia de la imprenta y librería en Barcelona (1474–1553)*, Barcelona, Gremio de editores, de libreros y de maestros impresores, 1955; Martin Lowry, *The World of Aldus Manutius. Business and Scholarship in Renaissance Venice*, Oxford, Blackwell, 1979.
4. On the *Articella* and its dissemination, see among others, Paul Oskar

Kristeller, *Studi sulla Scuola Salernitana*, Naples, Istituto Italiano per gli Studi Filosofici, 1986; G. Baader, 'Articella', in *Lexikon des Mittelalters*, Munich and Zurich, Artemis, 1980–, vol. 1, cols 1069–70; Nancy G. Siraisi, *Taddeo Alderotti and his Pupils. Two Generations of Italian Medical Learning*, Princeton, Princeton University Press, 1981, pp. 96–107; *eadem*, *Avicenna in Renaissance Italy. The Canon and Medical Teaching in Italian Universities after 1500*, Princeton, Princeton University Press, 1987, particularly pp. 49, 132–3; Luis García-Ballester 'Arnau de Vilanova (*c.* 1240–1311) y la reforma de los estudios médicos en Montpellier (1309): el Hipócrates latino y la introducción del nuevo Galeno', *Dynamis*, 2 (1982), pp. 97–158: pp. 99–102; Per-Gunnar Ottosson, *Scholastic Medicine and Philosophy: A Study of Commentaries on Galen's 'Tegni' (ca. 1300–1450)*, Naples, Bibliopolis, 1982, particularly pp. 28–34; Tiziana Pesenti, 'Editoria medica tra Quattro e Cinquecento: L'"Articella" e il "Fasciculus medicine"', in Ezio Riondato, ed., *Trattati scientifici nel Veneto fra il XV e XVI secolo*, Venice, Università Internazionale dell'Arte, 1985, pp. 1–28; *eadem*, 'Arti e medicina: la formazione del curriculum medico', in L. Gargan-Oronzo Limone, ed., *Luoghi e metodi di insegnamento nell'Italia medioevale (secoli XII–XIV)*, Galatina, Congedo, 1989, pp. 155–77; Jon Arrizabalaga, Luis García-Ballester and José Luis Gil-Aristu, 'Del manuscrito al primitivo impreso: la labor editora de Francesc Argilagues (*fl. ca.* 1470–1508) en el renacimiento médico italiano', *Asclepio*, 43, 1 (1991), pp. 3–49.

5. On the *Isagoge*, see Kristeller, *Studi sulla Scuola Salernitana*, pp. 109–10; Gregor Maurach, 'Johannicius, Isagoge and Techne Galieni', *Sudhoffs Archiv*, 62, 2 (1978), pp. 148–74; Danielle Jacquart, 'À l'aube de la renaissance médicale des XIe–XIIe siécles: L'"Isagoge Johannitii" et son traducteur', *Bibliothéque de la l'École des Chartres*, 144 (1986), pp. 209–40. On Johannicius, whose Arabic name was Hunain Ibn Ishaq, see George Sarton, *Introduction to the History of Science*, 3 vols, Baltimore, Williams and Wilkins for the Carnegie Institution of Washington, 1923–1948, vol. 1, pp. 611–13.
6. On Theophilos Protospatharios, and on his works, see Sarton, *Introduction*, vol. 1, p. 478; Kristeller, *Studi sulla Scuola Salernitana*, p. 112.
7. On *De Pulsibus* and its possible author, see Kristeller, *Studi sulla Scuola Salernitana*, pp. 112–13; John A. Pithis, *Περισφυγμων. Die Schriften 'Peri sphygmon' des Philaretos: Text, Übersetzung, Kommentar von ...*, Husum, Matthiesen, 1983; Piero Morpurgo, 'Il commento al "de pulsibus Philareti" di Mauro Salernitano. Introduzione ed edizione critica dal ms. Parisinus Latinus 18499', *Dynamis*, 7–8 (1977–78), pp. 307–46.
8. Fernando Salmón, 'Sources for a Galenic Visual Theory in Late Thirteenth Century', *Sudhoffs Archiv*, 80, 2 (1996), pp. 167–83.
9. According to Tiziana Pesenti, the name *Articella* sprang up in the Veneto during the second half of the fourteenth century and first appeared at the medical faculties of Padua, Pavia and Bologna during the early fifteenth century. Yet this designation originally referred to the Hippocratic *Aphorismi* with Galen's comments with which only the *Articella* in use at the Italian universities actually began. This 'Italian' *Articella* included in this order the Hippocratic *Aphorismi* with Galen's commentary, Galen's *Tegni* with 'Ali Ibn-Ridwan's commentary, and the Hippocratic *Prognostica* and *De regimine acutorum morborum* with Galen's commentaries.

However, it did not incorporate the triad *Isagoge – De urinis – De pulsibus* with which this collection began in other manuscript traditions, including the Salernitan one. Among them Pesenti points to the tradition of the *Ars commentata*, which included this traid along with the whole set of Hippocratic and Galenic works at the 'Italian' *Articella*, and that of the *Ars medicine* which presents a similar pattern except for the fact that the Hippocratic and Galenic writings are not accompanied by their commentaries. See Tiziana Pesenti, 'Le "Articelle" di Daniele di Marsilio Santasofia (+ 1410), professore di medicina', *Studi Petrarcheschi*, 7 (1990), pp. 48–92; *eadem*, '"Articella" dagli incunaboli ai manoscritti: origini e vicende di un titolo', *Mercurius in Trivio. Studi di bibliografia e di biblioteconomia per Alfredo Serrai nel 60° compleanno (20 novembre 1992)*, Roma, Bulzoni, 1993, pp. 129–45. Whether the *Ars medicine* represents a French canon while the *Ars commentata* a German one as Pesenti has claimed, is to the best of my knowledge an open question still to be substantiated. See Cornelius O'Boyle, 'Medical Teaching at the University of Paris, *ca.* 1200–1400. Scholars and Texts in the Classroom', paper presented at the First Meeting of the Articella Steering Committee, Cambridge, December 1994.

10. For a quite exhaustive account of early printed editions of medical and natural philosophical works, see in combination Arnold C. Klebs, *Incunabula scientifica et medica* [1938], facsimile reprint, Hildesheim, G. Olms, 1963 (henceforth, Klebs); Margaret B. Stillwell, *The Awakening Interest in Science during the First Century of Printing, 1450–1550. An Annotated Checklist of First Editions Viewed from the Angle of their Subject Content. Astronomy–Mathematics–Medicine–Natural Science–Physics–Technology*, New York, The Bibliographical Society of America, 1970 (henceforth, Stillwell). On the medical and philosophico-natural book in the early printing press, see among others William Eamon, *Science and the Secrets of Nature. Books of Secrets in Medieval and Early Modern Culture*, Princeton, Princeton University Press, 1994; Arrizabalaga, García-Ballester and Gil-Aristu, 'Del manuscrito al primitivo impreso'; Luis García Ballester, 'La nueva industria del libro médico y el renacer del humanismo médico latino', in Manuel Fernández-Alvarez et al., *La cultura del renaixement. Homentage al Pare Miquel Batllori*, Bellaterra, Universitat Autònoma de Barcelona [Monografies Manuscrits, I], 1993, pp. 111–28: 120–21; José Pardo-Tomás, 'La producción impresa de libros científicos en la Corona de Aragón (1475–1600)', in Esteban Sarasa and Eliseo Serrano, eds, *La Corona de Aragón y el Mediterráneo (siglos XV y XVI)*, Zaragoza, Institución 'Fernando el Católico', 1995, pp. 231–66.
11. From Stillwell's repertory we can tentatively conclude that none of the six medical works printed before 1470 was written by an identifiable living author; only 10 authors of 95 (= 10.5 per cent) during the decade 1470–79; 3 of 69 (= 4.3 per cent) during the decade 1480–89; and 24 of 61 (= 39 per cent) during the decade 1490–99.
12. Only three printers published two editions of this work, namely the brothers Johannes and Gregorius de Gregoriis (Venice, 1500 and 1502), Jacob de Burgofranco (Pavia, 1506 and 1510), and Jacobus Myt (Lyons, 1519 and 1527).
13. From 1477 onwards Liechtenstein printed books on his own in Treviso (1477), Vicenza (1478–80), and Venice (1482–94). On Petri's and

Liechtenstein's printing activities, see Konrad Haebler, *Typenrepertorium der Wiegendrucke*, 5 vols, Halle an der Salle, Leipzig and New York: R. Haupt – O. Harrassowitz, 1905–24, vol. 2, pp. 69, 108, 142, 201, 202. There was a partnership too in the case of the two Pavian editions (printed by Jacob de Burgofranco at the charge of [*impensis*] Bartholomeus de Morandis), and for four of the six Lyonese ones (Johannes de la Place for Bartholomeus Troth, Jacobus Myt for Constantinus Fradin, Antonius de Ry for Jacobus q. Francisci de Giunta, and Johannes Moylin for Jacobus q. Francisci de Giunta). By contrast, there was only one Venetian edition produced by a partnership, namely that of 1492 (printed by Bonetus Locatellus for Octavianus Scotus).

14. Arrizabalaga, García-Ballester and Gil-Aristu, 'Del manuscrito al primitivo impreso', pp. 29–30.
15. Arrizabalaga, García-Ballester and Gil-Aristu, 'Del manuscrito al primitivo impreso', p. 30.
16. Roger K. French, 'Teaching Aristotle in the Medieval English Universities: *De Plantis* and the physical *Glossa ordinaria*', *Physis*, 34 (1997), pp. 225–96.
17. On Argilagues see Mario E. Cosenza, *Biographical and Bibliographical Dictionary of the Italian Humanists, 1300–1800*, 4 vols, Boston, G. K. Hall and Co., 1962–67, vol. 1, p. 258; Arrizabalaga, García-Ballester, Gil-Aristu, 'Del manuscrito al primitivo impreso'. On Della Volpe, Cosenza, *Bibliographical ... Dictionary*, vol. 4, p. 3714; Pesenti, '"Articella" dagli incunaboli ai manoscritti', pp. 140–41. On Rustico, Cosenza, ibid., vol. 4, p. 3115; Alfonso Corradi, *Memorie e documenti per la storia dell'università di Pavia e degli uomini più illustri che v'insegnarono*, 3 vols, Pavia, Tip. Successori Bizzoni, 1877–78: vol. 1, p. 120. On Pomar, José María López-Piñero, Thomas F. Glick, Victor Navarro-Brotons and Eugenia Portela-Marco, *Diccionario histórico de la ciencia moderna en España*, 2 vols, Barcelona, Península, 1983, vol. 2, pp. 191–2. And on Salio, Cosenza, *Biographical ... Dictionary*, vol. 4, p. 3148.
18. Paul Oskar Kristeller, *Renaissance Thought and its Sources*, New York, Columbia University Press, 1979, pp. 29–30.
19. On humanism and, in general, on learned culture in late fifteenth- and early sixteenth-century Italy and Europe, see among others, R. R. Bolgar, *The Classical Heritage and its Beneficiaries*, Cambridge, Cambridge University Press, 1954; L. D. Reynolds and N. G. Wilson, *Scribes and Scholars. A Guide to the Transmission of Greek and Latin Literature*, 3rd edn, Oxford, Clarendon Press, 1991; Kristeller, *Renaissance Thought*; John Stephens, *The Italian Renaissance. The Origins of Intellectual and Artistic Change before the Reformation*, London and New York, Longman, 1990; Anthony Goodman and Angus MacKay, eds, *The Impact of Humanism on Western Europe*, London and New York, Longman, 1990; James Hankins, *Plato in the Italian Renaissance*, 2 vols, 2nd impr., Leiden, Brill, 1991; Walter Rüegg, 'Epilogue: The Rise of Humanism', in Hilde de Ridder-Symoens, ed., *A History of the University in Europe. Volume 1: Universities in the Middle Ages*, Cambridge, Cambridge University Press, 1992, pp. 442–68; Francisco Rico, *El sueño del humanismo. (De Petrarca a Erasmo)*, Madrid, Alianza, 1993. On the university medical and natural-philosophical culture in this period, see among others, Richard J. Durling, 'A Chronological Census of Renaissance Editions and Translations of

Galen', *Journal of the Warburg and Courtauld Institutes*, 24 (1961), pp. 230–305; Francis Maddison, Margaret Pelling, and Charles Webster, eds, *Linacre Studies. Essays on the Life and Work of Thomas Linacre, c. 1460–1524*, Oxford, Oxford University Press, 1977; Jerome J. Bylebyl, 'The School of Padua: Humanistic Medicine in the Sixteenth Century', in Charles Webster, ed., *Health, Medicine and Mortality in the Sixteenth Century*, Cambridge, Cambridge University Press, 1979, pp. 335–70; Roger K. French, 'Berengario da Carpi and the use of Commentary in Anatomical Teaching', in Andrew Wear, Roger K. French and Ian M. Lonie, eds, *The Medical Renaissance of the Sixteenth Century*, Cambridge, Cambridge University Press, 1985, pp. 42–74, 296–8; R. K. French, 'Pliny and Renaissance Medicine', in Roger K. French and Frank Greenaway, eds, *Science in the Early Roman Empire: Pliny the Elder, his Sources and Influence*, London and Sydney, Croom Helm, 1986, pp. 252–81; Nancy G. Siraisi, *Avicenna in Renaissance Italy. The 'Canon' and Medical Teaching in Italian Universities after 1500*, Princeton, Princeton University Press, 1987; Vivian Nutton, *John Caius and the Manuscripts of Galen*, Cambridge, The Cambridge Philological Society, 1987; Daniela Magnai-Carrara, *La biblioteca di Nicolò Leoniceno. Tra Aristotele e Galeno: cultura e libri di un medico umanista*, Florence, L. S. Olschki, 1991; Anthony Grafton, *Defenders of the Text. The Traditions of Scholarship in an Age of Science, 1450–1800*, Cambridge, MA, Harvard University Press, 1991; Jon Arrizabalaga, John Henderson and Roger K. French, *The Great Pox. The French Disease in Renaissance Europe*, New Haven and London: Yale University Press, 1997; Vivian Nutton, 'The Rise of Medical Humanism: Ferrara 1464–1555', *Renaissance Studies*', 11/1 (1997), pp. 2–19.

20. Richard J. Durling, 'A Chronological Census', *idem*, 'Corrigenda and Addenda to Diels' Galenica', *Traditio*, 23 (1967), pp. 461–76; 37 (1981), pp. 373–81; Stillwell, pp. 113–17, 125–31; Nutton, *John Caius*, pp. 19–49.

21 Pearl Kibre, *Hippocrates Latinus: Repertorium of Hippocratic Writings in the Latin Middle Ages*, revised edition, New York, Fordham University Press, 1985, pp. 29–90, particularly, pp. 50–61; Stillwell, no. 408. On Constantine the African, see Herbert Bloch, *Monte Cassino in the Middle Ages*, 3 vols, Cambridge, Mass, Harvard University Press, 1986, vol. 1, pp. 93–110, 127–34; Francis Newton, 'Constantine the African and Monte Cassino: New Elements and the Texts of the *Isagoge*', in Charles Burnett and Danielle Jacquart, eds, *Constantine the African and 'Ali ibn al-Abbas al Magusi. The Pantegni and Related Texts*, Leiden, Brill, 1994, pp. 16–47.

22. To the best of my knowledge, some unsolved difficulties remain in identifying the manuscript traditions reflected in these two versions. The catalogue of Thorndike and Kibre related the *incipit* of the first-placed version ('Omnis qui medicine artis studio seu gloriam ... ') to that of the Hippocratic *Prognostica* with Galen's commentary according to Constantine the African's translation, and that of the second version ('Videtur mihi ut sit ex melioribus rebus ... ') to Galen's commentary to this Hippocratic work according to the probable translation by Gerard of Cremona. See Lynn Thorndike and Pearl Kibre, *A Catalogue of Incipits of Mediaeval Scientific Writings in Latin*, London, The Mediaeval Academy of America, 1963 (henceforth, TK), cols 1002, 1694. Additionally,

they rightly identified the *incipit* of what actually seems to be the Galenic commentary itself ('Manifestum est quod Hypocrates non utitur ... ') (TK, col. 847). Kibre, who appears to have wrongly identified 'Omnis qui medicine ... ' with the *incipit* of the preface to the *Prognostica*, and 'Videtur mihi quod ... ' with the *incipit* of this book itself, claimed that both of them correspond to an Arabic–Latin translation of this Hippocratic text by either Constantine the African or Gerard of Cremona (+1187) (Kibre, pp. 199–221: particularly, pp. 199–213). While both versions appear one after another in all the *Articella* printed editions which add Galen's commentary to this Hippocratic text, only the former (*incipit* 'Omnis qui medicine artis ... ') is reported in those editions without Galen's commentary.

23. Some unsolved difficulties also remain here in identifying the manuscript traditions reflected in these versions. TK referred the first-placed *incipit* ('Qui de egrotantium accidentibus in singulis egritudinibus tractantes ...') to that of the Hippocrataic *De regimine acutorum morborum* without Galen's commentary, and the second one ('Illi qui sententias illis de assidis relatas scripserunt ... ') to that of the same text accompanied with Galen's commentary ('Non solum cum scripserunt rememorationes ... ') according to Gerard of Cremona's translation (TK, cols 660, 922, 1205). Although Kibre suggested that 'at least one or possibly two of the variant texts found in the manuscript may, in all probability, be assigned to the well-known translator from the Greek, Nicholas de Reggio', she was unable to properly settle this second manuscript tradition. Furthermore, she seems to have wrongly ascribed 'Qui de egrotantium' both to Gerard of Cremona and to Constantinus Africanus, and identified 'Illi qui sententias' with Galen's commentary (Kibre, pp. 5–25, particularly pp. 7–18). While both versions appear one after another in all the *Articella* printed editions including Galen's commentary to this Hippocratic text, only the former (*incipit* 'Qui de egrotantium accidentibus ... ') is reported in those editions not including it.
24. Durling, 'A Chronological Census', p. 282, and *passim*; Durling, 'Corrigenda and Addenda', 23, p. 463; 37, pp. 373–4.
25. Arrizabalaga, García-Ballester and Gil-Aristu, 'Del manuscrito al primitivo impreso'.
26. Arrizabalaga, García-Ballester and Gil-Aristu, 'Del manuscrito al primitivo impreso', pp. 39–40.
27. Arrizabalaga, García-Ballester and Gil-Aristu, 'Del manuscrito al primitivo impreso', pp. 40–41.
28. French, 'Berengario da Carpi'; *idem*, 'Pliny and Renaissance Medicine'.
29. Arrizabalaga, García-Ballester and Gil-Aristu, 'Del manuscrito al primitivo impreso', p. 41.
30. For a fifteenth-century manuscript copy of this work, which accompanied Gentile's commentary on Galen's *Tegni*, book 1, see TK, col. 1220.
31. Kibre, pp. 138–142, particularly pp. 140–42; Stillwell, no. 411; C. D. Pritchet, ed., *Johannis Alexandrini commentaria in sextum librum Hippocratis Epidemiarum*, Leiden, Brill, 1975.
32. Kibre, pp. 189–91; Stillwell, no. 659.
33. Kibre, pp. 182–86; Stillwell, no. 415.
34. Thomas Rütten, 'Receptions of the Hippocratic *Oath* in the Renaissance: The Prohibition of Abortion as a Case Study in Reception', *Journal of the*

History of Medicine and Allied Sciences, 51(4), 1996, pp. 456–83, esp. pp. 461–3, 479–80. Rütten's essential work has definitely settled Nicolò Perotti's authorship of this Latin version of the Hippocratic Oath. Its attribution to the early Hellenist grammarian Pier Paolo Vergerio, *il Vecchio* (1370–1444) was not only constant in all the printed editions of the *Articella* which included it, but has also been usual until now. See, e.g., Kibre, pp. 177–82; Stillwell, no. 414.

35. Pesenti, '"Articella" dagli incunabuli ai manoscritti', pp. 135–6. For more information see above under Note 9.
36. Contrary to what Kibre indicated (see Kibre, p. 62), the version of Theodore Gaza was included in no printed edition of the *Articella* before 1502.
37. There is no trace of this aphoristic series at TK.
38. There is no manuscript copy of these *Flosculi* at TK. According to Nicolò Comneno Papadopoli, *Historia Gymnasii Patavini*, 2 vols, Venice, 1726, vol. II, p. 185, Pietro Carrerio (died 1506), medical lecturer at the University of Padua, was the author of some *Scholia in Celsum* which might be identified with the *Flosculi*. See Tiziana Pesenti, *Professori e promotori di medicina nello Studio di Padova dal 1405 al 1509. Repertorio bio-bibliografico*, Padua, Lint, 1985, pp. 67–9.
39. On this work and its Latin transmission, see Yûhannâ ibn Mâsawayh (John Mesue), *Le livre des axiomes médicaux (aphorismi) (édition du texte arabe et des versions latines avec traduction française et lexique ...)*, Danielle Jacquart and Gérard Troupeau, eds, Geneva, Droz, 1980, pp. 1–140. On the Latin version upon which this text leaned, see pp. 13–88.
40. Siraisi, *Avicenna*, pp. 132–3. On the role of the *Canon* in medieval medical teaching, see ibid., pp. 43–76. As to whether these excerpts of the *Canon* were part of the *Articella* before the printed edition of 1506, for the moment I cannot go beyond Siraisi. Very cautious on this point, she merely said that 'The *Canon* excerpts were not part of the *Articella* as it existed in the twelfth or thirteenth century, and are not found in incunabular editions of the *Articella* (ibid., p. 132).
41. See Roger French's Chapter 12 in this volume.
42. Siraisi, *Avicenna*, pp. 188, 362.
43. For medieval manuscript copies of this work, see TK, cols 727, 857.
44. Sarton, *Introduction*, vol. 1, pp. 609–10; Klebs, no. 826; Stillwell, no. 689.
45. Ernest Wickersheimer, *Dictionnaire biographique des médecins en France au Moyen Âge*, 2 vols, Geneva, Droz, 1979, vol. 1, pp. 326–7; Danielle Jacquart, *Supplément* to Wickersheimer's *Dictionnaire* ... , Geneva, Droz, 1979, pp. 134–5; Klebs, no. 331. For medieval manuscript copies of this work, see TK, cols 323, 493, 1021, 1437, 1681. On Jacques Despars, see Jacquart, 'Le regard d'un médecin sur son temps: Jacques Despars (1380?–1458)', *Bibliothèque de l'Ecole des Chartres*, 138 (1980), pp. 35–86.
46. In full, *Liber Prognosticorum Hippocratis dictus Capsula Eburnea*. On the Latin transmission of this and other treatises under this common designation, see Kibre, pp. 110–23.
47. It had first been printed in an edition of Serapion's medical works in Venice in 1497.
48. Kibre, pp. 25–8; Stillwell, no. 658.
49. Kibre, pp. 110–123; Stillwell, no. 421.
50. Kibre, pp. 94–107; Stillwell, no. 416.

51. Kibre, pp. 192–5; Stillwell, no. 660.
52. Kibre, pp. 165–7; Stillwell, no. 417.
53. Kibre, pp. 175–6; Stillwell, no. 413.
54. The *Aphorismi* sive *Parabole Universales* was traditionally known as *Parabole Medicacionis*. For a critical edition and study of these aphoristic series by Arnau of Vilanova, see Juan-Antonio Paniagua, Lola Ferre and Eduard Feliu, eds, *Arnaldi de Villanova opera medica omnia. Vol. VI.1. Medicationis parabole. Pirqé Arnau de Vilanova*, Barcelona, Universitat de Barcelona, 1990; Juan-Antonio Paniagua, Pedro Gil-Sotres, Luis García-Ballester and Eduard Feliu, eds, *Arnaldi de Villanova opera medica omnia. Vol. VI.2. Commentum in quasdam parabolas et alias aphorismorum series ...* , Barcelona, Universitat de Barcelona, 1993.
55. Durling, 'A Chronological Census', pp. 250–51, 294.
56. Kibre, pp. 199–221; Durling, 'A Chronological Census', pp. 251, 295. Actually, both of them consisted only of Galen's *In Hippocratis Prognosticum III Comm. III.*
57. This version was first published as a part of Hippocrates's *Opera* (Rome, 1525). See Stillwell, no. 406; Durling, *A Catalogue of Sixteenth Century Printed Books*, no. 2320.
58. On Michel de La Chapelle, see Wickersheimer, *Dictionnaire biographique*, vol. 2, pp. 551–2; Jacquart, *Supplément*, p. 209.
59. Durling, 'A Chronological Census', p. 282; *idem*, 'Corrigenda and Addenda', 23 (1967), p. 463; 37 (1981), pp. 373–4.
60. On this work of Leoniceno, see Daniela Mugnai-Carrara, 'Una polemica umanistico-scolastica circa l'interpretazione delle tre dottrine ordinate di Galeno', *Annali dell'Istituto e Museo di Storia della Scienza di Firenze*, 8, 1 (1980), pp. 31–57.
61. Leoniceno, 'Prefatio in artem medicinalem Galeni', in *Articella*, Venice, 1523, f. 84rb.
62. The address prefaces Leoniceno's introduction to his translations of Galen. The enemy are *neroniores*, more and worse than Nero. See *Articella*, Venice, 1523, f. 80v.
63. *Articella*, Venice, 1523, f. 84rb.
64. *Articella*, Venice, 1523, fol. 157v.
65. Leoniceno's preface to the Galen translations. See *Articella*, Venice, 1523, ff. 81r–84r.
66. Armando Petrucci, 'Alle origini del libro moderno. Libri da banco, libri da bisaccia, libretti da mano', *Italia medioevale e umanistica*, 12 (1969), pp. 295–313: pp. 297–8.
67. The quotation cames from Argilagues' postface. See Arrizabalaga, García-Ballester and Gil-Aristu, 'Del manuscrito al primitivo impreso', p. 30.
68. Petrucci, 'Alle origini del libro moderno', pp. 298–9.
69. Petrucci, 'Alle origini del libro moderno', pp. 308–12.
70. Lowry, *The World of Aldus Manutius*, pp. 142–3.
71. Pesenti, 'Editoria medica tra Quattro e Cinquencento', pp. 25–8.
72. Walter Rüegg, 'Epilogue: The Rise of Humanism', p. 467.
73. *Articella*, Lyons, 1527, fol. 1r.
74. *Articella*, Pavia, 1506, signat. ii8r.
75. On the aphoristic genre in medicine see Paniagua, Gil-Sotres et al., *Arnaldi de Villanova Opera Medica Omnia. Vol. VI.2*, pp. 241–4, and the bibliography cited there.

76. French, 'Teaching Aristotle'.
77. See Arnau de Vilanova, *Repetitio super Vita brevis*, Bayerische Staatsbibliothek Ms. Clm 14245, fol. 31r (ed. Michael R. McVaugh). Quoted by Paniagua, Gil-Sotres et al., *Arnaldi de Villanova Opera Medica Omnia. Vol. VI.2*, p. 244.

CHAPTER TEN

Epidemics and State Medicine in Fifteenth-Century Milan

Ann G. Carmichael

Giovanni Catelano died in 1497, five hundred years ago. In medical circles he was known well only in Milan, but there he was prominent enough that advisers could beg Duke Ludovico Sforza to pay a visit to him before he died.[1] Through his involvement in civic projects advanced by Ludovico's father, the great Renaissance warlord Francesco Sforza, Catelano allied his training in medicine with the interests of early modern state building. The civic death registers of Milan are the primary witness to Catelano's dedication, and to the evidence of an important way that recurrent plague epidemics effected profound medical changes in urban Europe. Although Catelano died just before the French disease offered further challenges to a stable Galenic view of disease, the evidence of this Milanese physician's diagnoses of causes of death illustrates that new diseases were already a troubling feature of the late fifteenth-century medical world. Moreover the casual but necessary process of assigning an official cause to deaths privileged anatomical localization with attention to either the body's surface or to the patient's story.

Giovanni Catelano's name appears in 1452, linked to the first three cases of the earliest surviving register of the Milanese *Necrologi*.[2] A fierce and costly plague was ending, but the death registers stalwartly recorded details of each new plague death. Catelano reported a newly infected household on Friday, 21 July: an 18-year-old woman named Caterina fell ill on 19 July, and now evidenced a pestiferous 'dragonzello' or bubo in her left groin. At the 'Locus Montanee' (a temporary pest house)[3] a 29-year-old woman died of a pestiferous *dragonzello* in the right groin, by Catelano's judgement on 17 July. Finally, this day he also reported that in the convent of St Euffemia, 50-year-old Lucia, wife of lord Alesio Aliprandi, died from 'anthrax' in the left hip, of the pestiferous kind, according to Catelano's judgement on 13 July.

These earliest records do not always clarify the various dates involved, that is, the point at which Catelano actually made his inspection of the ill person, or the cadaver – nor if, in fact, he personally viewed the body rather than simply talked to one who had seen the deceased.

Instead the entries primarily seek to provide information about the length of time a person was incapacitated by illness, the place of residence (including both household and parish) and the primary cause of death. In this last component Catelano offered extraordinarily detailed observations: a case was not merely plague, but plague because a bubo (and not just any swelling but a 'pestiferous' one) bore witness to the underlying cause. Ambiguous evidence, such as 'anthrax' – probably referring to a blackened or discoloured skin lesion over the hip – is preserved in the report and left as a presumptive plague diagnosis. Catelano here and elsewhere meticulously notes the side of the body on which a lesion was visible. In other words, the information that Catelano provided, in this case to the clerk of the office that kept these registers, well exceeded local statutory requirements for cause-of-death reporting.[4]

Catelano probably arrived in Milan at the time Francesco Sforza seized control, for his name is first recorded in 1450 as a 'foreign' member of the prestigious College of Physicians.[5] Sforza favoured doctors in his retinue and quite a few were able to join this exclusive Milanese body during the 1450s. By the end of the century, no non-native physicians would be allowed in; by the 1530s even prominent native sons such as Girolamo Cardano would be refused if their social qualifications and connections were questionable.[6] The college controlled formal access to patients in Milan, thus collected fees and protected their long-standing privileges within the city even as their actual public responsibilities diminished. Catelano's career in 'public' health – his lifelong involvement with the *Sanità* (as the health office came to be called), his services to the existing hospitals, and his practical involvement with the early development and use of the *Ospedale Maggiore* (called the *Ca' granda* or great house) – is in many ways a testimony to his social distance from the native Milanese physicians of the college. When he worked with other physicians in making a diagnosis, it was typically either the surgeon of the *Sanità*, Dionysio of Nursia, or the duke's physicians, who were not usually hired from the local talent.

The college had nevertheless ensured their own relationship to the cause-of-death surveillance with civic statutes requiring that reporting and acting upon the reports of dangerous illnesses not be left to poorly educated healers. Milanese college physicians were university graduates (by this time almost exclusively from Pavia), were further examined and licensed, and then underwent a period of traineeship, with mandatory consultation (thus fee-splitting) with established senior collegians if an illness appeared dangerous. In addition to reporting causes of death, collegians had to be called to the patient's bedside if an unofficial healer's care exceeded three days. The system had obvious economic advantages, but equally obvious and unpleasant responsibilities in risky plague times. Most members of the college were away from Milan in 1452, while the plague still stalked new households.

In a typical entry of the fifteenth-century *Necrologi*, the sector of the city, identified by closest gate, the deceased's name and age – sometimes reported in days or hours if a newborn – and the parish church, appeared along with a cause of death. Burial of individuals older than two years at death required a written report of a cause of death, in every year, whether or not plague threatened. Occasionally the length of time a person was ill found mention in the reports, either linked to a plague diagnosis (because the illness and death were acute and unexpected), or to a firm refusal of plague suspicion (because the illness had lasted long and was all too expected). With most diagnoses the name of a physician appeared, to claim both credit and responsibility for the judgement.

Between 1452 and 1497, the years Catelano was active in Milan, surviving records attest his responsibility for a quarter to a third of all diagnoses of cause of death in the city (see Table 10.1). Many records are now missing, in part because a fire at the *Sanità* on New Year's Eve, 1502/03, claimed them, but even so Giovanni Catelano reported 12 065 deaths. In only twelve of these reports did he (or the clerk) fail to supply a diagnosis. In 13 per cent of the deaths that he reported, Catelano provided four or more primary or contributing causes of death. His successors – even as late as the nineteenth century – were never so meticulous nor concerned with much more than monitoring feared diseases. Table 10.2 shows the principal diagnoses of cause of death reported by Catelano, excluding the plague years, 1483–85.

Catelano lived an inglorious, work-centred life, often housed in properties controlled by the rich hospital trustees, who in turn worried that they might not be asking enough in return for their largesse.[7] Every major epidemic to hit Milan during his 45-year career found Catelano on the front lines – one of the few university-trained physicians to undertake the thankless task of surveillance, and survive. One plague year, 1468, he had to defend and justify nearly every decision that he made, because declarations of plague interfered with the elaborate summer marriage plans of Duke Galeazzo Maria Sforza.[8] In his reports Catelano described many trips, both pre-and post-mortem, to the lodgings of individuals who may have had plague. He looked over the bodies of victims for signs of the feared infection, and he clearly probed surviving family members or other doctors for details of the patient's sufferings. Catelano and other physicians were accused of stealing from plague victims; and his diagnoses and methods were challenged by the new, tyrannical, 22-year-old duke. The death of Catelano's housekeeper

Table 10.1 Catelano and Death reports,* 1452–1494

Year	Total deaths reported	Catelano's reports (%)
[1452] §	831	304 (36.5)
1453	787	252 (32.0)
1459	1 249	451 (36.1)
[1469]	1 626	656 (40.3)
[1470]	1 228	507 (41.3)
1471	1 556	660 (42.4)
1472	1 711	658 (38.5)
1474	1 677	612 (36.5)
1475	1 653	589 (35.6)
[1476]	1 873	696 (37.2)
[1477]	3 775	1 493 (39.5)
1478	2 878	716 (24.9)
1479	2 198	649 (29.5)
1480	1 927	529 (27.5)
[1481]	702	211 (30.1)
1482	2 394	621 (25.9)
1487	1 424	307 (21.6)
1488	1 515	265 (17.5)
1489	2 100	301 (14.3)
1490	1 986	326 (16.4)
1491	2 200	427 (19.4)
1492	2 083	399 (19.1)
1494	2 564	436 (16.6)

Notes:
* There are additionally scattered reports from years with fewer than 500 deaths reported.
§ Brackets [ ] indicate years for which surviving *Necrologi* are not complete.

from plague made him a plague suspect, so he had to walk the familiar streets with clear and visible indication that he himself was a source of contamination to others.

Three times during Catelano's half century at work in Milan bubonic plague appeared in the city: 1451–52, 1468 and 1483–85. The 1468 plague was quite mild in comparison to the other two plagues. Plague had a minor, cameo role again in 1506–07, and in the war-torn years of the early 1510s. Before 1450 the last great plague was in 1400–02; the next monstrous epidemic after 1485 levelled the city in 1524. Thus Catelano's life in service coincided with two punishing plagues in

Table 10.2 Diagnoses of Giovanni Catelano, non-plague years: percentage of all diagnoses coded (n = 20 917)

Diagnosis	Number	%
Continuous fever	2 640	12.6
Hectic fever	2 170	10.4
Other fevers	3 525	16.9
[Acute fever]	46	0.1
Chronic fever	620	3.0
Pleurisy	442	2.1
Catarrh	526	2.5
Asthma	488	2.3
Phthisis	278	1.3
Pneumonia	178	0.8
Dropsy	450	2.2
Cachetic, emaciated	344	1.6
Old age	475	3.9
Flux, diarrhoea, and dysentery	1 176	5.6
'Worms'	444	2.1
Chronic illness	220	1.1
Measles	486	2.3
Smallpox	95	0.5
Plague	184	0.9
Fistulae	246	1.2
Ulcers	92	0.5
Epilepsy	383	1.8
No diagnosis given	12	0.1

Milan, and he was primarily engaged in public service during both epidemics. His first-hand experience with two great plagues was atypical.

Modern demographic analysis of these later fifteenth-century plagues in Milan focuses on the cycles of war, famine and plague that moderated mortality as well as governmental response to crises.[9] In some ways little changed during this period because Milan had long before developed a state-of-the-art surveillance and management system in plague control. Compared to her neighbours, even among the advanced northern Italian city states, Milan was typically first in creating government offices dedicated to gathering information about plague occurrences outside and inside its domain, first in designating locations to which plague suspects, plague victims or the homeless were transported during epidemics, first in employing (usually by the Dukes of Milan) physicians who maintained that plague was a contagious disease best confronted with controls that minimized contact between the ill and the well.[10]

The overall effect of sustained governmental control of plague was, by 1450, a focused and dedicated health office derived from the earlier 'officials in charge of bulletins' (*officiali delle bollette*). Reports came to both the senate and to the duke.[11] Information was gathered at the parish level, and typically monitored both illnesses and deaths; permission to bury a body was linked to reporting. Probably as early as the 1430s, and certainly by the time of Francesco Sforza this system no longer relied exclusively on the parish elders for conveying information.[12] Rather, the College of Physicians asserted the value of its professional stature and expertise, as well as its justly privileged role in monitoring state health. When the physicians of Milan became associated with a humdrum, routine surveillance system that was becoming widespread in northern Italy is unknown – possibly many of the Visconti records now lost held some clues to their assertion of interest and privilege.[13] Whatever the reason they were incorporated into this sphere of civic activity, physician contributions to the record-keeping added a unique element to the civic death records in Milan. Here physicians reported causes of death for all individuals, not simply for disputed or worrisome cases. The health office consequently had to cope with and make sense of the massive amount of information that a physician-inclusive reporting system produced.

The *Necrologi* begin well after the worst of the current plague had passed. Plague was at a peak from July to September 1451, and the best-laid plans to minimize epidemic losses by shipping first the homeless, then plague victims and their families away from the city to Cusago (they were taken along a great canal to a villa 6 miles west of Milan) had failed.[14] The 'Locus Montanee', along the perimeter of the city to the southwest was hastily constructed to house more sufferers; monasteries and little-used hospital properties were conscripted as well. Even so, temporary cabins of wood and straw appeared outside all the gates of the city almost as mushrooms after a rain. Reacting to plague as an environmental problem, health officials focused on creating spaces where its effects could be circumscribed, diligently spending communal funds for transporting victims, burying the dead, and sanitizing abandoned dwellings.[15] Military and political advisors who wrote to the duke similarly tended to emphasize the spatial and familial relationships of putative plague victims.[16]

Physicians viewing cases and places one at a time instead focused on the outward manifestations of putrefactive processes within the bodies of victims. For example, there was the case of a 25-year-old retainer of one of the duke's associates. Two physicians working with the *Sanità* in 1468 reported that the man died of a 'draconzello in Inguine dextro' – a bubonic swelling in his right groin – but one due to ulceration of the area after application of constricting medications. The putrid matter reversed, that is it travelled inward rather than brought peccant material to the surface as intended, and this in turn caused a 'proportional tertian fever'. Their diagnostic reasoning excluded the possibility of plague, despite an acute swelling in the groin area.[17]

The pathological processes at issue here were central to Hippocratic–Galenic medicine. Leaving aside discussion of the predisposing causes of humoural imbalance, once that balance was disrupted the natural healing process was to expel putrefying humours through a variety of different mechanisms. An aposteme, roughly what we might describe as an abscess, represented localization and consolidation of putrefying humours. Naturally any one of the four humours could putrefy, so not all apostemes were the same. It also made a considerable difference in a patient's prognosis where the aposteme originated.[18] If too close to the heart, as happened with fulminant plague, the vital spirits generated by the heart could be overwhelmed and undermined, resulting in the patient's swift demise. A less precariously positioned focus of putrefaction could channel the aposteme's formation to one of the 'emunctories' or outlets for corrupted humours. (We generally associate clusters of lymph nodes with some of the principal sites of the emunctories, though no such anatomical correlation was made in the fifteenth century.) The axilla drained superfluities of the heart; excess or corrupted humour in the liver exited to the groin; putrefaction of humours in the brain led to an aposteme in the neck or behind the ears.[19]

Bubonic plague presented an anomaly to medical authorities. On the one hand it was clearly associated with a continuous fever that could not also be characterized as hectic (involving the solid parts), ephemeral (involving the spirits) or putrid (involving the humours). Pestilential fevers came from breathing corrupted air, which generated excess heat in the heart and surrounding region, suppressing the vital spirit.[20] On the other hand, buboes were a dramatic clinical feature in epidemics of plague, and buboes were understood usually with the term 'aposteme'. Unfortunately buboes and pestilential fevers could have different etiologies.

During the late fourteenth and fifteenth centuries, physicians were unwilling to assume that the plague was a 'new' disease, neither seen nor understood by Galen and Avicenna.[21] First they did not view diseases as entities but as humoural imbalances. Secondly, their predecessors had offered so thorough and overarching a synthesis of human pathophysiology (i.e., the description and explanation of disease) that it was difficult to wrest free and reconfigure discrete clinical phenomena.

Observations about apostemes and about fevers were based on centuries of logically elegant, clinically sophisticated observations.

Chase examined 25 plague treatises written by the medical faculty at Montpellier, a leading medical centre, between 1348 and the mid-fifteenth century, and found that medical educators increasingly differentiated pestilential fevers from 'apostemic diseases' by seeing some apostemes as caused by specific but invisible poisons.[22] The poison could be inspired, just as corrupted air incited pestilential fever, or it could be adsorbed in other ways. In the plague cases, internal apostemes were formed which then sought an exit at the emunctories. They thus hypothesized a material cause to plague swellings that might in turn resemble other non-plague apostemes.

The consequence of this idea was twofold. 'Pestilential fevers' became in theory distinguishable from glandular plague, permitting individuals who carried a less stigmatized diagnosis an escape from the increasingly severe public health protocols during plagues. Secondly, 'apostemic' diseases included both plague and non-plague categories, so that even the sudden appearance of a bubo did not necessarily mean that the plague poison was at work; appearances on the body's surface could deceive. To distinguish one kind of aposteme from another required either a detailed clinical history or some physical means of differentiating among swellings in the emunctories. The clinical history helped to distinguish the original, inciting events, and thus whether the swelling was an 'accident' (a following, consequential event) from humoural disturbances, or was a primary cause (expanding, redirecting poisonous matter). The poison theory also permitted an explanatory model for 'contagion', or spread of the plague through contact.

Caught in this diagnostic nexus, physicians in Milan during the late fifteenth century honed their clinical and anatomical skills to meet the demands of evolving state medicine. The best and most direct example I have found comes from 1468, when the commissar of the *Sanità*, Hector Marchese, confronted Catelano and other college physicians about their failure to diagnose plague early enough in the course of an illness to make segregation of plague victims and suspects straightforward. Marchese wrote to the duke the answer that he received:

> in the beginning they neither know nor could have known from the urines [alone], because they do not visit the sick nor touch them ... ; so they report only such-and-such fever. In time the situation changes and the urines appear subjugated and pestilential, and only then do we learn who has plague; only then can we next determine who visited the sick and who touched whom.[23]

The duke and his commissars sought unambiguous evidence, and tended to privilege signs read directly from the body, if necessary, postmortem. Then, at least, all discussion and doubt about the clinical prognosis was over. When new cases of plague occurred despite effective sanitary management, individuals were seen to 'throw out' or expel the signs of pestilence from their sequestered, hidden sites within their bodies.[24] Likewise the health officials expelled the infected from the body of the city. In September the duke's spies tracked down a young boy who roguishly escaped, only to die in the suburbs. The duke ordered the local constable to refuse burial until a team could get out to the place and view the body. 'Then,' the Duke Galeazzo Maria Sforza told Hector Marchese,

> we'll know the extent to which it was a suspect death, and whether we have to take further precautions. I tell you that at the Pillastrello, which is along the road and just opposite the church [where the boy was found] someone will be waiting for you to inform you about it all.[25]

Building a permanent lazaretto – an emunctory to drain the putrefactive plague stricken away from the heart of the city – was the firm intention of Galeazzo Maria and his councillors. The issue was decided by a will and architectural plans, given to the city in the midst of plague.[26] After 1468 the next important epidemic in Milan coincided with a famine sweeping over most of northern Italy. Not only was this epidemic not a plague epidemic, evidenced in retrospect by its slow but steadily rising mortality rates, but the deaths did not involve many teenagers and young adults, as was common in Milanese plagues. Giuliana Albini has elegantly analysed the demographic differences between this epidemic and the plague of 1483–85 that followed.[27] As others noted before, the principal symptoms reported make this mortality most likely one of epidemic typhus fever. To show what that meant to a stable health department relying on bodies to betray hidden contagion alongside physicians eager to assist their paying patients from an over-zealous application of draconian plague controls, I offer one long case report filed by college physician Matteo dei Busti:

> 23 March 1479. Concerning the case and the judgement of Donato di Giochario, on the Saturday just past, in the morning when he wanted to get out of bed, where he had remained since the preceding Friday, he was seized by a fainting spell, with diarrhoeal flux [caused] by corrupt yellow bile. Summoned that morning, I applied some cordials and other stomach remedies and he quieted, such that at the hour of vespers when I visited him again he told me he had rested well even with the shortness of breath he had, and he ordered dinner and syrups for the following day, which was Sunday. Then that morning I visited him and he said he had slept well and slept through the night. The urines were fully laudable although he was assailed by fever, and after a full meal he seemed to rest well. Then he confessed

his sins and in the evening took a bit of *phthisana ordeaca* and having a little coughing when he wanted to sleep, the whole night could not rest. His fever rose sharply during the night such that by morning his urine was turbid and, in the upper part, livid. Seeing this I said that this was a bad sign, showing the mortification of natural heat. And when he wanted to eat he began to vomit, choked by some part, though he did retain a small part, probably even a whole dish. And then in the evening of this same day, Master Absalom and I came again. We saw the urines were of very small quantity, were turbid, and his evacuations were corrupted diarrhoea, whence we began to suspect measles [*morbilis*] or other signs. And so, bringing the candle to the bedside, we saw a great quantity of red measles. Holding his pulse from that hour all the way until he had a remission, we judged him to be almost moribund. And these things all took place from Sunday evening until Monday vespers, whence Master Absalom and I deliberated together about this case and decided that this was a continuous choleric fever with a great quantity of venomous matter generated close to the heart, and with red signs of the type which appeared with that fever of 1477, from which [people] died quickly because the great quantity of [putrefactive] matter and its proximity to the heart accelerated death. Knowing these things I, Matteo, made a denunciation to the lord deputies, and even to Hector [Marchese] lest any evil arise in the city and so that they would send Catelano before [the patient] died. With all our might we [tried to report] to the deputies ... the judgement we had made about the appearance of what we had found in [Donato's] axilla. The servants, his sisters, and his wife, who all knew about this thing, said that he had extra flesh there for more than twenty years, though it was presently enlarged. Not knowing whether or not this was so, I debated to myself whether to believe his wife and sisters that the swelling was long-standing, because that Monday, the day he died, I witnessed his sudden decline, the livid urines, and manifold signs. I asked him if he was in pain anywhere and he answered not once but six times that he didn't hurt anywhere except his head, and that for the entirety of this illness he had had pain in his stomach and chest such that he thought he was suffocating, and that elsewhere he was not suffering. Thus he had no pain in any other place, neither in that aposteme nor elsewhere, of recent origin. Because this fever can signify its sudden alteration or steady resolution by such pain, and especially with a choleric aposteme, thus it must have been that this swelling not only was not contracted with the malady [i.e., the present illness] but also that if it had been it would have been accompanied by pain. That he was not suffering there nor even felt this matter [in the axilla] and because [the area] was continually intact [*boni intelectur*], thus it seemed to me that this aposteme was not resultant from the present illness but was an old lesion, because the overlying skin and its natural color had changed. Thus, by these reasons I say that I was unwilling to doubt Donato's story and even that I had full confidence: neither the aposteme nor the pain issues escaped me – By the judgement of Matheo dei Busti.[28]

In late fifteenth-century Milan it was commonplace to allow the appearance of a patient's urine to guide the physician's diagnosis, prognosis and therapy. And so in this heatedly argued case, a university-trained physician defended his judgement that he did not suspect his patient suffered from plague or any other dangerous disease until the man's urine became cloudy and discoloured (probably 'livid' meant it was blood-tinged). Observing that, he and a colleague moved closer to the patient for a look at the skin, where the by-products of a putrefactive process would also be registered. At this point they saw the 'measles' or red blotches, not well described in the testimonial. In the process they also saw a worrisome lesion under his arm. They concluded first that they were in no danger, that is, that this was not plague and, second, that they had seen the particular form of measles before – in 1477. Matteo dei Busti and Absalom were resolutely convinced that this was not plague, because in seeing the measles we must conclude that they had removed Donato's garments, making visible the swelling in his left axilla; they probably touched him.

Their eyes and ears meanwhile were being sharpened by the vital need to distinguish plague from non-plague. While they acknowledged that choleric fevers could also produce apostemes, they relied on the family's testimony that the lesion was not recent. When called to account for their faulty diagnosis – the reason this report was written – they further argued that the appearance of the skin overlying the affected axilla, as well as the patient's clear and repeated testimony that he did not feel any pain in this part, showed this was not plague. They argued that he surely would have complained of the swelling had this been a plague bubo. Instead he suffered a splitting headache and continued gastrointestinal distress – nausea, vomiting, diarrhoea. The fever of 1477, the one this 'choleric fever' recalled to the attending physician, had been a killer, for the same basic (humoural) reason that plague killed swiftly: putrefaction close to the heart.

Notified of the case, Giovanni Catelano went to see for himself, taking with him the young surgeon of the *Sanità* with whom he had worked closely for at least eight years.[29] They saw instead a restless, disoriented man, fearful and near death, with 'purplish and black measles from toe to top, and with a notable bubonic swelling, discoloured and corrupt, in the left axilla'. (Typically Catelano noted the side on which the swelling occurred; Matteo did not.) They examined the corpse three hours after death finding it 'much worse than before', and decided that this was plague and that the patient lied about being ill before Saturday (3½ days before his death), when he had summoned Matteo.

Time appeared to vindicate their official diagnosis of plague. On 1 April, Donato's 20-year-old son died, ill six or seven days in the sequestered house, and his body revealed 'five blackened pustules [*antracibus*] over his shoulders and back, with a slight pestiferous rash'.[30] Eight days later, a 36-year-old female servant, one of the people testifying earlier to the antiquity of Donato's bubonic swelling, died with a measly rash and a bubo in the groin. Finally, Donato's 85-year-old mother died 19 April, however, of 'senile debility'.

Fever accompanied by a rash, headache and delirium, together with a resemblance to the fever of 1477, all suggest the retrospective diagnosis of typhus fever. The epidemic quickly acquired a vernacular name in Lombardy, 'mal mazzucco', a popular defiance of the authority embedded in physicians' neat, Galenic explanations. While the regions south of Bologna tended to merge all illnesses into a generic diagnosis of 'plague' during these years, in Lombardy, the Veneto, and the Piedmont of northern Italy, the fever of 1477–79 was not plague.[31] Moreover, many claimed the disease was new, unfamiliar to practitioners. In fact twenty individuals in Milan during the late spring of 1478 – for relatively few records survive to document the severe epidemic of 1477 – died with what the doctor's described as 'puntilli' or lesions resembling pinpricks.[32] Girolamo Fracastoro would later characterize these lesions as typical of typhus or 'lenticular' fever – a rash resembling lentils – in his classic work *On Contagion and Contagious Diseases*.[33] In addition to the evidence of chroniclers, there is ample support in the Milanese records for deaths from typhus. We could count hundreds of deaths as related to an epidemic of typhus fever if we included the deaths from non-pustular rashes, headaches and 'alienation' (probably referring to delirium), never mind the fact that the 'choleric' fever was the only symptom most would notice, probably even then as a refinement of the more typical continuous fever. See Table 10.3.

Table 10.3 Selected diagnoses of cause of death reported from August 1477 to December 1478 compared to three non-epidemic periods

Diagnosis	1477–78	1470–72	1480–82	1487–89
Continuous fever	2 567	729	731	579
'Acute' fever	213	21	216	78
'Choleric' fever	85	1	10	8
'Measles' or 'red measles'	707	51	18	9
'Alienation'	61	10	17	3
'Urines' reported	178	1	5	1
'Worms' and 'flux'	451	146	235	139
[Total deaths reported]	10 625	5 954	7 333	6 651

In other words, the narrative description of Donato's last illness by Matteo dei Busti can be neatly and forcefully assimilated to a retrospective diagnosis of epidemic typhus fever, but just as easily the corporeal evidence provided by Catelano could lead us to a retrospective diagnosis of plague. It is not important to resolve the matter. Rather the point is that the problem of plague control for urban health departments on the one hand, and individual physicians diagnosing individual clinical cases on the other, elicited both anatomical–pathological evidence visible pre- and post-mortem, and begged full, storied attention to the different meanings that could be attached to bodily signs. The historical timing of the controversy, defining and understanding a new non-plague epidemic in the 1470s and 1480s, places it contemporary with the proliferation of anatomical studies in northern Italy, and to the curious search for wondrously hidden signs of disease or sanctity in the bodies of recently dead individuals.[34]

Matteo dei Busti's reflections on a later case, during the waning months of the great plague of 1483–85, show how the traditional medical diagnosis of plague in Milan continued to challenge simple determinations from physical, post-mortem findings. Physical evidence for plague or non-plague affliction was linked to urinalysis. Thus on 2 June 1485, Matteo reported that

> Margarita, wife of Francisco da Campo, 30 years old, was being cared for by Master Niccolò da Niguarda, when in the fullness of her infirmity she had a continuous fever that came to the point of alienation [or mental confusion], and her urine was sent to me. It was confused at the base, but tended toward clear, or possibly white and confused, as I judged by the rising of the material to the top. I ordered those coming to me that they should see whether or not *morbilli* (measles) were present. First they said that some had appeared, afterwards that they had not. Instead the disorientation had not ceased, from which I predicted from all that I could gather, that she was suffering from *carabito* or a sudden parafrensy, and would either die or begin to recover on the seventh day. As I understand from their account, two days later, on the seventh day, she died.
>
> [Presumably the next was added to the original report to the scribe:]
>
> In the judgement of Matteo dei Busti the above Margarita might have been cured by her doctors if her illness had been recognized earlier. It was questioned whether their decisions were true or, at least, reasonable. We, however, saw her corpse with a certain swelling in the right groin, which could have resulted from something other than plague, as from a crisis or strong accident of the spirits. In the judgements of Catelano and Dionysio.[35]

Possibly a rash, certainly mental disorientation and the appearance of a bubo all in a plague year – the right signs for the *Sanità* and yet this case was not judged to be plague. Moreover, the foundational judgement was made on the basis of a flask of urine and the testimony of servants who had both cared for Margarita and carried her urine to the prestigious physician. Three collegians (Catelano himself, Matteo dei Busti, and Niccolò da Niguarda) and the health department's surgeon agreed about the cause of death.

Urine flasks were a familiar sight to fifteenth-century patients.[36] Basically, whatever issued from the body permitted conclusions about the state of the internal, invisible humours. Most of the body's fluids became critical indicators of the processes under way within, and it was not possible for there to be a serious imbalance of the humours without the urine reflecting the pathology. The flask itself was hefty, usually called a matula or 'jordan', and it held a good quantity of urine in order to give the physician who analysed it ample knowledge of the patient's condition that could not be acquired otherwise. The flask had a bowled, full bottom, a short, narrower neck, that rapidly curved out again to contain the 'circulus' or head of the flask. Sediment collected on the bottom (*fundus*), other substances floated to the top, and colour and overall consistency revealed the humour responsible for a patient's illness.

One also read the flask anatomically, as if the matula were a totem of the patient's body, once it contained her urine. The bottom sediment revealed problems in the lower half of the body including the genitals, the middle region showed the state of vital organs such as the liver and spleen (the *substantia*) or the heart and lungs (*superficies*). The top revealed the head's condition, including both sentiments and sensorium, thus matter rising to the top of Margarita's urine flask mirrored her disordered state of consciousness.[37] Turbidity in the urine belied incomplete 'digestion' or 'coction', the process by which digestive tract and liver converted food into healthy, nourishing humours.

For medieval physicians extensively trained in the subtleties of all possible permutations of urinary odours, colours, consistencies and inhering solids, the purpose of diagnosis was to understand the underlying pathological process in individual patients. The subject's age, sex, social station (from which both nutrition and activities could be understood), influenced understanding of urinalysis. So what was causing Margarita's confused urine? In the account, Matteo was obviously looking for 'measles', mental alienation, 'parafrensy', and *carabito* as companion indicators of the character and severity of the underlying humoural imbalance. They were all phenomena produced in the same logical way the urine became an indicator, and they allowed him to anticipate a 'crisis' in her condition, at which point she would either die or begin a fitful recovery. This time for Catelano and Dionysio, the swelling in the right groin was subsequently understood in the same way, that is, produced in the course of her body's desperate effort to expel the putrefying humour.

The mutability of the urine, while it could be defensibly seen as a sensitive clinical indicator of the patient's course of illness, was effectively undermined as a robust and reliable indicator of plague and, hence, as useful evidence for a cause of death. Moreover, since physicians in Milan were by this time convinced that plague was contagious, urinalysis was not only ambivalent information, it logically should have prompted questions about the dangers presented by urine and other body products.

Reports about urines disappear from the *Necrologi* in the late 1480s. In fact, in most respects detailed arguments about the patients' last sufferings disappeared in the wake of Milan's next, catastrophic bubonic plague. As the plague crept into Milan, Catelano valiantly applied the standard methods of medical diagnostics, as these cases illustrate:

> 9 September 1483. A new case. Margarita Pagani, 55 years old, died of a continuous fever with measles. On the fourth day of her illness she had confused urines, and she died on the sixth day, according to Master Baptista Bernadigio. She was seen post-mortem and found with various measles and two plague pustules, one on the right, the other on the left, between the neck and the humerus, in the judgement of Master Dyonisio, confirmed by Catelano. *Plague.*

> 24 September 1483. A new case. Ambrogio, son of Martino Plenio, 20 years old, died after about 4 days ill. He was found dead, with violet and lead-coloured measles on his sides. In the judgement of Catelano and Dyonisio, however, there is another judgement as [provided] below. Ambrogio, son of Martino Plenio, 20 years old, died from continuous fever with one reddish sign on his tibia, because he got in a fight with someone outside the city and was pressed up against a gate. In the judgement of Master Bertolo Syroni. *Visited by our doctors and found to have plague.*

> 19 October 1483. Zacharina, daughter of Antonio Nizia, 7 years old. Yesterday at 24 hours when she was eating at a tavern (*locus potus communi*), she unwittingly consumed mercury (*aqua argenta sublimata*) mixed with wine. She immediately became agitated (*cepti anxiari et inquietari*), was nauseated, and had other accidents stemming from the ingestion of mercury and other extrinsic poison. Considered post-mortem, she was found to have signs of poison ingestion, such as a blackening of the tongue and palate, [but] with a notable, partly blackened swelling in the groin that was ascribed to ulcers in the fingers on that side. In the judgement of Master Giovanni Catelano.[38]

But the magnitude of the plague overwhelmed even Giovanni Catelano. Albini emphasizes three features of the 1483–85 plague. First, it was proportionately less costly in lives than any of the fourteenth-century epidemics, but even so overall mortality reached the 10 per cent level, and the population to confront it was already thinned by a decade of famines and fevers. Secondly, the patterns of mortality by age and sex were characteristic of Milanese plagues, with 5- to 25-year-olds suffering the highest mortality levels, females dying more than males. Thirdly, the health office dramatically intensified its policing agency and its conflation of control and order with public health maintenance.

These systems of reporting deaths reflected an impressive bureaucratic efficiency for so brutal a plague. Records kept of deaths occurring inside sealed houses were automatically assumed to be plague deaths, but otherwise all were counted by name, age, parish and sector. On most days 100 or more deaths (females again dying more frequently) were added to a few cases judged as non-plague. Similarly a register of deaths and recoveries was made at the temporary pest house outside the Porta Orientale. Finally, the duke received notification of new cases each day, a mix of deaths and illnesses verified.[39] Of 51 individuals listed on 8 October 1485, for example, eight were reported by the surgeon Dionysio of Nursia; all of the rest were reported by Catelano.[40] All the individually noted new cases provided the specific bodily evidence of plague, whether bubo, *glandula, dragonzello, tumore* or *antracibus*, the site and the side of the body, and the accompaniment of other signs, such as red or black 'measles', pregnancy, or fever. Diagnostic standards did not fall, but neither did the plague relent.

Albini's analysis of this plague reveals that until the full force of the plague arrived in August, 1485, over 60 per cent of the individuals sent to the lazaretto survived. After that point the record-keeping was suspended, and health conditions worsened there. Entire families were relocated, with disproportionately high numbers of women and children confined because the male heads of household had died or fled. Suddenly economically marginal families became targets of mixed public assistance and public control. Up until the murderous phase of plague their chances of survival in the lazaretto were enhanced, for control in the initial fear-driven stages undoubtedly confined many who were not infected. At the same time food and reasonable hygienic amenities protected many of the poor. But in the brutal months of August, September and October minimal assistance slipped toward maximal control. Those confined to their own houses had a better chance of surviving.

Shifting our own gaze from the minutiae of diagnosing apostemes, rashes and urines, to the global costs of a dramatic urban plague is to make the adjustment Catelano made every minute of these months in Milan. Effectively the health office, together with the duke and his advisers, determined and decided what physicians saw. Controlling the spaces in which plague could be observed enhanced the verification of plague as a contagion. More directly the directors of the *Sanità* applied pressure when necessary to confirm their model of the causes of pestilence. To the duke one wrote 8 December 1485 that the health deputies and members of the duke's Secret Council met in the Castello to discuss what more they needed to do to eradicate plague. Each deputy took a sector of the city, going house to house personally to observe the state of cleaning and purging, and burning objects that had touched plague. They believed that the only reason that plague still existed was that either goods and cloths had not been adequately handled or judgements about causes of death were falsified. A mandatory meeting the next morning of 'those few doctors who can be rounded up' would select two to review all their judgements.[41] With the strength of such corrective lenses Catelano and others doubtless began to see contagion as a diagnostic feature equal to the body's wounds or the patients' stories.

In early 1486 Count Galeotto Bevilacqua died without male heir, so the conditions of his uncle's will in 1468 could finally be applied to the building of a lazaretto (see Figure 10.1). The will imposed two changes on the original plans, which envisioned a vast structure at some distance from the city. The pest house would claim permanently the nearby location at San Gregorio, and the city had to commence building within two years. The architect-engineer's plans were quickly subjected to a group of physicians, who debated the potential this locale had for spreading plague back into the city with the winds or by wicked inmates. Wisely bending to the will of the state, physician advisers concluded that the proposed plans included rooms that retained most of the vapours of plague.[42] When such did escape through the high windows, they would be rectified by the heat of the sun by day and mist of the stars by night. Moreover, placed northeast of the city, the lazaretto would receive, rather than pass along the putrefactive western winds. They praised the plans for a double water source, carrying polluted water away from the city and its canals. All in all, it was a proper asylum for the poor plague-stricken.

From this point on, I believe, much of the collegiate physicians' tedious advisory work was over. The health office's duties separately matured in a brave new world of focused cause-of-death assessment and focal isolation of plague. The one-time medical contributors to Milanese state medicine retreated to what Guido Panseri has described as a 'corporate refuge'.[43] Elite college physicians, as Catelano had been, gradually withdrew their presence and voice from the routine surveillance of causes of death. A tabulation (Table 10.4) of the diagnoses of Catelano's successor, Antonio di Arona Catelani, points out the general

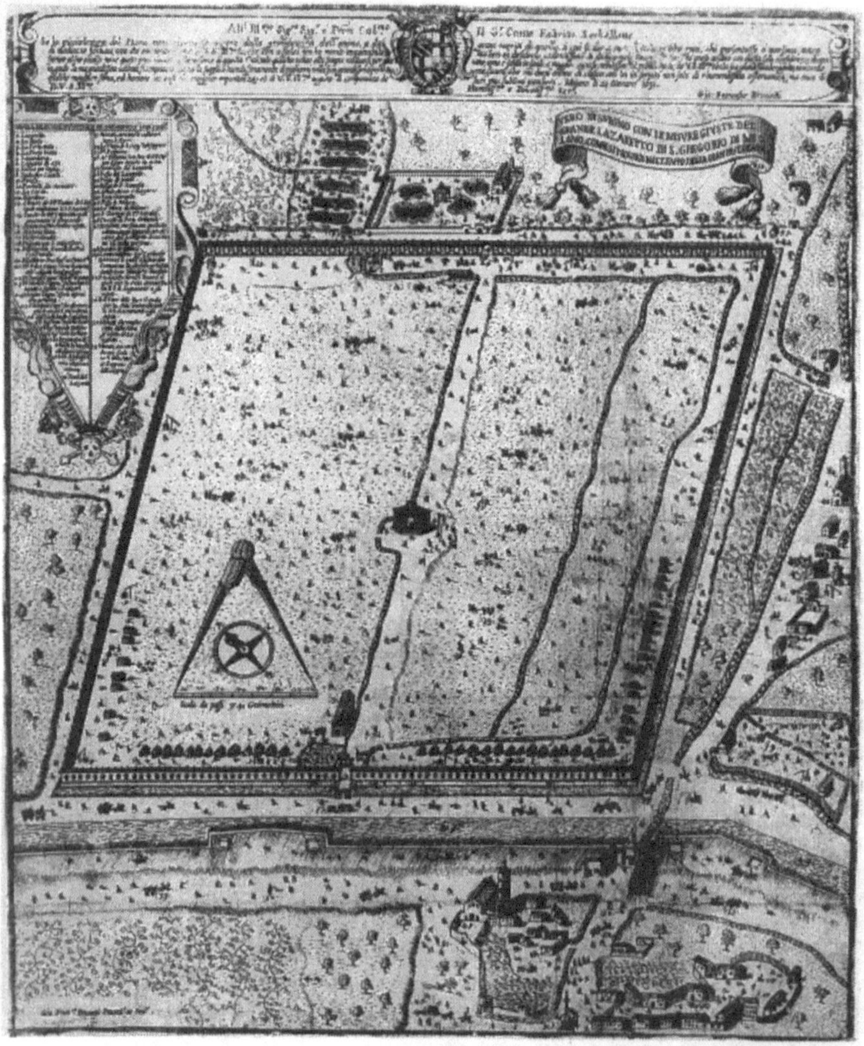

10.1 The Lazaretto of Milan (1488) in 1630; an immense hollow square of 288 contiguous cells with an octagonal church in the middle. By permisson of Civica Raccolta delle Stampe Achille Bertarelli, Castello Sforzesco, Milan.

direction of change. From the surviving register of 1503 until the massive, unfolding plague of 1523–24, Antonio provided 20 917 diagnoses. While there are no dramatic differences in his diagnostic habits during these two decades when compared to Catelano's years, Antonio was almost eight times more likely to report a non-specific 'chronic illness' as

Table 10.4 Causes of death reported by Antonio di Arona Catelani, 1503–1522: percentage of all coded diagnoses (n = 20 917)

Diagnosis	Number	%
Continuous fever	2 981	18.6
Hectic fever	880	5.5
Other fevers	482	2.9
[Acute fever]	46	0.3
Chronic fever	463	2.9
Pleurisy	208	1.2
Catarrh	404	2.5
Asthma	395	2.5
Phthisis	552	3.4
Pneumonia	24	<0.1
Dropsy	522	3.2
Cachetic, emaciated	90	0.6
Old age	301	1.9
Flux, diarrhoea, and dysentery	578	3.7
'Worms'	116	0.7
Chronic illness	1 234	7.7
Measles (red)	239	1.4
Black or purple measles	613	3.8
Smallpox	75	0.5
Plague	796	5.0
Fistulae	205	1.3
Ulcers	89	0.6
Epilepsy	588	3.7
No diagnosis given	12	0.1

the cause of death than was Catelano; Antonio spent less time discerning types of fevers; Antonio never reported the evidence of urinalysis. What the tables by comparison do not reveal is the extent to which the *Sanità* became far less concerned with official, medical diagnosis of accidents, trauma and wounds in general. In the period after 1500, and only then, the nameless certifier 'in the public judgement' (*iudicio publico*) appears in the records whenever street battles led to deaths.

Statutes relevant to the health office were revised in 1534, after the plague of 1523–24, and the pan-Italian famines and fevers of the late 1520s. Collegiate physicians retained their privilege of adjudicating causes of illness and death, but the statutes now allowed an alternative, the 'surgeon of the *Sanità*'. Additional clauses, such as 'no physician may touch the ill until after the fourth day of the physician's first visit', suggest protective legislation for the physicians, rather than the imposing, restrictive state others have noted about the health office's expanding powers over medical corporations.[44]

Dante Zanetti sampled the annual *Necrologi* data from three centuries: 1503, 1616, and 1783. The first of these years, as we have seen, occurs after the intensive burden of diagnosing cause of death had been transferred from the collegiate doctors to a health department. Over the course of three centuries the basic format of reporting did not change.[45] Throughout the sixteenth and early seventeenth centuries, the descriptions of various maladies varied considerably from one diagnostician to the next. Individual physicians seemed to have favourite diagnoses. Some of the variation appeared to depend upon the rapport of the physician with the patient or his/her family before death, or upon the dominant medical preference for either Galenic or Hippocratic diagnoses. But overall, the early period had the greatest number of different diagnostic formulations; complexity and variance among diagnoses decreased over time. In 1606–07, two additional years Zanetti studied, there were 34 physicians reporting causes of death, plus one surgeon employed by the *Sanità*: In 1606, 2 886 deaths were reported; 4 020 in 1607. Over 77 per cent of all the reports were made by one poor surgeon, a fellow who of necessity and economic constraints submitted the 'briefest and most schematic of diagnoses'.[46] He was 48 times more likely to report 'epilepsy' or 'fever and epilepsy', 25 times more likely to cite merely 'long illness'; 51 times more likely than the collegiate physicians to report simply 'newborn'.

Because Zanetti remained convinced that in later years the data more faithfully represented a modern reality of causes of death, he was most impressed that in the later centuries fewer individuals escaped the diagnostic process altogether (18.5 per cent of the entries had no accompanying cause in 1503; fewer than 1 per cent did in 1616; and there was virtually no entry without a cause supplied in 1783). The 'progress' evident in the records was not medical, but bureaucratic – that of the state's enforcement of reporting and, by the eighteenth century, the suppression of the importance of individual diagnosticians. A greater absolute value thus accrued to the diagnoses themselves, which had, in his view, an increasingly more sophisticated, less 'symptomatic' medical formulation wherever they did not report specific diseases. To reinforce this argument, Zanetti noted the steady increase in the diagnostic category 'acute fever', which displaced the complex Galenic classification of fevers.

At the same time the prestige and well-being of collegiate physicians did not suffer from their distancing themselves from public health opportunities for a steady income.[47] Instead the increasing interest they assumed in detailed clinical narratives seems to have offered them expert status in advocating the exemptions their privileged patients required.[48] Increasing state controls over the poor during epidemic times created new needs for patients and physicians within privileged medical settings. This tacit separation of spheres of activity even during dangerous epidemic times gave élite university physicians good reason to expand the role of narrative in medical practice. At the same time the health office could pursue a corporeal model of diagnosis, more evident, less negotiable, and in perfect harmony with their strategies for confining the poor and the ill.

Acknowledgements

Research for this study was sponsored generously by the National Endowment for the Humanities, RH–20835–87. I would also like to thank Leah Shopkow and Michael McVaugh for helpful comments on parts of this paper.

Notes

1. Archivio di Stato di Milan [hereafter ASM], *Miscellanea storica*, 2, letters numbered 594 to 603.
2. ASM, *Fondo Popolazione*, parte antiqua, reg. 73. The general contents of the *Necrologi* are described by Emilio Motta, 'Morti in Milano dal 1452 al 1552', *Archivio storico lombardo* [hereafter *ASL*] 18 (1891), pp. 241–86. In general see Carlo M. Cipolla, 'I libri dei morti', in *Le fonti della demografia storica in Italia*, vol. 1, pt 2 (Rome, CISP, 1972), pp. 851–952; and Dante Zanetti, 'La morte a Milano nel secoli XVI–XVIII: appunti per una ricerca', *Rivista storica italiana* [hereafter *RSI*] 88 (1976), pp. 803–51.
3. Carlo Decio, *La peste in Milano nell'anno 1451 e il primo lazzaretto a Cusago* (Milan, Coglieti, 1900), p. 23; Giuliana Albini, *Guerra, fame, peste: crisi di mortalità e sistema sanitario nella Lombardia tardomedioevale* (Bologna, Cappelli, 1982), p. 122.
4. A. Bottero, 'I più antichi statuti del collegio dei medici di Milano', *ASL*, n.s., 8 (1943), pp. 72–112; and A. Francesco La Cava, 'Igiene e sanità negli statuti di Milano del sec. XIV', *Collano di studi di storia della medicina*, diretta da N. Latronico, vol. 3 (Milan, Hoepli, 1946), pp. 21–89.
5. Sforza made appointments to the health office one of the first orders of business. Governing élites in every Lombard city were in charge of an office relaying information. In Milan the office proper in 1451 consisted of a commissar in charge, a 'medico fisico' [already Catelano?], a surgeon, a barber, a notary, and service personnel – two horsemen, three servants, a person to carry the lists, a cart driver and two gravediggers.

See Albini *Guerra, fame, peste*, pp. 29–30, and p. 90. The earliest documentation I have found regarding Catelano in Milan is printed in Decio, *La peste in Milano*, p. 30n: Catelano attended the secretary of the Duke's Secret Council. On the College of Physicians and Milanese physicians generally see Luigi Belloni, 'La medicina a Milano sino al Seicento', in *Storia di Milano*, vol. 11, pt xii, (Milan, Treccani degli Alfieri 1958), pp. 597–646 for the extensive section on physicians.

6. Cardano, of illegitimate birth, was eventually admitted. On Cardano see Belloni, 'La medicina a Milano', pp. 628–32; on the general point, see Richard Palmer, 'Physicians and the State in post-medieval Italy', in Andrew Russell, ed., *The Town and State Physician in Europe from the Middle Ages to the Enlightenment*, Wolfenbütteler Forschungen, Band 17 (Wolfenbüttel, Herzog August Bibliothek, 1981), pp. 47–62, here, pp. 51–3.
7. On the Ospedale Maggiore in general see Salvatore Spinelli, *La Ca' Granda* (Milan, 1958); A. Francesco la Cava, 'Le scuole medico-chirurgiche dell'Ospedale Maggiore di Milano', *Ospedale Maggiore*, 44 (1956), 157–74; and G. C. Bascapé, 'L'assistenza e la beneficenza a Milano dall' Alto medio evo alla fine della dinastia Sforzesca', in *Storia di Milano*, vol. 8, pt iv, pp. 391–420.

   Catelano's remuneration and obligations appear in the *Deliberazioni* of the Ospedale Maggiore's archives, especially in registers, 2, 3 and 4 (1456–69). Register 2, f. 47v, 6 March 1458, applauds Catelano's service: 'Attenda etiam eius modestia et patientia, qua visus est'. But by the late 1470s, Catelano was deemed too busy with general civic tasks, and the directors moved to sever his connection to the hospital; see *Deliberazioni*, reg. 6, f. 24v and f. 59r (November 1477).
8. For discussion of the progression and importance of this plague in Milanese history see A. G. Carmichael, 'Contagion Theory and Contagion Practice in Renaissance Milan', *Renaissance Quarterly*, 44 (1991), pp. 213–56, here p. 224.
9. G. Albini, 'La mortalità in un grande centro urbano nel '400: il caso di Milano', in R. Comba, G. Piccini, and G. Pinto, eds, *Strutture familiari, epidemie, e migratione nell' Italia medievale* (Naples, Edizioni scientifiche italiane, 1984), pp. 117–34, here summarizing and extending her *Guerra, fame, peste*.
10. Richard Palmer, 'The Control of Plague in Venice and Northern Italy: 1348–1600', PhD thesis (University of Kent at Canterbury, 1978), pp. 27–45; and Carlo Cipolla, *Public Health and the Medical Profession in the Renaissance* (Cambridge and New York, Cambridge University Press, 1976), pp. 14–18.
11. Albini, *Guerra, fame, peste*, pp. 81–90.
12. Antonio Pasi Testa, 'Alle origini dell'Ufficio di Sanità nel Ducato di Milano e Principato di Pavia', *ASL*, 102 (1976), pp. 376–86; and Albini, *Guerra, fame, peste*, p. 89. Surviving legislation refers to the *commissario sul'offitio della conservazione della sanitade de Milan e del Ducato*.
13. Albini, *Guerra, fame, peste*, p. 86, cites 1438 proclamation that all illnesses had to be reported to parish elders if the patient was in the care of a collegiate physician. Moreover, every 'medicus, ciroychus, barberius, herborarius' must send notice in writing of patients in his care. The ordinance was reconfirmed in 1447.

14. Albini, *Guerra, fame, peste*, pp. 72–5; Decio, *La peste in Milano*. The 'Locus Montanee' became the site of the Ospedale Maggiore, begun in 1456 and opened to patients by 1476.
15. ASM, *Miscellanea storica*, 3, no. 332, 23 October 1451: 'sotteratori et speciatori et nettegiatori de le case et casse morbose non uscino ne prseumano uscire fuora et partirsi da li suoy loci ordinati ... '. If they were in public spaces, they had to wear 'el signo ordinato de la croxeta' on both the front and back of their garment, so that the well could recognize them at a distance.
16. For example, ASM, *Miscellanea storica*, 2, 2 October 1463, from Bellinino at the Castello in Cotignolo to Francesco Sforza. Eight days before in the house of Andrea Porto

    > outside the walls, but abutting the castle, two died of *morbo pestifero*, the which was not known until yesterday, when a cousin of this Andrea, in his household, died and the case was thus revealed as pestiferous. I commanded the said Andrea that he and his whole company in the household must clear out of the area.

    The dead woman's kinsmen, however, first begged to let them bury her at the castle, and when Bellinino refused, said they would bury her 'whether or not I permitted, because I was of little threat'. Negotations with a local priest to find suitable burial space failed, and the confrontation degenerated into a full test of power, Andrea's company winning.
17. ASM, *Carteggio interno*, 1468, dated 5 August: 'Emanuel famulus dni. Uberti de Flisco [decessit], annorum xxv a draconzello in Inguine dextro propter ulceratione propoltii (?) ex indebita applicatione medicinarum constrictinarum. Reversa est materia putredi ad Intus. Et sic causata est febris tertiana continua proportionale sine suspectu. Iudicio Magistri Stephani de Trivultio et Dionysii de Cerutis cirugici.'
18. E.g., Baverio Baviera's [d. 1480] recommendations to poor men:

    > Ma se pur ad alcuno sopravenisse la infettione et si ammorbasse o havendo fatto le cose dite o non si debbe considerare dove sia lo apostema se ello appare. Perche molte siate e ammorbato l'huomo et non li appare apostema essendo lo apostema o antrace overo bubone overo carboncello overo ademenul overo giandula o codesella o chiamala come tu voi. Et non se maraviglia alcuno se io non distinguiro al presente la cura della giandola dalla cura del carbone o dalla cura dello antrace o altra apostema. Ne delli carboni generadi da diversi humori piu adusti e manco adusti fra si. Ni ancora da humore corrosivo o non corrosivo; perche communamente non sono medicate queste egritudine da persone che sapesse distinguere simile cose. Ma sotto una generalita metero la cura perche tutti communicano in questo che sono venenosi et hanno bisogno o di tutte o di parte de le cose che se diranno

    originally published in 1478; reissued, *Trattato mirabile contra peste composto per ... misser Bavera ... Uno conseglio famoso promulgato a Venesie contra la peste* (Bologna, 1523), f. 12v.

19. Bloodletting was deemed the most effective intervention, but the site from which blood was taken depended upon the original anatomical site of the aposteme (whether visible or invisible at the bedside); and it depended upon the length of time the patient had been ill – for example, drawing from the same side as the lesion was more appropriate early in an illness. See Pedro Gil-Sotres, 'Derivation and Revulsion: The Theory and Practice of Medieval Phlebotomy', in L. García-Ballester, R. K. French, J. Arrizabalaga, and A. Cunningham, eds, *Practical Medicine from Salerno to the Black Death* (Cambridge, Cambridge University Press, 1994), pp. 110–55.
20. On the speciation and pathology of fevers, especially from the putrefactive process, see Iain M. Lonie, 'Fever Pathology in the Sixteenth Century: Tradition and Innovation', *Medical History*, suppl. no. 1 (1981), pp. 19–44.
21. On medieval medical diagnosis in general and physicians' reluctance to see plague as a new disease, see Nancy Siraisi, *Medieval and Early Renaissance Medicine* (Chicago, Chicago University Press, 1990), pp. 123–33; and Jon Arrizabalaga, 'Facing the Black Death: perceptions and reactions of university medical practitioners', in García-Ballester et al., *Practical Medicine from Salerno to the Black Death*, pp. 237–88.
22. Melissa P. Chase, 'Fevers, Poisons, and Apostemes: Authority and Experience in Montpellier Plague Treatises', in Pamela Long, ed., *Science and Technology in Medieval Society* (New York, Annals of the New York Academy of Sciences, 1985), pp. 153–69.
23. This translation is freer than the version I supplied in my 'Contagion Theory and Contagion Practice', p. 245. The text of the letter, in ASM, *Miscellanea storica*, 2, no. 70, 5 June 1468, is provided there. Giovanni Simonetta, much closer to the duke than Hector Marchese, repeated the explanation 23 June 1468; now in the ASM, Sforzesco, *Carteggio interno*, no. 844.
24. E.g., ASM, *Miscellanea storica*, 1, no. 229, 22 May 1468 'hebbemo noticia de una Jacomina nominata nel iudicio qua incluso quale in moret *butoe* il signo pestifero ... ', emphasis added.
25. ASM, *Carteggio interno*, 885, 2 September 1468.
26. Luca Beltrami, 'Il lazzaretto di Milano', *ASL*, 8 (1882), pp. 403–41; and Pietro Canetta, *Il lazzaretto di Milano* (Milan, 1881). The specific idea was presented in a 10 August 1468 letter to the duke. Notary Lazzaro Cairati offered his idea and design for an enormous structure (26 hectares) to be built in Cresenzago, like Cusago at some distance from the city. Cairati and his engineer partner, Elia Reina, envisioned a structure rivalling the Duomo, the Castello and the Ospedale Maggiore. While these plans never materialized, and are now lost, in October 1468 the property that would become the lazaretto site was left to the city in the will of Count Onofrio Bevilacqua, should his sole heir die without male issue. Bevilacqua's heir died childless in 1488.
27. Albini, 'La mortalitá in un grande centro urbano nel '400', in R. Comba, G. Piccini and G. Pinto, eds, *Strutture familiari, epidemie, e migratione nell' Italia medievale* (Naples, Edizioni scientifiche italiane, 1984), pp. 117–34.
28. ASM, *Miscellanea storica*, 2, no. 420, 23 March 1479.

29. Ibid.:

> Postscript: The aforesaid Donato was considered in life, though scarcely living, having almost succumbed with the restlessness and disorientation fearing death, and with purplish and black measles throughout from toe to top [*a calce usque ad apicem*], and with a notable bubonic swelling, discoloured and corrupt, in the left axilla. Returning to him three hours after his death, I examined him again, finding the body much worse than before. The illness began, as was said, on last Saturday, sickening from choleric [fever], for he could have lied and claimed to have been [recently released from other fevers?] ... by the judgement of Catelano and Dyonisio.

30. The present case represents the common use of the term in the fifteenth century, to refer to 'pestilential pustules'; for a case resembling modern anthrax (Milan, 1492), see Gonario Deffenu, 'Storie cliniche del passato', *Castalia*, **11** (1955), pp. 75–7.
31. Alfonso Corradi, *Annali delle epidemie occorse in Italia*, 5 vols (repr. Bologna, 1974), vols. 1, 4 and 5, *ad annum*. And see Anna Maria Nada Patrone and Irma Naso, *Le epidemie del tardo medioevo nell'area pedemontana* (Turin, Centro studi piemontesi, 1978), p. 49, for brief discussion of 'mal di friole'. The chronicle of Tommasino Lancellotti of Modena, spanning the period from 1480 to 1530, shows that the name 'male mazucho' was in continuous use, that 1528 was an epidemic year of this disease, and that it had yet another popular name, 'el begon'. See Corradi, *Annali*, vol. 1, p. 394.
32. Corradi, *Annali*, vol. 1, pp. 319 ff.

> L'anno 1477 ... la Petecchia penetrò in Italia, e penetrovvi quando i Turchi fecero sanguinosa irruzione nel Friuli, e della quale già abbiam tenuto parola. Ma se dir non puossi donde e quando que' barbari pigliassero cotal morbo, ci conforta almeno, soggiunge l'Omodei, il pensare, che si può negativamente determinare l'epoca storica della petecchia presso altre nazioni, dal non incontrarsi in nessuna di queste verun documento che essa regnasse in un periodo antecedente a quello di cui si tratta.

Ficino's 'Consiglio contro la peste', written in the late 1470s, describes the petecchiae, however as part of the special plague symptoms that year ['subita debilità di polso, gravamente di tutta la persona, massime di capo, farnetico, scorticamenti, arsioni, sete, macchie di sangue in vari luoghi, orina grossa et torbida ... ' quoted in Corradi, *Annali*, vol. 1, pp. 320–21], as well as chroniclers [the anonymous of Parma, and Jacopo Melga of Brescia, who report the name of 'mal mazzucco']. Giusseppe Ferrario, *Statistica medico-economica di Milano*, 2 vols (Milan, 1840–50), vol. 2, p. 38, also summarizes the contemporary evidence: 'da alcuni registri dei morti in Milano rilevasi che dall'anno 1477 al 1478 qui si ebbe una grande mortalità per *Febbre Petecchiale*. In molti certificati di morte trovansi le seguenti parole: *Obiit ex febre cum morbilis rubeis, violatis, fuscis, morelis, etc.; cum pontilis nigris, etc.*'.

33. In 1546: *De Contagione et Contagiosis Morbis et Eorum Curatione, Libri III*, trans. and ed. W. C. Wright (New York, Putnams, 1930), 100–103.
34. See Katharine Park, 'The Life of the Corpse: Division and Dissection in Late Medieval Europe', *Journal of History of Medicine and Allied Sciences*, [hereafter *JHM*], 50 (1995), pp. 111–32; *idem*, 'The Criminal and the Saintly Body: Autopsy and Dissection in Renaissance Italy', *Renaissance Quarterly*, 47 (1994), pp. 1–33; L. R. Lind, 'Introduction', *Studies in Pre-Vesalian Anatomy* (Philadelphia, American Philosophical Society, 1975), pp. 3–19; and Jerome J. Bylebyl, 'Interpreting the Fasciculo Anatomy Scene', *JHM*, 45 (1990), pp. 285–316.
35. 2 June 1485: ASM, Fondo popolazione, reg. 77, at the date'.
36. Antonio dal Canton and Maria Castellano, 'Theory of Urine Formation and Uroscopic Diagnosis in the Medical School of Salerno', *Kidney International*, 34 (1988), pp. 273–7; Lorrayne T. Baird, 'The Physician's "Urynals and Jurdones": Urine and Uroscopy in Medieval Medicine and Literature', *Fifteenth-Century Studies*, 2 (1979), pp. 1–8. In general see Siraisi, *Medieval and Early Renaissance Medicine*, p. 125.
37. If heated, urine containing protein will turn cloudy. See Meryl H. Haber, 'Pisse Prophecy: A Brief History of Urinalysis', *Clinics in Laboratory Medicine*, 8 (1988), p. 417. However, few of the accounts would lead one to the optimistic conclusion that the urine studied was 'fresh'. Thus cloudiness of the urine may well reflect bacterial growth.
38. ASM, *Fondo popolazione*, reg. 77, at the dates.
39. ASM, *Fondo popolazione*, reg. 76 and 77.
40. ASM, *Miscellanea storica*, 1, no. 613.
41. ASM, *Miscellanea storica*, 2, no. 521, Thomas Torniellis to the duke.
42. Beltrami, 'Il lazzaretto di Milano', pp. 407–13; and Canetta, *Il lazzaretto di Milano*, pp. 7–9. The latter includes few physicians on the committee, however; only Ambrogio Rosati, at that point head physician of the Ospedale Maggiore, was an official medical member. Élite, citizen representatives from each sector of the city consulted with unnamed physicians; Govanni Giacomo da Vaprio, commissar of the *Sanità*, and deputies of the Ospedale Maggiore foundation were also members.
43. Guido Panseri, 'La nascità della polizia medica: l'organizzazione sanitaria nei vari stati italiani', in *Scienza e tecnica nella cultura e nella società dal Rinascimento a oggi*, Storia d'Italia, Annali, vol. 3 (Turin, 1980), 155–96.
44. Nicola Latroncino, 'La medicina e l'igiene nei libri e nei documenti del Magistrato di Sanità dello stato di Milano', *Atti e memorie dell' Accademia di Storia dell'Arte Sanitaria*, ser. 2, a. 4, n. 6 (1938), pp. 273–92; and Palmer, 'Physicians and the State in Post-Medieval Italy', in Andrew W. Russell, ed., *The Town and State Physician in Europe from the Middle Ages to the Enlightenment*, Wolfenbütteler Forschungen, vol. 17 (Wolfenbüttel, Herzog August Bibliothek, 1981), pp. 47–62.
45. Dante Zanetti, 'La morte a Milano nel secoli XVI–XVIII: appunti per una riceras', *RSI*, 88 (1976), pp. 803–51.
46. Zanetti, 'La morte a Milano', pp. 819–20.
47. Palmer, in 'Physicians and the State', makes this point well.
48. Nancy G. Siraisi, 'Girolamo Cardano and the Art of Medical Narrative', *Journal of the History of Ideas*, 52 (1991), pp. 581–602, supplies an authoritative overview of the use of narrative in clinical texts of the late Middle Ages and Renaissance, illustrating the growing interest in

Hippocratic texts, typically for their narrative style, with a case study of Milan's Girolamo Cardano. I would only add that cause-of-death diagnoses were effectively a form of medical, clinical narrative outside the text tradition that Siraisi examines.

CHAPTER ELEVEN

Coping with the French Disease: University Practitioners' Strategies and Tactics in the Transition from the Fifteenth to the Sixteenth Century

Roger French and Jon Arrizabalaga

Introduction

Among the many threats to health in the late Middle Ages, the French Disease was distinctive. Since the disastrous advent of the Black Death in 1348 there had been epidemics of greater or lesser impact and of different diseases, the most recent of them (although confined to the north) being the English Sweats. Most of these diseases were acute and when fatal killed quickly, in days or sometimes hours. But although the French Disease spread rapidly, it was a lingering disease. It is true that some very early reports of the French Disease's arrival attributed to it a high mortality, but a few years' experience soon showed that it was a chronic disease, condemning its victims to years of pain. It was also a disfiguring disease, which cut its sufferers off from normal social lives: the civic reaction to the disease was as much about clearing the streets of victims disgusting to look at as about medical help. There is a parallel with leprosy – indeed many medical men at first argued that it was a form of leprosy – and it carried a similar social stigma.[1]

The sufferers turned wherever they could for help – to the Church, to unlicensed practitioners, some with specific remedies, to surgeons (with or without university training) and to university-trained physicians. It is from the last group that we have most evidence for the medical reaction to the French Disease (prayers, surgery and specifics leave little written trace of themselves). Communities, too, reacted to the disease with measures directed towards prevention and care. They, too, turned to medical sources in order to take appropriate action, and the university-trained physician figures large as a source of advice.

This chapter seeks to understand that disaster historically; that is, to reconstruct as far as possible how the disease was perceived and what actions were taken. In other words the identity of the disease is for us the fifteenth- and sixteenth-century identity: we are not in the least concerned with arguments about 'syphilis' and whether it was pre- or post-Columbian. Syphilis is a modern concept, giving false explanatory power within history by the success of the germ theory of infectious disease in the nineteenth century. This attached the ontology unshakeably on to the infective organism and gave historians of medicine a powerful hindsight that has proved difficult to remove. We shall not call the disease 'syphilis' but 'the French Disease',[2] as a translation of the very generally used *morbus gallicus*, and we shall examine how it was seen in its first years.[3] Our chapter will be mostly focused upon university-trained practitioners' strategies and tactics in the face of the French Disease during the late fifteenth and early sixteenth centuries.

Renaissance perceptions of the French Disease

To highlight the difference between the modern understanding of syphilis and fifteenth-century understanding of the French Disease let us begin with an aspect of the French Disease that is not now familiar. Although it is still sometimes possible to catch a flavour of a moral perception of illness when a disease is thought to be due to bad habits or even poverty, we do not now think in religious terms about disease. In the fifteenth and sixteenth centuries, in contrast, the divine origin of the disease was fundamental to perceptions and reactions to it. The doctors had a professional reason for declaring that their own business was only with secondary causes, but nothing they wrote could be construed as denying the reality of the first cause.

For lay people, great and small, it was not that the disease had religious 'significance', as we might be tempted to say, but that it was a religious event. In 1495 the emperor Maximilian thought that the disease was God's punishment for blasphemy.[4] Or at least that is what he thought until he caught it himself, when his mind turned to how it could be cured. (The delegation he sent to make enquiries about how the guaiac wood was being used in Spain and Portugal reported back to his chancellor, Cardinal Matthew Lang, at the end of 1517.) At about the same time (before the end of the fifteenth century) the court physician to the dukes of Ferrara, Coradino Gilino, thought that the French Disease was a divine punishment especially for Italians.[5] In fact the court at Ferrara and the disputation staged there is a useful case study in perceptions of the French Disease. Let us take a brief look at it.

Some mood of millenarianism was abroad in Italy as the year 1500 approached. In the 1490s there were floods, pestilences, famines and earthquakes.[6] These reached a height as Charles VIII of France invaded Italy and effectively changed the nature of life in the city-states.[7] The rivers flooded, it was exceptionally cold, famine and disease were everywhere, and when the French went, they left behind the French Disease. It seemed that something was fundamentally wrong. Prodigies appeared. The Virgin Mary appeared miraculously on 2 January 1496 announcing famine and war to come. Lesser persons prophesied worse events. In Rome pope Alexander VI presided over penitential fasts. In Ferrara the new order of friars of St Lazar urged the same course of action. The pious duke, Ercole d'Este, complied, nervous too of reports of a monster seen on the banks of the Tiber.[8]

By the middle of 1495 Ercole had become a fervent follower of the Dominican Girolamo Savonarola, who saw himself as God's envoy to warn Italians of their critical position in the eyes of God. Ercole with Savonarola behind him set about reforming Ferrarese society. Severe measures were taken in respect of blasphemy and of a variety of crimes related to sexual activity.[9] But in 1496 rumours were abroad of a new scourge, the disease the Italians called the *mal francese*. Before the year was out, the disease was in the court. During 1497 Ercole's daughter and daughter-in-law died from other, different, causes. Between 1497 and 1499 at least three of Ercole's sons had become its victims.[10] It must indeed have seemed that Savonarola had been right and that God's vengeance had been enacted.

Not only was the disease seen primarily as divine retribution, but it was perceived as the disease of St Job. His disease, too, had been sent by God and was unknown to man; both were incurable and of long duration. It was incurable because God had given it and only God could take it away. The cult of Job was strong by the end of the fifteenth century; and when on the advice of his physician the stricken Alfonso d'Este cut off his hair, it was an enactment of the story of Job at his crisis. It was to Job too that was dedicated the religious confraternity that Ercole gave a patent to in 1502 – later ratified by the new duke Alfonso in 1505 – to collect funds for the establishment of a hospital for the victims of the French Disease.[11] The model of Job's afflictions allowed a double interpretation of the French Disease. On the one hand it could be argued that the disease had been sent by God to innocent people as a test of their faith; this is perhaps what Ercole preferred to think. On the other the disease was soon perceived as connected with sinful sexual practices, one of the very things that Savonarola had warned them all about. Undoubtedly in that case one characteristic of the French Disease in terms of lay perceptions was that it was a moral stigma. Everyone knew that the Este court was riddled with the disease; but only outsiders named it or suffered from it.

Problems

When the French Disease appeared, many different groups of people became involved and each had their own problem. The general reaction by those uninfected was one of fear and disgust. Their problem was to avoid infection and the sight of the infected. The biggest problem of course was that of the victims. They wanted desperately to find a cure for their frightful disease. The poor had the special problem of finding the price of a potion from an unlicensed practitioner or a fee for an apothecary or surgeon, and the rich had the problem of finding the best physician. While the rich could be treated at home, the poor could not afford it. Nor were there suitable hospitals to house them. Earlier hospitals, meeting the problems of their own time, were largely places for victims of acute disorders, where they died, were cured or got well quickly, thus manifestly using charitable support efficiently. City authorities became worried about the spread of the disease and sought medical advice. Some of them maintained a city physician, whose duties included treating the poor without a charge.[12]

The growth of corporations was a characteristic of Europe during the period covered by this book, and their involvement in medicine is a change characteristic of the medicine of the time. The learned and rational physician owed his power to the university faculty, a comparatively recent institution at the time of the Black Death. The professional medical colleges and their relationship with the faculties were also comparatively recent, and in England came into being only after the French Disease. Confraternities based on religious models and concerned with the spiritual and physical health of the poor sick appeared in Italy in response to the French Disease; and special hospitals were built for those ill with the 'incurable' French Disease. The hospitals were staffed partly by physicians or surgeons, and as charitable institutions dependent on private and public funds they became a characteristic feature of medicine – another change within its structure. The hospitals' problems were to secure funding for administering expensive medicines to very many poor patients.

The learned physicians of the faculties and colleges were in a difficult position. They had for two centuries or so consolidated their position at the top of the medical ladder, arguing that their medicine, being rational and learned, was the best. They claimed a monopoly of practice of internal medicine, at least where the power of the *studia generalia* and professional colleges was enforceable. They accordingly licensed other practitioners at an appropriate level. It was an extremely important part of their professional code not to use empirical remedies, for these were used by unlicensed practitioners on a basis of either experience or fraud. Of its nature an empirical remedy had no justification in reason or learning, the two principle characteristics of university medicine. The physicians also claimed that their craft subsumed that of the apothecary and surgeon, and asserted their right to examine and license them. But it was professionally important – it was ethical – not to associate with apothecaries or surgeons and not to practise their trades: the learned and rational physician had to be socially, intellectually and financially superior.[13]

Their difficulty was that they were suddenly faced with a huge and disastrous epidemic. They were being pressed on all sides for help, from patients and cities. Yet the disease was unknown. It did not have a proper name. Within the rational and learned system it was therefore without identity. It was not possible to read about it or argue about it. That did not worry the unlicensed, who did not rationalize about their empirical treatments or specifics. The surgeons were trained to deal with appearances, like the pustules and ulcers that appeared in many diseases as well as the French Pox, and lack of precedent in the literature was less important for them than for the physicians. Apothecaries too claimed a knowledge of what substance was good for which appearance, like pustules and ulcers. Part of the physicians' difficulties was that one of the distinguishing features of the disease was the reluctance of its symptoms to disappear.[14]

The physicians thus had two pressing tasks. They had to respond to the calls made upon them. They had to maintain the professional *status quo* at a very disturbing time and when the unlicensed and lower levels of practitioner had every justification for claiming the disease as their business. The French Pox was in addition often seen as a cutaneous disease, manifested in the pustules and ulcers, and thus a traditional disorder within the surgical realm. Above all, then, the physicians had to make the disease both a rational and a learned business in order to bring it into their professional preserve and so maintain their claim that they alone had an understanding of it, and also the authority that came from both rational understanding and ancient writings. Only in this way could they keep their part of the tacit agreement with the civic authorities that allowed them a monopoly of practice and higher fees on the grounds that their medicine was better for the public. Undoubtedly they believed that it was better, and we need not doubt that their motivation was also humanitarian and pious.

To achieve their aims the physicians had certain resources they could turn to, certain strategies they could adopt and certain conditions that limited what they did. These three things give shape to this chapter.

Resources

University practitioners first had to give the French Disease a proper name. This meant identifying it with something within the medical literature, so that its nature, its causes and treatment could be discovered. In doing this they were in fact medicalizing the French Pox, bringing it into the culture of the university-trained physician. Even at the level of giving it a name, the mechanisms that kept the physicians as a coherent profession came into play, for it would be a technical name, one that related it to parts of the medical apparatus but which impressed and rather confused outsiders.

The resources available within the medical literature for naming a disease were considerable. Some argued that names did not matter, for the important thing was the essence of the disease. Others held that real names signified the essence and it was accordingly important to get them right. Others again thought that a meaningful name would allow the disease to be 'capitulated', that is, put into the right 'chapter' of Avicenna's scheme of classification of disease. 'Establishment' physicians were inclined to do this; it was partly a device to seek advantage over the empirics by having an 'official' medical name for the disease. To press home the advantage such physicians called their practice 'canonical'. By this they meant proceeding by a series of rules that embodied the rationalism and learning of their medicine, but it also implied the importance they gave to Avicenna's *Canon*. Other physicians qualified their practice as 'methodical', to express the rules of properly conducted practice and to recall the importance of the *Methodus Medendi* of Galen.[15]

An alternative way of medicalizing the French Pox was to argue that it was a new disease. It was then necessary to construct a new name for it. This would be taken from parts of the literature where something similar seemed to be described. A compound name could provide access to different parts of the literature to better fit the perceived characteristics of the disease. It is striking that almost all authors of the late fifteenth and early sixteenth centuries in fact gave very few characteristic features of the disease. Most of their surviving works are not clinical descriptions written for the purpose of identifying the disease, but are addressed to people who knew very well what it was. There are two important corollaries to this. First, the disease was recognized in practical terms by those less-qualified practitioners mentioned above who were greater in number but produced less historical evidence than the physicians. The disease had a word of mouth reputation that identified it to patients and practitioners of all kinds, and it must be this that we mean when we try to see through the writings of the learned physicians. Second, we cannot hope to try to identify the French Pox with a modern disease.

So, to give the French Pox a formal name, new or old, was to gain access to the technical stock in trade of the rational physician, his traditional learning. The main resource for the learned and rational university physician was the apparatus of medical theory. This was largely Galenic at root. Although sometimes respected less than Hippocrates, Galen was seen as the great commentator on Hippocratic medicine who had explained the master's terse wisdom on the basis of a natural philosophy that was mostly Aristotelian in nature. The learned physician thus had at his fingertips an apparatus whose authority was recognized by everyone who had been through a university arts course and by everyone who knew the phrase 'where the philosopher finishes the physician begins'. The physicians recognized the power of a system of knowledge that had authority, and seemed to explain medical particulars in terms of an entire world-picture, and which was complex enough to slightly dazzle the lay person, if pitched at the right level.[16] The elements, causes, matter, form, privation, qualities, complexion, the naturals, non-naturals and contranaturals all formed an interlinked and undeniable system of the body and the world.

While medical theory of this kind was largely physical in the Aristotelian sense, another apparatus available to the physician was astrology.[17] This had been allied to medicine for more than a century and a new kind of authority was given to it by the cosmic sympathies evident in the exciting new Platonism of some of the Hellenists. Although it soon came to be seen as pagan, astrology offered another system of belief about the world which employed a mathematical rather than physical apparatus and offered a kind of prediction different from the usual prognosis of the physician.

Strategies

Unlicensed strategies

The learned physicians had some advice in the case of dangerous and widespread diseases. 'Go away quickly, stay a long time and come back reluctantly', they said. It was good advice, and they took it. In fact the physicians shared the general reaction of fear and disgust to the French Disease, and often refused to attempt to deal with it when it first appeared. By the time the disease was better known in the sixteenth century, the physicians themselves saw that their early professional neglect of it had opened the way for unlicensed practitioners.[18] Some physicians held that the first to treat the French Disease were empirics who like the disease itself came from France.[19] Others wondered at the rashness with which such people threw themselves into a dangerous situation. Many saw that by some combination of determination, good fortune and God's will some of the unlicensed practitioners were successful in their treatment while even the slowly returning physicians were not. Lastly, all physicians combined in condemning the ignorance of the unlicensed and the consequent danger of their uncontrolled remedies. Apart from surgeons and apothecaries, who had a recognized place in the medical hierarchy and earned only muted criticism from the doctors, the learned physicians poured rhetorical scorn on the heads of the bath-house keepers, barbers, oil massagers, wrestling-masters and little-old-women-of-the-bedside.[20]

Perhaps these were indeed the groups who had first offered advice and help to the early victims of the French Disease and who continued to do so for those who could not afford professional help and who could not find a place in a hospital. Their advice drew upon a folk culture in which there was a simple correlation between diseases, or parts of the body, and natural products, mostly herbs. It was from this culture and these groups that the two standard treatments for the French Disease came. The first was mercury, which had long been in use by the surgeons and even those treating animals as a remedy for skin diseases. The swellings and ulcers of the French Disease looked like a disorder of the skin and invited the same treatment.[21] The second empirical remedy was guaiac wood. This, the empirics liked to point out, came from the same part of the Indies as the disease itself, a land without learned physicians. It was agreeable to 'empirical' thinking and to some shades of religious opinion that a natural remedy should be found close to the disease it was to be used for.[22]

The unlicensed practitioners had a number of advantages over the learned physicians. There were, in the first place, many more of them. Moreover, the university physician maintained his monopoly of practising internal medicine – and often with difficulty – only where the power of his faculty or college reached, generally within cities. Secondly, unlicensed practitioners could act quickly, coming to be seen as experts in the field while the learned doctors were still wondering how to fit the French Disease into the learned apparatus. They were not encumbered with the lengthy regimen and individualism that characterized the learned physician's approach to the patient, and could announce at once a 'specific' remedy. This was one that was directed at the disease rather than at the individual patient and so was the same for everyone. As in the case of guaiac, it seemed likely that God or nature had put an antidote close to the disease, as docks are said to grow by nettles.

Some unlicensed practitioners had the advantage of opportunism. While the physician was wholly committed to his trade (although he could of course teach in addition) the spice-sellers and collectors of herbs could readily become medical advisers, especially at a time of crisis. This infuriated the physicians, who argued that such people were secretly practising internal medicine while hiding behind another trade.[23] In the terms we are using in this chapter, for the unlicensed practitioner, the knowledge of the surgeon, apothecary, the collector and retailer of herbs and spices, the barber and the midwife, all denounced by the physicians, was a resource from which they could draw strategies for their own advantage in the absence of a learned physician. Empirical medicine was directly advertised, cheap and quick. It was a threat to learned medicine.

Learned and rational strategies against the empirics

One century and a half after the Black Death, another medical disaster made physicians feel themselves to be going through another crisis of confidence in the community. It was not just that many refused to inspect, visit or treat the victims,[24] bringing themselves into society's contempt,[25] but that because the disease was apparently new they at first could give no rational and learned explanation of it.

The physicians later saw this as an opportunity for the empirics, who either with rash courage or with God's help[26] hastened to treat the victims. It worried the physicians that with some apparent successes the empirics were dangerously close to making the disease their own specialty. It became important for the physicians to fight back. They did so by employing their own resources and taking over those of the empirics. Contemporary professional ethics of the physicians made them distance themselves from unlicensed practice. But if the empirics were successful, it must be because of their mercury and guaiac. The physicians' strategy, therefore, was to take over these two remedies and medicalize them by making them rational. They had to transform them from empirical specifics, directed to the disease, to rational cures, applied in a lengthy regimen and qualified in use by the age, sex, strength and so on of the patient, and by the season, time and place. These were the physicians' traditional concerns, centred on the patient, and all their learning and rationality went into demonstrating them.

The physicians hastened to explain that while the empirics had the occasional success (for the physicians accepted that mercury and guaiac were powerful substances) yet more often they had damaged their patients or had been quite ineffective. This, insisted the physicians, was because the empirics did not know how the body worked or how one body differed from another and so did not know how to control the use of the remedies. In this way too the physicians transformed the empirical one-to-one relationship between disease and cure into a complex relationship between a diseased and idiosyncratic patient and a regimen of treatment. While there is no need to doubt the sincerity of most physicians in believing that they were improving the situation by doing this, yet the change undoubtedly had beneficial effects for their kind of medicine. Every patient was different and needed continuing advice as his case progressed. Essentially, the learned and rational physician advertised his rationality and learning by allowing the patient a limited insight into the technical apparatus of this kind of medicine.[27] Certainly he maintained the place of this kind of medicine in the world at large, which was administered by men who had also been to a university, by reference to a world-system which was agreed by all educated men and which supported the apparatus of theoretical medicine. None of this was available to the 'illiterate' empirics, who were truculent when faced with physicians and 'impious' about the great authors of medical learning, lacking the medical faith that bound the learned tradition together.[28]

These things are illustrated by the story of the introduction of the guaiac treatment.[29] When the French Disease became a matter of concern to the emperor Maximilian and his chancellor, Cardinal Matthew Lang, the latter set up a commission of enquiry to go to Spain and probably Portugal to find out how the disease was treated there. It was known that the Spaniards had control of that part of the Indies from where the disease had come and perhaps a rumour had reached the imperial court that a new remedy had recently been found there. The rumour would have been about a Spanish nobleman who contracted the disease in the New World – *Hispaniola* – and who had subsequently discovered the local remedy, which he brought home to Spain. The team dispatched by Lang included the emperor's physicians Nicolaus Pol (1470–*c*.1532) and Paul Ricci (*fl*. 1512–32). (Both came from Augsburg, where the local administration was seriously concerned about the spread of the disease.)

Pol wrote up his report in 1517. It was not published until 1535,[30] but the findings of the commission soon became known. In 1518 Leonard Schmaus of Salzburg published a tract on the French Pox addressed to German leaders and based on nineteen reports from the Indies and

Portugal: almost certainly, then, from the original commission of enquiry.[31] The earliest recipe using guaiac was published a few days before Schmaus's tract by the same publisher; it is probable that the guaiac wood was first known in Germany in 1516, and a contemporary chronicle says that it first came to Augsburg, from Lisbon, in 1518.[32]

The doctors were ready when it came. It was an empirical remedy and, like the French Disease itself, was new and without a proper name. It came from a distant and scarcely known land without doctors. It worked without doctors. The doctors had to make sure that treatment of the French Disease with guaiac became their affair. Pol's own tract shows how this medicalization was done. He asserts that his business was not simply to report on the practices from the Iberian Peninsula, but to adapt them for the German people. At once this brings in the physicians' traditional approach to the patient and draws away from the empirics' attack on the disease. Pol points to the differences between the Indians, the Spaniards and the Germans in terms of their complexions, their bodies and the climates in which they live. Clearly, what works naturally and empirically in the West Indies needs medical care and adjustment in Spain and even more in Germany.[33] Pol the physician asserts himself here even before describing how guaiac is applied. Again, his advice centres on the individual patient, who is to be purged before the treatment begins. The administration of purges was a characteristic act of the learned physician in giving internal medicines. He held that only his learning and knowledge of the patient could arrive at the correct dose; and that excessive purging by empirics was highly dangerous. Pol is at pains to point out that the purging should be under the supervision of a learned doctor, who will judge with skill how to proceed, from the age, sex, strength and habits of the patient and the nature of his surroundings. Some will be too weak to be purged, says Pol (and again, by implication, only a true physician can know this).[34]

The purpose of purging, according to Pol, is to remove a salty and melancholic humour that is involved in the disease. This is another way of medicalizing the disease, by inserting traditional causality into it. Deciding the doses of guaiac to be given is also part of the medicalization process, and Pol repeats what he said about what has to be considered in purging. The Indians, slightly built and living in a hot country on a sparse diet, are very different from the Germans, and the treatment must be modified accordingly, again taking into account the individual's age, sex, complexion, habits and the non-naturals that surround him.[35]

With this professional apparatus established, Pol comes to the treatment. The normally robust German regimen, particularly diet, is to be reduced a little every day. After four days the patient must start taking the decoction, remaining well covered in bed so that he sweats. The unspoken theory is that the sweat evacuates a poison involved in the disease, and Pol knew that this would be recognized as proper by his peers and their patients. By now the patient was living on a quarter of his usual food and sweating for three hours a day. He continued to do so for a further ten days, after which he was allowed a little increase in his rations; the whole process lasted about 30 days, depending of course on the nature of the individual.[36] Pol makes much of this traditional concern of the learned and rational doctor: not only do the differences between men explain how the Indians are cured in ten days and the Spaniards twice or even six times as long, but the length of necessary treatment depends on the expulsive powers of the individuals.[37] Pol concludes his medicalization of the guaiac with the recommendation that the whole treatment should be supervised by a faithful *medicus* (i.e., one who is rational and learned). Such a physician, like Pol himself, believed that many Germans had been so weakened by mercury treatment that the guaiac cure took a long time.[38] In other words, the medicalization of guaiac emphasized the empirical nature of mercury, and Pol is scoring a point for his own group of physicians and their individual-centred medicine. He expressly claims that his modifications of the remedies for the particular nature of the Germans is in imitation of the ancients, that is, where the patient, not the disease, is the entity.[39]

The Augsburg merchants, like the doctors, welcomed the coming of the guaiac. Indeed, they may have been behind it. Paracelsus seems to have believed that Lang's mission to Spain was financed by the important merchant family, Fugger. Jacob Fugger ('the Rich') of Augsburg not only built houses for his workers, but hospitals in which to treat them with guaiac when they caught the French Disease. Having control of the guaiac trade,[40] it was in the interest of the merchants that the doctors should continue to prescribe it. The doctors probably benefited by assuming control over treatment with guaiac in their competition with unlicensed practitioners. And at least some patients benefited by what they saw as successful treatment. Ulrich von Hutten (1488–1523) in the same breath thanked Christ and the Fuggers when he thought he had been cured of the French Disease in Augsburg in 1518. He thought that the experts in the disease were Paul Ricci, the emperor's physician, and Heinrich Stromer (1482–1542).[41] Stromer was Dean of the Leipzig medical faculty and helped Hutten to write his report on his own case in 1519. But it has been argued that Stromer was in the pay of the Fuggers, promoting the use of the guaiac wood, and Hutten may have unknowingly provided advertising for both the doctors and the merchants.

Tactics in the physicians' civil war

The combatants

The physicians not only fought the unlicensed practitioners, they fought each other. Those who thought about the learned profession of medicine as a whole, like Gabriele Zerbi in Padua, urged all university-trained doctors to close ranks against the other kinds of practitioner. For Zerbi the most unethical thing a learned practitioner could do was to argue on substantial medical points with another of his kind in the hearing of those lower down the medical scale. Such a display would above all bring into suspicion the learning of the physician, the learning on which he depended to maintain his claim to superiority.

But within the group of learned physicians as a whole, there were different kinds of learning. Different groups of physicians believed that their particular kind of knowledge was that which had to be defended and not opened to the suspicion of those lower down the medical ladder. They also believed of course that their particular knowledge made them better doctors. When we look at the early battles over the nature and treatment of the French Disease between learned doctors we see the different groups. These were the Hellenists, who wanted medicine to be a Greek business, centred on Hippocrates and his interpreter Galen. The Hellenists had drawn inspiration from the Greek culture of Byzantium and claimed a cultural superiority over the Latins. They were opposed by a group that may have formed in reaction. These, the Latin humanists, developed what they called the *res Latina*, the Latin tradition to which they belonged and had helped to bring to a state where it rivalled the important Greek culture of the Hellenists. Both of these wide cultural movements had medical partisans, who were opposed within medicine by a third group. This was less clearly defined and perhaps is marked out only in terms of disagreement with the Latin humanists and above all the Hellenists. Often 'establishment' medical teachers belonged to this group, with a fondness for Avicenna's *Canon* as the most comprehensive and tightly organized teaching text. For them it was Avicenna, not the Greek, Galen, who was the 'Prince of physicians'. They often prided themselves on their grasp of the technical detail of medicine and pictured the Hellenists and humanists as merely literary or grammatical. They sometimes called themselves 'scholastics' in the period before the word gained a pejorative sense. The different intellectual allegiances of these groups provided them with different resources when in dispute.

Disputations

Learned and rational medicine of the late Middle Ages was a creature of the universities. The authority of medical knowledge of this kind came from the fact that in broad terms it was agreed by doctors who had been to universities. It was agreed because it was arrived at by an open and formal discussion, the disputation. The agreement was not of course complete, or disputations would not have been possible. The teaching masters agreed that medical knowledge should be – first – authoritative, where authority lay primarily in the Greek authors Hippocrates and Galen (we have seen that the authority of Avicenna varied from one group to another). Secondly, they agreed that medical knowledge should be dialectical, that is, rational in the sense of consisting of arguments. Medical knowledge of this sort included true demonstrative knowledge – knowledge of final causes – and rested largely on Aristotle's logic. Thirdly, a considered place in medical knowledge was given to the doctor's own experiential knowledge, gained and needed in actual practice – for instance it was argued that only experience could give knowledge of the action of some drugs and the shape of some parts of the body. The difficulty here was that the doctor as a modern was not an authority and that experiential knowledge was dangerously close to empirical. Nevertheless the doctor was in touch with the real physical world and knowledge of it was a legitimate part of his professional knowledge.

These features of medical knowledge relate closely to the nature of the disputation. Disputations were central to university life. Not only did they sharpen the dialectical skills of students but at the magisterial level they established what knowledge was to consist of. The bachelor intending to be a master incepted by disputation; that is, he demonstrated his ability to be a master. Disputations were sometimes ceremonial, celebrating the characteristic action of the academic. They allowed the full use of the disputant's grasp of logic and of his knowledge of the literature in his field: in medicine, the attributes of what we are here calling the rational and learned physician.

A thesis which survived the attacks of its opponent had been confirmed by the full rigour of academic examination. Potentially at least a successful thesis represented established knowledge; at the very least it could lead to further refinements. Change in medical thinking came about by such mechanisms. When the medical men tried to understand the nature of the French Disease, therefore, it was not surprising that they disputed formally about it. For, to emphasize the point again, it was by such a formal examination of knowledge that the full weight of academic examination – the use of reason and learning – that truth could be established. A number of disputations were held on the French Disease. We shall briefly look at two, those in Leipzig and Ferrara.

The French Disease spread rapidly in German-speaking countries. It was in Zurich by May 1496, and by the summer had reached Frankfurt and Nuremberg. It was clearly an epidemic of large proportions and the medical faculties were worried. They did not know whether the disease had a real name or what caused it. Without such knowledge they would be powerless to advise about it or treat it. In Leipzig Martin Pollich of Mellerstadt (1450–1513) thought that the cause of the French Disease was a corruption of the air. Pollich thought strongly enough about the matter to defend a thesis on it.[42] The process began with the defendant of the thesis publishing it by posting it in a public place (perhaps on the door of the university church). This gave time for the opponent to marshal some arguments against the thesis and the reasoning that would support it in disputation. The attack would be mounted on the logical form of the thesis, on the validity of the arguments used in its support, or on the authorities selected by the defendant.

The arguments used by Pollich have been preserved, and it is worth noting the form they took because it was by means of such processes that the medical men of the time decided what the French Disease was. He actually starts with a *conclusio*, not a 'conclusion', but matters to be included. This is a general statement, of which the thesis is a particular case. Here it is that changed dispositions of the air do indeed produce diseases; and that the heavenly bodies have a weakening effect on the human body. As a general principle this was so widely held as to be unassailable. In practice, it was the first stage in bringing a disease thought by many to be new into the extant theory of medicine. Pollich then proceeded to his first 'corollary', which was a device to show how the general principle of the 'conclusion' applied in the special case under review. It said simply that whenever the air became putrescent, the body changed. There was a second corollary, which defined the picture further in asserting that not all bodies changed in the same way. This was a way of saying that even though the disease was epidemic (and thus apparently the same thing in many people) yet the careful physician could see differences between his patients. This too had the effect of drawing the disease in from the territory of the empirics and their specifics (aimed at the disease) and giving it to the learned physicians (who aimed their treatment at the individual patient). In further conclusions and corollaries, Pollich demonstrated how the corrupt air affected the liver and caused the disease in a person, and how it was then spread to other people.

No doubt Pollich's argument contributed to the way the French Disease was perceived in Leipzig. Something similar had happened in Ferrara;

we shall look at it in a little more detail below and here we need note that the apparent victor there, Nicolò Leoniceno, had written up the disputation and published it, in 1497.[43] There was an edition printed in Leipzig and Pollich read it. He found that he agreed with Leoniceno and consequently he set up another disputation to defend Leoniceno's opinion. But this time he ran into stiff opposition. It came from another member of the faculty, the Leipzig physician Simon Pistoris (1453–1523).[44] Pistoris presented his objections formally in his own thesis, conclusions and corollaries in the next year, 1498.

Pistoris's arguments included the following important points. First, since air is an element, with a pair of manifest elementary qualities, it cannot become corrupt, as Pollich claimed. Nor could manifest qualities – air was wet and warm – cause disease. Pistoris argued that air must instead owe its dangerous nature to a hidden, *occulta*, property. Second, Pistoris argued that the French Disease was new. He denied that it had been included in the section of the *Aphorisms* where Hippocrates describes summer diseases and those arising from a change in the air. Pollich's strategy, in contrast, had been to make the French Disease a business for the learned physician by drawing it into the apparatus of learning. This necessarily meant that the disease obeyed ancient rules and had been known to the ancients (even though the name had since been lost).

Faced with opposition, Pollich became angry. In the pamphlet war that followed, we can find traces of the actual arguments used in the earlier disputations (not represented in the published theses); and we can see why the dispute should have become so bitter.[45] To be sure, to understand the French Disease aright was an important matter in dealing with it medically. But this was an argument about much more than the technical aspects of medicine. It was ultimately about what was to be allowed as medical knowledge and from what sources it should be drawn.

Pollich and Pistoris belonged to opposite ends of a cultural spectrum. Pollich was a humanist with great sympathy for the Italian Hellenists.[46] Pistoris was one of a larger number of men of the schools. He was a busy teacher and practitioner, well read in his field, convinced of its utility and autonomy, and businesslike about its technical details. When Pollich tried to insult him by calling him a 'scholastic' he did not seem to resent it and may even have felt that the term implied mastery of techniques of pedagogy and practice. He certainly used the term 'scholastic certainty' for examination of a topic by disputation. He thought that the place where the question of the nature of the French Disease should be settled was in medical faculties, and particularly his own, where his thesis had been defended. He constantly refers disputed points to his professional colleagues and promoted an image of himself as a pious and experienced physician. The insults he offers to Pollich are of course parts of an opposing image: Pollich is a mere grammarian, an orator; a *dilettante* doctor with only two patients; a mere philosopher in thrall to his Italian heroes Pico della Mirandola and Nicolò Leoniceno, swept along by their prose and forgetting the essence of things in a game with names.

Pollich was certainly a humanist. He belonged to a German literary sodality and was the friend of a number of notable German humanists (they called him *lux mundi*, the light of the world). He wrote to other humanists with a clear sense of their joint superiority over the common vulgarity of the crowd. But Pistoris was right. Pollich's heroes were the Italian Hellenists. He may well have shared with his own circle the distinctive features of German humanism: in contrast to the Italians, German humanism was an affair of the universities, emphasized a Christian rather than pagan piety, sought to glamorize a German golden age (including the inheritance of the power of the Caesars) and rather resented the cultural superiority affected by the Italians. Pollich did not resent it. In the pamphlet war with Pistoris, he calls Leoniceno 'the master' whose doctrines Pollich felt the urge of a missionary to spread among German doctors. He wrote with passion and elegance, if not always with clarity, to Leoniceno himself and to Giovanni Manardi of Ferrara (1462–1536), who answered with a comfortingly humanist reply. The greatest compliment he could pay to the German humanist Bohuslaus de Hassentain was to call him the 'Pico of the Germans'. When he read Pico's attack on astrology he gave up the beliefs of a lifetime and turned savagely to attack Pistoris's claim that astrology, while not part of medicine, was extremely useful to the doctor.

In other words Pollich was a convert to Italian Hellenism. This meant that it was unthinkable that the French Disease had not been described by the ancients. It was a common Hellenist position to argue that the ancient name of the disease had been lost in the intervening period, the much maligned Latin Middle Ages, by the carelessness of its scholars. It followed that the Hellenist task was to identify the French Disease among the descriptions and categories of disease made by the ancients and either to recover its name or to construct a suitable one for it. For decades the Hellenists continued to talk of the pure streams of knowledge flowing down from the Greeks, and how they were constantly in danger of being muddied by the barbarians of Latin culture. What made Pollich so angry about Pistoris was he was such a person, muddying the water with Arabicisms from Avicenna, who had been the object of 'master' Leoniceno's criticism, and denying that the Greeks had experienced or described the French Disease.

The disputation at Ferrara was a rather different kind of event. It took place in a princely court and not a university and may not have been structured as rigidly as the disputation in Leipzig, with thesis, conclusions and corollaries. But like that in Leipzig it was prompted by the arrival of the French Disease and an urgent need to understand it in order to be able to react appropriately. While German humanism was a recognizable movement with strong connections with the universities, it makes little sense to talk of 'humanism' in late fifteenth-century Italy, at least in respect to medicine. Humanism had been an active force in the universities and elsewhere for a long time and certainly medicine had become as humanized as the nature of the subject allowed by now.[47] The vigorous minority movement corresponding to German humanism was Hellenism, and where the Hellenists could not proselytize in the universities they often succeeded in the princely courts.

Another way in which a disputation at a court differed from one in a university was that it was promoted by the grandee of the place, who wanted to raise matters of interest to himself or his circle. Above all he wielded patronage, and his clients, real or potential, no doubt had this in mind in what they said and did.

The patron at the Estense court in Ferrara was probably duke Ercole I. The disputation took place in April 1497 and the disputants were Nicolò Leoniceno,[48] Sebastiano dall'Aquila (a teacher in the medical faculty of Ferrara)[49] and, probably, the Estense court physician, Coradino Gilino.[50] Leoniceno was the arch-Hellenist. He had been born into Latin culture before the fall of Constantinople. The Council 'of Florence', in which the beseiged Byzantines asked for military help against the Turks, first met in Ferrara, the city where he later spent most of his days. During his lifetime Constantinople fell, and a tide of refugees, manuscripts and teachers reached Italy. The young Nicolò learned his Greek in such a manner and became a dedicated Hellenist. The refugees called first for military help and second for the establishment of a new Greek state. The political nature of their own Hellenism was never entirely lost and played its part as the Hellenists worked to persuade the politically powerful of the superiority of Greek culture. They did so – and this is one of the reasons why Leoniceno was now in the Estense court – by denigrating the contemporary Latin culture. So in convening the disputation Ercole was providing an arena for a battle between medical men with different cultural allegiances.

Intellectually Leoniceno's Hellenism looked to Paduan Aristotelianism for authority. Dall'Aquila, on the other hand, had made a name for himself as a Hellenist with a decided taste for Neoplatonism of the kind becoming well known in Florence.[51] He actively promoted the *pia philosophia* of Marsiglio Ficino in Ferrara and there was much on which he must have disagreed with Leoniceno. Both, as Hellenists, would have liked to see the medical curriculum reformed, but in different way.

Hellenists of any kind were comparatively small in number in contrast to the physicians who felt themselves to be part of the late medieval Latin tradition. Since the Black Death, when Gentile da Foligno had completed a commentary on the *Canon* of Avicenna, this text had had an authority, based on its comprehensiveness and regular structure, that could not be easily matched. The statutes of the universities continued to specify its use for many years.[52] It was, to be sure, full of technical terms derived from the Arabic that were inelegant to humanists' eyes and unbearable to Hellenists', and when the *De medicina* of the classical Latin writer Cornelius Celsus was discovered in the fifteenth century, many of the more humanistically inclined physicians of the Latin tradition turned gratefully to it. The elegance of Celsus's Latin – he became known as the *Cicero medicorum* – was helpful to those who rather resented the *graecitas* of the Hellenists and who wanted to emphasize their own tradition, the *res Latina*. All that we can say of Gilino, who was no Hellenist, was that he had no hesitation in using Avicenna.

In giving his account of the disputation, Leoniceno presents it as his systematic destruction of a series of alternative identities of the French Disease. We saw that it had no real name, and the business of understanding it and working out a treatment began with finding a name in the literature that was considered identical, or finding a generic name of which the disease could be a perhaps new species. Dall'Aquila held that the French Disease was the *elephantiasis* of Galen, and Leoniceno's principal task in the disputation was to destroy this opinion. Gilino in contrast, and as we might expect from what we know of his allegiances, turned to Celsus as a resource and claimed that the French Disease was Celsus's 'sacred fire', *ignis sacer*. This was the same as the 'Persian fire', *ignis persicus*, of the late medieval Latin tradition. In destroying all these identifications Leoniceno was leaving room for his own interpretation, that the French Disease was among the diseases described by Hippocrates, which arose during the heat and damp of summer.

This interpretation by Leoniceno was entirely consistent with the rest of his beliefs and actions. He had spent years teaching and translating Greek medicine. The centre of his notion of Greek medicine was Hippocrates, an author already venerable to Galen, much of whose work could be seen as an interpretation or commentary on that of Hippocrates. Leoniceno saw Arabic medicine and especially that of Avicenna as little better than stolen and mutilated Greek medicine, and he savagely attacked the inaccuracies and inelegancies of the *Canon*. He also attacked Pliny for his medical errors; and no doubt also because Pliny's attitude to Greek medicine and doctors was that the former was a tissue of plausible lies and the latter little better than criminals threatening the lives of imperial Romans. No devoted Hellenist physician could read Pliny without indignation.

The medical arguments used by all three authors in the reports of the disputation are too technical to be followed in detail here. What is important is that they all follow from the fundamental positions taken by the authors as a result of their cultural positions. Dall'Aquila favoured Galen's arguments partly at least because his own Neoplatonism was sympathetic to Galen's sometimes obvious Platonism. Dall'Aquila put emphasis on the 'accidents of the soul' in the treatment of the disease in a way that also reflected his and Galen's Platonism. Gilino in contrast relied on Avicenna because he held that all diseases had their 'chapter' in the *Canon*. The term he uses, *capitulatio*, seems to be part of Avicennan scholarship and implies that the genera–species relationship of disease and Avicenna's systematic treatment gave extra understanding to the Avicennan doctor. The Latin tradition in medicine of which Gilino was part also relied on astrology, as we saw in the case of Simon Pistoris. But for the Hellenists astrology was coming under suspicion, both because no Greek author had anything like the highly elaborate and predictive astrological techniques of the medical tradition and because astrology could be seen as impious, infringing the free will of man or even god. When Pico attacked astrology, it began to fade; in this disputation at all events the two Hellenists give it less attention than did Gilino.

Patronage, Rome and medical practice

We have seen in the last part of the previous section that when a prince wanted a topic aired he could call a disputation; and that the advice and information offered to him varied with the cultural allegiances of the participants. There was urgency in the matter when the topic was the French Disease, and the advice offered would determine the nature of medical practice in which the disease was treated. In this section we examine a related situation, where the pressures on the doctors in terms of gaining or maintaining patronage, finding good medical advice to give and of putting their theoretical understanding of the disease to the practical test of developing a treatment, were extreme.

There can hardly have been greater problems for physicians than for those at the papal court. Like all problems, these needed resources and strategies: we are still considering the ways (and the whys and hows) in which university-trained physicians battled with each other, and in this case we shall see the practical outcome. It was at the court of pope Alexander VI, Rodrigo Borja ('Borgia' in its Italianized form).[53] His *familia* was attended by seven physicians,[54] of whom we are concerned with two, Gaspar Torrella (*c*.1452–*c*.1520)[55] and Pere Pintor (*c*.1423–1503).[56] The problem with the French Disease was the common one that a lot of people – here, important people – caught it. Joan Borja and Joan Borja-Llançol and four other cardinals were stricken (one of whom became pope Julius II), and so was cardinal Cesare, Rodrigo's son.[57] To maintain the patronage they enjoyed the physicians had to do something.

What our two physicians did was determined by their background. Like Rodrigo himself, both came from Valencia, and both had secured the protection of Rodrigo when their families, converted Jews, suffered at the hands of the Inquisition. The difference between them was that Torrella had studied medicine in Italy, at Siena and Pisa, while Pintor, a full generation older, had remained in Spain, learning his medicine at Lérida, the *studium generale* of the Crown of Aragon. Torrella was then in Tuscany in the 1470s when Marsiglio Ficino was active in Florence, and one of Torrella's teachers was a member of Ficino's circle. There were other significant differences. Torrella was a priest who secured a medical degree only with the help of Rodrigo Borgia and some years after having finished studying. In contrast, Pintor, who had been born in the late 1430s, had been practising medicine since 1445, had served as a civil examiner of physicians and was instrumental in the setting up and in the later reorganization of the Valencia school of surgery, where he also taught.

These differences between the two men were reflected in what they published. Both were interested in epidemics, perhaps not surprisingly at a time of the French Disease, the English Sweats, the 'modorrilla' – an epidemic which spread across the Iberian Peninsula in the 1500s – the petechial fever and, of course, the plague. But Pintor's conservative training made him believe, with Guy de Chauliac, that progress in medicine was a collaborative and cumulative affair, following the principle of 'aggregation'. Pintor had put this principle into practice by systematizing the opinions of earlier authors on epidemics in an *Agregator* on plague he had published in 1499.[58] Pintor accordingly thought that he could best solve the problem of the French Disease and one year later he published his *De morbo foedo et occulto his temporibus affligente*, although on this occasion he merely referred those readers interested in more information to his previous volume. He solved the problem of the name of the French Disease by identifying it with a disease he found in the literature, *aluhumata*,[59] an obscure third species of the generic title *variola*. Torrella in contrast coined a new name for the disease, calling it *pudendagra* because it began in the *pudenda*.[60] Both strategies served the interests of learned physicians in labelling the disease with a technical name and making possible a discussion about it by placing it in the learned apparatus.[61] Both men gave the appearance of refining the apparatus, by expansion or insertion, and this gave them authority to the reading public and to their patron. Indeed publication in a printed format was itself a strategy for personal promotion, and a comparatively new one: books printed within the lifetimes of their authors formed a small category of early printed books. Most medical books printed at the time of Pintor and Torrella were those of the scholastic masters of previous generations and of the ancients. Both of our authors were therefore taking very unusual steps, and were clearly in some sense successful, for they were rewarded by their patron.

We shall see that these different backgrounds and strategies led ultimately to different practice in cases of the French Disease. Indeed all practice in the case of learned and rational physicians depended on the learning and reason of the practitioner and so what happened to the patient was determined in a cultural way. Let us follow the beliefs of Pintor and Torrella down to the details of practice. Like Pistoris in Leipzig, Pintor held that there was something hidden, *occultus*, about the French Disease. Both authors thought that astrological circumstances were a direct cause of the French Pox and that the hiddenness of the disease was the unknown mode of action of the heavenly causes on terrestrial effects. Like other doctors Pintor worked out which conjunction must have been responsible. Torrella too was at first prepared to accept this kind of explanation. But Pico's attack on judicial astrology had appeared in 1496[62] and Torrella may have read it, for by 1500 he was sceptical. One of his complaints was that the astrologers were all working back from the effects of conjunctions – that is, the French Disease itself – to its cause; what they should have done was to predict the effect of the conjunction. Pico's attack could be represented as a pious reassertion of Christian free will. If it now seemed appropriate to some to make judicial astrology superstitious, it could be done better by making it seem a characteristic activity of some other group. Torrella, who came from a family of converted but persecuted Jews, held that his doubts about astrology began when he saw that the Jews, who claimed excellence in astrology, predicted neither the French Disease nor their own persecution[63] (which began at almost the same moment as the conjunction held to have caused the French Disease). Like Leoniceno, Pico[64] thought that astrologers had wormed their way into powerful positions close to political magnates by means of tricks. Probably they had; the Hellenists after all had adopted a similar strategy, using their learning to promote their aims.

These differences between Pintor and Torrella were developed as they began to think about the way in which the French Disease was spread. If the cause of the disease was astrological, or God's anger, would it go away when the first cause no longer operated? Experience was showing that the disease passed from one person to another by what looked like secondary causes, and the problem was to find out how this happened and what could be done about it. Pintor gave much more attention to astrology than Torrella.[65] The universality of the French Disease seemed good evidence of a universal cause. The sophistications of astrological theory could explain (with hindsight, Torrella said) why the conjunction of 1483 had taken over ten years to produce its effects and why it affected some people and regions more than others. Pintor believed that it was astrological reasons that determined that the symptoms should first appear in the genitals. It was a one-to-one relationship: the configuration of the planets has a 'whole property' or 'specific power' of generating the disease. We cannot know this power in the same way as we know the manifest action of the elementary qualities of standard school natural philosophy: herein lies their occultness. On this basis Pintor believed that the French Disease would disappear in the year 1500.[66]

But the theory of medicine available to Pintor did not deny contagion, and he had the resources to join the dialogue between the doctors and the civic authorities, whom the spread of the disease was teaching some severe lessons. He explained it by claiming that an infected person corrupts the air around him in just the same way as the stars do, and that proximity to such a person doubled the chance of contracting the disease. His practical advice on avoiding the French Disease was to go away from centres of its occurrence, and seek out low-lying spots where the air is thicker and less open to celestial influence.[67]

Torrella in contrast emphasized contagion. He held that some material was passed from one victim to the next, either by skin contact or indirectly, for example by means of bedclothes. He denied that there was any general corruption of the air, as Pintor had said, but allowed an airborne contagion on an individual basis. Wet-nurses could transmit the matter of the French Disease to their sucklings, he held, but as his name for the disease testifies, he thought that most infection came about from sexual contact. His main advice on avoiding the disease was to avoid infected women (all his advice is directed to men). He also argued political and civil action, that is, that the prostitutes suffering from the disease should be rounded up and kept in a hospital until cured.[68]

So the main difference between the two physicians was that Torrella emphasized the material nature of the disease. The French Disease had its own matter, passed on in contagion. Pintor in contrast, emphasized the hidden nature of the cause of the disease. Neither author wanted to avoid the standard medical explanation that disease was an imbalance or corruption of the humours, and Pintor held that it was this that was caused by the occult influences and in turn caused the symptoms of the disease. It was also common medical practice to attempt to modify and evacuate the 'peccant' humour by bleeding or encouraging one of the body's natural evacuations. In an eruptive disease like the French Disease it was held that what was discharged from the pustules or ulcers was the modified peccant humour, so the appearance and opening of the swellings in the French Disease was welcomed. The physician then helped nature's evacuation by attacking the pustules with abrasive and corrosive substances.

But their different theoretical positions led to very different kinds of practice. Pintor, in elaborating on the third species of *variola* that constituted his *aluhumata*, made the pain of the French Disease its chief distinguishing characteristic. He believed that the pain alone could kill the victim and was not, therefore, simply a symptom or sign of the disease; it was part of its essence. Accordingly Pintor advocated the use of narcotic and sedative remedies. In practice these were ointments containing mercury in some form. In some the mercury was prepared by burning and was extinguished by the 'saliva of a fasting person'. Sometimes the danger of the mercury was lessened, thought Pintor, by an admixture of medical simples. His authorities here are not the classical writers but the Latin and Arabic and surgical writers (we can recall that he had a partly surgical background). Some of his narcotics were taken internally by his patients. He knew very well that there were great dangers in this, but it was absolutely central to his position as a learned and rational physician. The mercurial remedies were surgical in origin and continued to be used by empirics. For professional reasons a physician like Pintor denigrated the empirical use of mercurials as dangerous. He had to maintain it was only with the knowledge of the physician that mercury could be used safely. Knowledge of its powers, knowledge of the patient, of doses, times, seasons and all the apparatus of learned medicine, was what made mercury safe in the doctor's hands, argued Pintor. Internal application of mercury was a final resort, after the failure of external remedies and when the patient is beginning to weaken: when the skill of the physician is most needed.[69]

Pintor believed that pains of *aluhumata* were partly due to a deficiency of innate heat. He accordingly recommended 'partial baths' in which the painful limb could be bathed in hot water or olive oil. The expectation was that the external heat increased the natural heat to the point where it could again begin to expel the morbid matter.[70] If the matter was particularly recalcitrant and the pain extreme, then Pintor proceeded to cautery. This was an attempt to destroy the morbid matter directly in the pustules, which were attacked either by 'actual' cautery – an iron hot from the fire – or 'potential' cautery: caustic ointments.[71]

Torrella's beliefs led him to another direction. Like Pintor he believed that the morbid matter had to be evacuated. But because he had made the morbid matter of *pudendagra* something outside the normal spectrum of disturbed humours, it needed a different technique of evacuation. From 1497 Torrella used the 'dry stove', the *stufa sicca*. At first it was simply a hot fire to make the patient sweat, by which Torrella hoped to evacuate the peccant humour. By 1500 he was recommending that the stove should be purpose built: it consisted of a wine barrel big enough for the patient to sit in. Hot stones were placed on a bed of sand at the bottom and the whole was covered with cloth. Torrella made his patients sweat 'for five days without any breakfast' to get rid of the poison and prevent more being formed from ingested food. In fact the regimen consisted of one or more sessions of an hour or so every day for a period perhaps as long as a week. It depended entirely on Torrella's belief that the morbid matter was humid and would come away in the sweat.[72]

In contrast, Pintor believed that the matter of the disease was dry and cold, like a melancholic humour, and that a dry heat would simply make it even drier and more difficult to move. He urgently warned against the use of the dry stove at any stage of the disease.[73] We have seen that he preferred a local bath, a half-barrel of warm oil. He also used his mercurials to promote sweating, taking care that they were applied in moist ointments to avoid drying the morbid matter further. With this precaution Pintor, too, could seat his patients close to a fire to encourage them to sweat. For eight days at a time he anointed the painful parts of the patient twice a day, warming his hand before the fire before doing so to open the pores and allow the ointment to reach the membranes round the bones.[74]

We have now looked briefly at Pintor's and Torrella's cultural allegiances and the differences that arose from them as they faced the French Disease and evolved strategies to deal with it, to maintain their own position and the professional image of the learned and rational physician and, in short, to solve the problems they faced. We can usefully end with a glance at an actual case history that illustrates all these points.

It is the case of Bertomeu Martí. Born in the same Valencian town as his friend Rodrigo Borgia, he was made a cardinal in 1496, during Rodrigo's pontificate as Alexander VI.[75] By March 1499 he was ill with the French Disease and in the hands of the Pope's doctors. Pintor was impressed by the cardinal's terrible pains, which may have some bearing on the doctor's later thinking on the nature of the disease. Clearly there was the pressure of expectation on the Pope's doctors. What they did at first is not clear; but the cardinal accepted from a Portuguese visitor an ointment consisting in part of pig's fat, pine resin, mastic, litharge and quicksilver. It was given with some secrecy and probably the visitor was not medically qualified. At all events the cardinal took the precaution of asking some physicians, including Pintor, what they thought of it. They thought that it contained too much mercury: the physician's usual reaction to empirics and their remedies. But the cardinal was desperate and the Pope's physicians were unsuccessful, so he used the ointment, with fatal results.[76]

The physicians disagreed about what killed the cardinal. Pintor, who was in favour of mercury without reservations, argued that as unlicensed practitioners often did, the cardinal had inappropriately used this and another ointment so that his radical moisture had been damaged and his natural faculties destroyed.[77] Torrella, who had already condemned some mercurial remedies, was rapidly abandoning others because Pintor was claiming success with them, and now he behaved in a more cautious way about the use of this remedy than he used to do before, simply blaming the mercury.[78] Both thought that the secrecy associated with the remedy smacked of empiricism and as learned physicians might, attacked the promises held out by the visitor. As combatants in the physicians' civil war, both used even death to promote his own views.

Post-mortems and anatomical rationality

One of the principal characteristics of medieval western medicine was its anatomy. Perhaps no other culture practised systematic dissection of the dead human body for teaching purposes. Whether or not his knowledge of the inside of the body made him a better doctor, there were a number of advantages to the medieval and Renaissance physician in basing his medicine on anatomy. It was consistent with the practice of Galen, the great rationalist interpreter of Hippocrates. The public dissections were dramatic statements about the kind of medicine practised by and limited to university-trained physicians. It gave them a special kind of rationality, based on Aristotelian and Galenic doctrines about the relationship between form and function. It marked them off from the empirics, apothecaries, often even surgeons and those who had not had a university medical education with its anatomies. The physician, who had always used his professional learning to secure business, now had a special kind of learning to add to his special rationality.

Anatomically minded doctors found that they were expert witnesses in the law courts. Indeed the legal need to know the cause of death, for example, may have been one of the reasons why dissection began, probably in the late thirteenth century; it presupposes that something physical can be found in some sort of causal relationship with the outcome.

This remained part of medical doctrine at the time when practitioners were thinking about the French Pox. One of them recalled a case given by Gentile da Foligno in the first half of the fourteenth century, where a patient had died through an accidental overdose of mercury. Perhaps the story was now repeated because mercury was a treatment for the French Disease, and many held it to be dangerous; at all events in Gentile's story the doctors dissected the body and attributed death to the congealed blood they found near the heart.[79]

The doctors of the late fifteenth and the sixteenth-centuries stoutly maintained that it was only their detailed knowledge of normal anatomy, learned by dissection, that gave them the knowledge of pathological appearance. Their particular kind of rationality and learning was a resource and their strategy was to secure professional advantage over other kinds of practitioners by making obvious the superiority of their resources. It was customary for the university physicians to berate the 'empirics' for their failures and the danger they presented to the public. One of their arguments was that the nostrums, specifics and secret remedies of the empirics had no known means of action. It was in the interest of the physicians to make manifest the means of action of their medicines in terms of their rationality and learning. Since the latter were partly anatomical, the doctors found it good to be able to find in the body a material, visible cause for the French Disease.

Many found such a thing in a pathological material discovered in the dissected body where the pains had been in life. We know that a convicted criminal was executed in Ferrara on 11 April 1497, just after the dispute there. He had suffered from the French Disease and was dissected soon after his execution.[80] This much was known to one of the contenders in the dispute, Dall'Aquila, but we do not know the result of the dissection, nor what the anatomists' expectations were.[81] There were dissections too in Rome, for many patients at the Incurabile hospital of San Giacomo died from the illness. Pietro Andrea Mattioli (1500–77) (speaking as the physician 'Andreas' in his dialogue) dissected a number of victims, looking for a viscid material that he called *virus*. He did not always find it.[82]

Others were more positive. They were looking for a viscid or phlegmatic matter for two reasons. First, the resistance of the French Disease to cure invited them to believe that its material cause must be very difficult to purge, and a phlegm with some characteristics of melancholy was traditionally difficult to remove. Second, it seemed that nature was attempting to expel this substance through the pustules and sores of the disease. The same matter then, was the inner cause of the disease and the exudation of the pustules, where its character could be recognized. It seemed plain that this material cause of disease was located where the pains were in life, that is, the bones and especially joints and in fibrous parts. The anatomists therefore had a fairly good idea of what it was they were looking for and where to find it. Nicolò Massa (d. 1569), dissecting in 1524, found what he was looking for in a hard or sometimes soft viscous matter on the membrane of the bone of the leg. Nicolò Massa was a well-known anatomist and physician, and had a good knowledge of normal anatomy. He therefore felt obliged to recognize the unnatural white substance as the material cause of the disease.[83] The same expectation of finding a material cause is apparent in the works of another well-known author, Gabriele Falloppio (1523–62) (and in those of the lesser-known Giovanni Pascale (*fl.* 1534), both writing on the French Disease).[84] The connection between the matter expelled in the running pustules of the disease and its inner material cause were strong enough for authors like Leonhard Schmaus and Antonio Scanaroli (*c.*1450–1517) to declare that when no pustules were visible on the surface they could be found within the body, revealed by dissection after death.[85]

But while the learned physicians agreed enough within their anatomical rationality to present a united front to the empirics, their civil war continued with the strategies they were able to draw from their resources. Traditionally diseases had been regarded as imbalances of the elementary qualities of the humours and parts. A complexional disease of this kind did not presuppose the presence of a special matter of disease, for the changed qualities inhered in extant matter.

Trapolino, a major teacher of medical theory at Padua, did not give much attention to what was found close to the bones at post-mortem examination (and he denied that it was phlegmatic) and pointed instead simply to the attenuation to be observed as a symptom in the limbs. A matter of disease was less important to him and he accordingly denied the existence of internal pustules. For Trapolino, the physical matter of disease and the manifest qualities of complexional change were inadequate as the basis of a comprehensive account of diseases and their cures. His orientation was towards 'subtlety', powerful forces that acted in unknown and unAristotelian ways: we met them above as 'occult' forces. He suspected that there might be a whole unknown practice of medicine still to be discovered and based on the wonderful properties of plants and minerals. He had seen half-healed ulcers in a sheep's lung, and concluded that the sheep had begun to cure itself by eating a particular herb; but the doctors did not know what it was. Nor did the doctors know why epilepsy was cured by paeony, or why a leper should have been cured by wine in which a viper had drowned. The mechanism of such actions was unknown – it was *occultus* – and the effects could only be learned by experience (rather than being predicted by reason).

Trapolino was aware that the empirics too relied on experience (rather than reason), used medicines that were specific to the disease (rather than to the patient) and which had an unknown means of action. Like other rationalist and learned physicians, Trapolino wanted his kind of medicine to be seen to be better than that of the empirics, but his strategy was not to condemn the empirics out of hand. Instead, he thought that rational medicine should embrace whatever was valuable in empirical practice and 'medicalize' it by using it in conjunction with rationalist practice. He even accepted that sometimes barbers and empirics treated the French Disease more successfully than the most learned man. But Trapolino the learned and rational physician, knew why this should be so: there are wonderful powers of natural things, some quite unknown. The ancients (and therefore the learned physician) could not have known all these, nor their mode of action (who knows how lettuce juice reduces a swelling of the tongue?). Many such effects are accidental or contingent and therefore impossible to know *a priori*. They cannot be known *certitudinaliter* or *scientifice*, that is, with Aristotelian causality.

In a word, Trapolino thought that the traditional medicine of the ancients was incomplete and could be added to. His rationalism was wider than that of the conventional doctor who confined himself to the manifest qualities and causes of the Aristotelian–Galenic learned apparatus. Among the moderns he admired Pietro d'Abano, from whose *Conciliator* came some of his examples of 'subtleties' in action. He also admired Gentile da Foligno as a theoretician – *speculator* – and quotes from him some modern observations of things unknown to the ancients, like a worm generated between the skin and the flesh, discharge of stones from the gut and the little animals in the lungs that cause coughing as they creep about. The French Disease, he said, was of the same order of things, a new disease quite unknown to antiquity. In a medical world like Trapolino's, in which specific remedies could act in hidden ways, their results knowable only by experience, where the daylight hours might reveal new healing powers in things and the night might contain revelations about such things by angels or demons, the French Disease was not to be limited to traditional explanations.[86]

Subtleties and infections

In these ways Trapolino was exhibiting a medicine that added a new dimension to the anatomical and manifest-quality rationality that was traditional. The key word was subtlety, specifics with unknown modes of action. Astrological causes were a species of subtle action, and Trapolino gave serious and sympathetic attention to the views of Pistoris on the astrological causes of the French Disease and on the astrological times for giving drugs. Again, where the mode of action was unknown, traditional reason could not predict the effect. Trapolino and Pistoris asserted that only experience could tell: practical medicine was a *habitus experimentalis*, and some doses, some kinds of medicine, the times and places of their use, cannot be demonstrated or taught in speech or writing. Trapolino again turns to the high scholastics – Gentile de Foligno, Jacopo da Forli and Turisianus, known as Plusquam Commentator – for an elegant demonstration that practical medicine consists of an infinite series of particulars of observation. But infinity is unknowable and the particulars belong to sensation, not reason (and they cannot be built up into universals, with which true knowledge deals). This is why, says Trapolino, the admirable Simon Pistoris declares that such things do not appear in books.[87]

It was not always to the advantage of the learned and rational physician to argue that there were parts of medicine that could not be written in books (and were therefore not available to the whole of the Western rationalizing tradition). To argue that experience alone could teach certain things and that medicines could act in an unknown way and specifically to a disease, looked close to empiricism. It is arguable that the physician – whose strategy had always been based on his learning and rationalism – was forced into a position like Trapolino's by experience of infectious diseases. The Black Death, the English Sweats and the French Disease were all things that swept out of some known part of the world and affected large numbers of people. In contrast, Galenic medicine centred on the individual patient and on how all his idiosyncrasies reacted with the environment to make him ill or well. Although pestilences were not unknown in the ancient world and could be found in the literature, it was the model of the individual patient, his exercise, diet, sleeping, age, sex, complexion, vigour, and the season of the year, time of day, geographical location and so on, on which the physician could employ the full extent of his learning and rationality.

But to see the French Disease as a thing created an entity and provided an ontological perception of a disease. It was a natural view and the empirics, as the physicians knew to their cost, had taken advantage of the situation with their disease-specific remedies and were often seen as more successful than the physicians. Again, the physicians had to do something about it. They had to bring the French Disease into rational and learned medicine. They had to accommodate the view that the French Disease was an entity, and had a capacity, like the Black Death and the English Sweats, to pass rapidly from one person to another. The ontological view of the disease was expressed when a number of physicians came to say that the disease passed through people, and even that it was made weaker in doing so.

The strategy employed by the physicians to do these things was to develop a piece of Galenic theory that had been rather neglected. Galen, in rationalizing the pithy wisdom of Hippocrates, had used a natural philosophy that was largely Aristotelian. It dealt largely with the four causes, accidents and essence, matter, form and elementary qualities. All of these were open to observation and reason and in the sixteenth century were called 'manifest'. But as a doctor Galen knew that some things had effects on the body that were out of all proportion to their manifest qualities. Small amounts of poisons for example could produce results that by their speed and scale could not be due to the action of normal qualities. Galen said that in those cases the material acted not by its complexion but by some virtue inherent in its 'whole substance'. He did not offer a detailed explanation of why this was so.[88]

There were a number of other things that acted in related ways. The reputed stare of the basilisk, the poison of the scorpion, the stupefying effect of the electric eel and the bite of a mad dog were all of this nature. These things were well known to doctors and were increasingly of interest to natural philosophers who were not content with an Aristotelian view of things. The doctors began to think that if infectious diseases were entities, then they too could have 'whole substance' action. It meant of course that they had to have substance, a term that still implied some sort of Aristotelian combination of matter and form. It was not difficult to imagine that the 'matter of disease' which was both evacuated from the body in the living pustules and found in the dead body where the pains had been, was related to or was the same as the 'substance' of the disease. A third correspondence was sometimes also found, that the matter of disease, its substance or entity, was the means of infection. Some writers treat on this matter as a sort of yeast, passing from body to body and converting their substance into its own. Others used the image of seeds, so that the disease was like a plant, coming to maturity and spreading itself by means of forms of its own substance. Others again, like Falloppio, took the Galenic doctrine of 'whole substance' and applied it to the disease and also to the body, in its reaction to the disease. Since whole-substance action was explicitly an exception to normal natural-philosophical explanation, Falloppio effectively freed himself from the need to follow 'manifest' arguments and qualities in the whole subject of infectious diseases.[89]

Conclusion

It is arguable then that experience with infectious diseases from the Black Death to the French Disease forced doctors to find new explanations and so changed the nature of medicine. To a certain extent they practised in the medical marketplace and needed theory as they traditionally had, but now of a new kind. But we have seen that not all physicians were the same. The Hellenists urged the superiority of Greek medicine, which centred on the patient, had little about infectious diseases and nothing about strategies to control them like quarantine, hospitals or locking up a town's prostitutes, all live issues in the Western Middle Ages. The Hellenists did not succeed in driving the Arabic authors Avicenna and Rhazes from the medical curriculum, and these authors provided the doctors of the medical establishment with different resources – they contained more on infectious diseases – with which to further the claims of university medicine. Doctors who believed in astrological causes had a further example of 'subtle' or hidden action and another strategy with which to negotiate their medicine into the marketplace; but by the end of the period covered by this book this strategy was beginning to fail, for astrology came to look like an impious encroachment on God's power and man's free will. Yet another group of doctors were those who were impressed by the new Platonism, which gave a whole new world picture, of which cosmic sympathies and antipathies were one feature. Neoteric theories based partly on such doctrines sometimes included arguments about immaterial infection which ran counter to the general perception of disease entity and material transmission; but these ideas did not figure large in practice. Doctors giving advice to individuals or to groups like hospitals and towns needed a theory that was intelligible at a fundamental level. People understood about seeds, yeast and poisons. They knew that tinder needed but a spark to create a fire and understood medical theories that spoke of *fomes* within the body set alight by an infective spark.[90] They accepted that a material poison could remain dangerous when inactive in a container, and so understood that infection could be indirect, lurking in a victim's clothes or possessions. The doctors controlled the theory and the situation as they did traditionally, by asserting that their own mastery of the detail of the theory gave them the unique right to offer practical action and advice; but they had to have some such theory by the collective experience of epidemic infections.

Notes

1. On the arrival and early years of the French Disease in Europe, see Jon Arrizabalaga, John Henderson and Roger French, *The Great Pox. The French Disease in Renaissance Europe*, New Haven and London, Yale University Press, 1997, particularly pp. 20–170.
2. The term 'pox' is also used, as a vernacular term that flourished in the absence of a formal name. The term was early used by Thomas Paynel, a canon of Marten Abbey, who translated Ulrich von Hutten's tract on *morbus gallicus*: his translation became one of the few books in English on what Paynel called 'the frenche pockes': Ulrich von Hutten, *Of the Wood called Guaicum*, trans. T. Paynel, London, 1536.
3. Historians have tended to accept uncritically the term 'syphilis' since the important studies on the earliest printed and manuscript literature about the French Disease that Karl Sudhoff published during the first quarter of this century. See among others his works, *Graphische und typographische Erstlinge der Syphilisliteratur aus den Jahren 1495 und 1496*, Munich, C. Kuhn, 1912; *Aus der Frühgeschichte der Syphilis. Handschriften- und Inkunabelstudien epidemiologische Untersuchung und kritische Gänge*, Leipzig, Barth, 1912; *Zehn Syphilis Drucke aus den Jahren 1495–1498*, Milan, R. Lier, 1924 (English version adapted by Charles Singer: *The Earliest Printed Literature on Syphilis, being Ten Tractates from the Years 1495–1498*, Florence, R. Lier, 1925). For the argument about the issue of relating pre-germ theory plague to post-germ theory plague, see Andrew Cunningham, 'Transforming Plague: the Laboratory and the Identity of Infectious Disease', in Andrew Cunningham and Perry Williams, eds, *The Laboratory Revolution in Medicine*, Cambridge, Cambridge University Press, 1992, pp. 209–44.
4. On the German religious perception of the French Disease see Paul A. Russell, 'Syphilis, God's Scourge or Nature's Vengeance? The German Printed Response to a Public Problem in the Early Sixteenth Century', *Archive for Reformation History*, 80, 1989, pp. 286–307, p. 293.
5. Coradino Gilino, *De Morbo quem Gallicum Nuncupant*, Ferrara, *c.*1497/98, fol. 1v.
6. On this see Alfonso Corradi, *Annali delle Epidemie Occorse in Italia dalle Prime Memorie Fino al 1850*, 5 vols, Bologna, Memorie della Società Medico-chirurgica di Bologna, 1865–92 (facsimile reprint: Bologna, Forni, 1972), vol. I, pp 338–60; vol. IV, pp. 212–54; vol. V, pp. 265–74.
7. On Charles VIII's invasion of Italy, see Ludwig von Pastor, *The History of the Popes from the Close of the Middle Ages*, 40 vols, London, Kegan, Paul, Trench, Trubner and Co., 1891–1953, vol. V, London, 1898, pp. 434–81; Cecilia M. Ady, 'The Invasions of Italy', in Denys Hay, ed., *The New Cambridge Modern History. Vol. I: The Renaissance, 1493–1520*, Cambridge, Cambridge University Press, 1961, pp. 343–67; Lauro Martines, *Power and Imagination. City-States in Renaissance Italy*, Harmondsworth, Penguin, 1979, pp. 387–415.
8. On all these events see Nicolò Leoniceno, *Libellus de Epidemia quam Vulgo Morbum Gallicum Vocant*, Venice, 1497, sigs. d1r–drv; Antonio Benivieni, *De Abditis Nonnullis ac Mirandis Morborum et Sanationum Causis*, Paris, 1528, *Observatio* 57 (*Fames Valida*), fol. 12v; Corradi, *Annali*, vol. I, pp. 349–3; *Diario Ferrarese dall'Anno 1409 sino al 1502*

di Autori incerti, ed. G. Pardi, in L. A. Muratori, ed., *Rerum Italicarum Scriptores*, Città di Castello-Bologna, N. Zanichelli, 1928–33, vol. 24/27 (henceforth *DFA*), pp. 165–208 (*passim*); Francesco Rococioli, *Libellus de Monstro Romae in Tyberi Reperto anno Domini MCCCCLXXXXVI*, Modena, 1501; and Pastor, *The History of the Popes*, vol. V, pp. 480–81.

9. On the relationship between the Duke of Ferrara and the Dominican friar, see Luciano Chiappini, 'Ercole d'Este e Girolamo Savonarola', *Atti e Memorie della Deputazione Ferrarese di Storia Patria, serie II*, 7 (3), 1952, pp. 45–53; Werner L. Gundersheimer, *Ferrara. The Style of a Renaissance Despotism*, Princeton, Princeton University Press, 1973, pp. 197–9; Jacob Burckhardt, *The Civilization of the Renaissance in Italy: An Essay*, London, Phaidon Press, 1965, pp. 301–3. For the letters exchanged between them see Antonio Cappelli, 'Fra Girolamo Savonarola e Notizie Intorno il suo Tempo', *Atti e Memorie delle RR. Deputazioni di Storia Patria per le Provincie Modenesi e Parmesi*, 4, 1868, pp. 301–406 (*passim*); Roberto Ridolfi, *Le Lettere di Girolamo Savonarola*, Florence, Leo S. Olschki, 1933, pp. 75, 104–5, 110–13, 117–19, 156–7, 180–81, 219–20, 228–31, 235–9; and Chiappini, 'Ercole d'Este'.

10. The earliest evidence from this city was a ducal payment order on 13 October of four marchesina pounds to the master surgeon Giovanni Giusti 'as a stipend for curing and liberating from the French Disease' (Archivio di Stato di Modena, Archivio Segretto Estense, Camera Ducale Estense, Mandati, Registro 36, fol. 163r). Ercole's sons were identified as sufferers from the French Disease among others by the *DFA*, pp. 204–5, 219, 224, 240.

11. On the settlement of the Confraternity of Saint Job at Ferrara, see Archivo Archivescovile di Ferrara, Compagnia di S. Giobbe di Ferrara, A4 (20 March 1502), A5 (20 March 1505). For the peculiar medical treatment prescribed to Alfonso, see Archivio di Stato di Modena, Archivio Segretto Estense, Archivio per Materie, Medici e Medicina, 19 [letter of 29 March 1498]. On the figure of Job in the Jewish and Christian religions, see S. Terrien, 'Job', in Mircea Eliade, ed., *The Encyclopedia of Religion*, 16 vols, New York, Macmillan, 1987, vol. 8, pp. 97–100; J. R. Baskin, *Pharaoh's Counsellors. Job, Jetho, and Balaam in Rabbinic and Patristic Tradition*, Chico, Cal., Scholars Press, 1983, pp. 7–43, 129–43; C. Kannengiesser, 'Job (Le Livre de)', in M. Viller, assisted by F. Cavellera and J. de Guibert, eds, *Dictionnaire de Spiritualité Ascétique et Mystique. Doctrine et Histoire*, Paris, Béauchesne, vol. 1– (1937–), vol. 8 (1974), cols 1201–25, p. 1201; L. L. Besserman, *The Legend of Job in the Middle Ages*, Cambridge, Mass., Harvard University Press, 1979, pp. 64–5; L. Menzies, *The Saints in Italy; a Book of Reference to the Saints in Italian Art and Dedication*, London, The Medici Society Ltd, [1924], pp. 137–8.

12. During the first five years of the sixteenth century at least two medical practitioners were employed by the authorities of Ferrara as 'specialists' on the French Disease, namely Maestro Ferrante da S. Domenico in 1501 'to operate on many and diverse diseases, above all on the disease of those who have been infected through their lower parts'; and Zan Jacomo da Padoa, medico del Mal Franzoso, in 1505. See Alfonso Corradi, 'Nuovi documenti per la storia dell malattie veneree in Italia dalla fine del quattrocento alla metà del cinquecento', *Annali Universali di Medicina e Chirurgia*, 269 (808), 1884, pp. 289–386: p. 347; Giulio Bertoni, *La*

Biblioteca Estense a la Cultura Ferrarese ai Tempi del Duca Ercole I (1471–1505), Turin, E. Loescher, 1903, p. 192.

13. See R. K. French, 'The Medical Ethics of Gabriele de Zerbi', in Andrew Wear, Johanna Geyer-Kordesch and Roger French, eds, *Doctors and Ethics: the Earlier Historical Setting of Professional Ethics*, Amsterdam, Rodopi, 1993, pp. 72–97; see p. 74.
14. Whether or not the physicians' inability to cope with the disease lessened public confidence (which has been disputed) it could hardly have increased their reputation. Contemporary diaries repeatedly echoed the notion that doctors were unable to treat the disease. See, e.g., *DFA*, pp. 198–9, 204–5, 219; Luca Landucci, *Diario Fiorentino dal 1450 al 1516* ..., Iodoco del Badia, ed., Florence, Biblioteca di Carteggi, Diarii, Memorie, 1883, pp. 132, 141.
15. 'Methodical' and 'canonical' modes of practice were discussed later in the sixteenth century and so take us beyond the purposes of this chapter in discussing the arrival of the French Disease. For an extended discussion on these modes of practice see Arrizabalaga, Henderson and French, *The Great Pox, passim.*
16. For the image of the doctor, created by his learning, see French, 'Medical Ethics'.
17. On astrology, see D. Kurze, 'Popular Astrology and Prophecy in the Fifteenth and Sixteenth Centuries', in P. Zambelli, ed., '*Astrologi Hallucinati*'. *Stars and the End of the World in Luther's time*, Berlin and New York, Walter de Gruyter, 1986, pp. 178–93: p. 180. See also H. R. Hammerstein, 'The Battle of the Booklets: Prognostic Tradition and Proclamation of the Word in Early Sixteenth Century Germany', in Zambelli, *Astrologi*, pp. 129–151: pp. 129, 131. On astronomical terminology see for example J. Tester, *A History of Western Astrology*, Woodbridge, Boydell Press, 1987; W. Shumaker, *The Occult Sciences in the Renaissance*, Berkeley and London, University of California Press, 1972, pp. 1–59.
18. See P. Borgarucci, *Methodus de Morbo Gallico*, Chapter 2, in Luigi Luigini, *De Morbo Gallico Omnia Quae Extant apud Omnes Medicos Cuiuscunque Nationis*, 2 vols, Venice, Zilettus, 1566–67, vol. 2, p. 150.
19. Lorenz Friese, *De Morbo Gallico Opusculum*, in Luigini, *De Morbo Gallico*, vol. 1, p. 299.
20. See Borgarucci in Luigini, *De Morbo Gallico*.
21. Mercury was already recognized as an efficient remedy for skin disorders by Arab medical authors like Rhazes and Avicenna. See, e.g., Rhazes, *Ad Regem Mansorem*, lib. 5, cap. 28; lib. 6, cap. 15 (Basel, 1544, pp. 125, 153); Avicenna, *Canon Medicinae*, lib. 2, tract. 2, cap. 47 (*argentum vivum*), lib. 4, fen 7, tract. 3, cap. 7 and 27 (Venice, 1527, fols 77v, 386r–v, 388r) Since the twelfth century its therapeutical effectiveness in this kind of complaint had been endorsed in Latin Europe by many university-trained physicians and surgeons, among them Petrus Hispanus, Guglielmo da Varignana, Arnau de Vilanova, Bernard de Gordon, Guy de Chauliac and Valescus de Taranta. On the history of mercury and of its therapeutical applications, see Erna Lesky, 'Die Arbeiter und das Quecksilber', *Ciba Zeitschrift*, **96**, 1959, pp. 3191–200; J. Schroeter, 'Quecksilber – und Quecksilberverbindungen im Wandel der Zeit', *Ciba Zeitschrift*, **96**, 1959, pp. 3202–6; L. J. Goldwater, *Mercury: A History of Quicksilver*, Balti-

more, York Press, 1972. On the treatment of the French disease with mercurial remedies, see Jean Astruc, *De Morbis Venereis*, Paris, 1736, pp. 131–232; G. S. Brock, 'An Early Account of Syphilis and of the Use of Mercury in its Treatment', *Janus*, 6, 1901, pp. 592–5, 645–7; Owsei Temkin, 'Therapeutic Trends and the Treatment of Syphilis Before 1900', *Bulletin of the History of Medicine*, 29, 1955, pp. 309–16, p. 311; Erna Lesky, 'Von Schmier- und Räucherkuren zur modernen Syphilistherapie', *Ciba Zeitschrift*, 96, 1959, pp. 3174–89; Juan Antonio Paniagua, 'Clínica del Renacimiento', in Pedro Laín-Entralgo, ed., *Historia Universal de la Medicina*, 7 vols, Barcelona, Salvat, 1972–75, vol. 4, p. 100.

22. On the guaiac wood see Robert S. Munger, 'Guaiacum: The Holy Wood from the New World', *Journal of the History of Medicine*, 4, 1949, pp. 196–229.
23. See Arrizabalaga, Henderson and French, *The Great Pox*, p. 253.
24. See Borgarucci in Luigini, *De Morbo Gallico*, vol. 1, p. 299; Friese in Luigini, vol. 1, p. 299.
25. See Antonio Benvieni, *De Morbo Gallico Tractatus*, in Luigini, *De Morbo Gallico*, vol. 1, p. 345.
26. See Borgarucci in Luigini, *De Morbo Gallico*, vol. 2, p. 150.
27. See French, 'Medical Ethics', p. 81.
28. See Johannes Benedictus, *De Morbo Gallico Libellus*, in Luigini, *De Morbo Gallico*, vol. 1, p. 148.
29. Munger, 'Guaiacum'.
30. Nicolaus Pol, *De Cura Morbi Gallici per Lignum Guaycanum Libellus*, Venice, 1535. For a critical edition and English translation of this work, see Max H. Fish, *Nicolaus Pol Doctor 1494. With a Critical Edition of his Guaiac Tract Edited with a Translation by Dorothy M. Schullian*, New York, The Cleveland Medical Library Association, 1947, pp. 56–93.
31. Leonhard Schmaus, *Lucubratiuncula de Morbo Gallico et Cura eius Noviter Reperta cum Ligno Indico*, Augsburg, 1518.
32. Munger, 'Guaiacum', pp. 42–4.
33. Pol, *De Cura Morbi Gallici*, pp. 56–9, 62–9.
34. Pol, *De Cura Morbi Gallici*, pp. 60–61.
35. Pol, *De Cura Morbi Gallici*, pp. 74–7.
36. Pol, *De Cura Morbi Gallici*, pp. 64–75.
37. Pol, *De Cura Morbi Gallici*, pp. 80–81, 74–7.
38. Pol, *De Cura Morbi Gallici*, pp. 80–81.
39. Pol, *De Cura Morbi Gallici*, pp. 74–7.
40. On the Fuggers and the trade of guaiac, see Fish, *Nicolaus Pol*, p. 46; Munger, 'Guaiacum', pp. 209–10; Walter Pagel, *Paracelsus. An Introduction to Philosophical Medicine in the Era of the Renaissance*, Basel, Karger, 1982, p. 24.
41. Ulrich von Hutten, *De Guaiaci Medicina et Morbo Gallico Liber Unus*, Mainz, 1519, sigs. c3r, d2v, d3r, d4v, e3v, g4r. Hutten's attitude to the medical profession and other monopolies was consistent with his Reforming beliefs. See, for example, Sam Wheelis, 'Ulrich von Hutten: Representative of Patriotic Humanism', in Gerhart Hoffmeister, ed., *The Renaissance and Reformation in Germany. An Introduction*, New York, Ungar, 1977.
42. On the Leipzig Faculty see K. Sudhoff, *Die medinische Fakultät zu Leipzig im ersten Jahrhundert der Universität*, Leipzig, J. A. Barth, 1909.

Some biographical details of Pollich are given in August Hirsch, ed., *Biographisches Lexikon der hervorragenden Ärzte aller Zeiter und Völker*, 5 vols + supplement, Berlin and Vienna, Urban and Schwarzenberg, 1929–35: vol. 4 (1932), p. 648. For Pollich's first thesis, see Karl Sudhoff, *Aus der Frühgeschichte der Syphilis. Handschriften- und Inkunabelstudien epidemiologische Untersuchung und kritische Gänge*, Leipzig, J. A. Barth, 1912, pp. 43–4.

43. Nicolò Leoniceno, *Libellus de Epidemia quam Vulgo Morbum Gallicum Vocant*, Venice, 1497. A facsimile of this text is reproduced by K. Sudhoff, *The Earliest Printed Literature*, pp. 119–82. On Leoniceno see among others Domenico Vitaliani, *Della Vita e delle Opere di Niccolò Leoniceno Vicentino*, Verona, Tip. Sordomuti, 1892; Daniela Mugnai-Carrara, 'Profilo di Nicolò Leoniceno', *Interpres*, 2, 1979, 169–212; Mugnai-Carrara, *La Biblioteca di Nicolò Leoniceno. Tra Aristotele e Galeno: Cultura e Libri di un Medico Umanista*, Florence, Leo S. Olschki, 1991.
44. Simon Pistoris, *Positio de Morbo Franco*, Leipzig, 1498. On Pistoris, see Hirsch, ed, *Biographisches Lexikon*, vol. 4 (1888), p. 617.
45. These tracts were collected and published by Conrad Heinrich Fuchs, *Die ältesten Schrifsteller über die Lustseuche in Deutschland von 1495 bis 1510, nebst mehrerer Anecdotis späterer Zeit, gesammelt und mit literarhistorischen Notizen und einer kurzen Darstellung der epidemischen Syphilis in Deutschland*, Göttingen, Dieterich, 1843. The sequence of theses and publication was as follows: (i) Pollich, *Utrum ex Corrupcione Aeris Causetur Francosica, Morbus Pestilencialis et Invadens*, 1496; (ii) Pollich supports Leoniceno, perhaps by thesis; (iii) Pistoris, *Positio de Morbo Franco*, 1498; (iv) Pollich, *Defensio Leoniceniana*, 1498; (v) Pistoris, *Declaratio Defensiva cuiusdam Positionis de Malo Franco Disputatae*, 1500; (vi) Pollich, *Castigationes in Alabandicas Declarationes D. S. Pistoris*, 1500; (vii) Pistoris, *Confutatio Conflatorum circa Positionem quandam Extraneam et Puerilem de Malefranco*, 1501; (viii) Pollich, *Responsio in Superadditos Errores Simonis Pistoris*, 1501.
46. On German humanism see for example Lewis W. Spitz, *The Religious Renaissance of the German Humanists*, Cambridge, Mass., Harvard University Press, 1963, particularly pp. 17 and 113; P. Joachimsen, 'Humanism and the Growth of the German Mind', in Gerald Strauss, ed., *Pre-Reformation Germany*, New York, Harper and Row, 1972, p. 162, Morimichi Watanabe, 'Gregor Heimburg and Early Humanism in Germany', in Edward P. Mahoney, ed., *Philosophy and Humanism. Renaissance Essays in Honor of Paul Oskar Kristeller*, Leiden, Brill, 1976, pp. 406–22; James H. Overfield, *Humanism and Scholasticism in Late Medieval Germany*, Princeton, Princeton University Press, 1984. On the difference between Hellenists and humanists see Roger K. French 'Berengario da Carpi and the Use of Commentary in Anatomical Teaching', in Andrew Wear, Roger K. French and Ian M. Lonie, eds, *The Medical Renaissance of the Sixteenth Century*, Cambridge, Cambridge University Press, 1985, pp. 42–74, 296–8; Roger K. French, 'Pliny and Renaissance Medicine', in Roger K. French and Frank Greenaway, eds, *Science in the Early Roman Empire: Pliny the Elder, his Sources and Influence*, London, Croom Helm, 1986, pp. 252–81.
47. See, for instance, Paul Oskar Kristeller, *Renaissance Thought and its Sources*, New York, Columbia University Press, pp. 29–30.

48. On Leoniceno see Note 43, above.
49. For Dall'Aquila's tract, which was written about 1497/98, although not published until more than a decade later, see Sebastiano Dall'Aquila, *Interpretatio Morbi Gallici et Cura*, in Marco Gatinaria, *De Curis Egritudinum Particularium Noni Almansoris Practica Uberrima* ... , Pavia, 1509 (henceforth *Interpretatio*), fols 184r–202v. On Dall'Aquila, see Jon Arrizabalaga, 'Sebastiano dall'Aquila (*c.*1440–*c.*1510), el "mal francés" y la "disputa de Ferrara" (1497)', *Dynamis*, 14, 1994, pp. 227–47, and the bibliography there referred to.
50. Coradino Gilino wrote his *De Morbo quem Gallicum Nuncupant* in 1497, soon after the disputation. On Gilino see Giuseppe Pardi, *Titoli Dottorali conferiti dallo Studio di Ferrara nei secoli XV e XVI*, Lucca, A. Marchi, 1901 (facs. repr.: Bologna, Forni, 1970), pp. 32–3, 48–9, 66–7, 84–5, 88–91, 94–5, 104–5, 110–11, 114–15; G. Pardi, *Lo Studio di Ferrara nei secoli XV e XVI*, Ferrara, Tip. Zuffi, 1903 (facs. repr.: Bologna, Forni, 1972), pp. 142; G. Pardi, ed., *Diario Ferrarese dell'anno 1476 fino al 1504 di Bernadino Zambotti* (henceforth *DFZ*) in Muratori, ed., *Rerum Italicarum Scriptores*, Città di Castello and Bologna, N. Zanichelli, vol. 24, pt 7 (in appendix) pp. 207, 261; See also Sudhoff, *The Earliest Printed Literature*, pp. XL–XLI; Cyril C. Barnard, 'The "De morbo quem gallicum nuncupant" [1497] of Coradinus Gilinus', *Janus*, 34, 1930, pp. 97–116.
51. On the Florentine Neoplatonist circle of Marsilio Ficino, see Arnaldo della Torre, *Storia dell'Accademia Platonica di Firenze*, Florence, Tip. G. Carnesecchi e figli, 1902; James Hankins, *Plato in the Italian Renaissance*, 2 vols, Leiden, Brill, 1990; Hankins, 'The Myth of the Platonic Academy of Florence', *Renaissance Quarterly*, 44 (3), 1991, pp. 429–75.
52. On the long career of this text, see Nancy G. Siraisi, *Avicenna in Renaissance Italy: the 'Canon' and Medical Teaching in Italian Universities after 1500*, Princeton, Princeton University Press, 1987.
53. On Rodrigo de Borja before and after becoming pope Alexander VI, see Pastor, *The History of the Popes*, vol. 5 (1898), pp. 375–523, vol. 6 (1898), pp. 3–181; Lacy Collison-Morley, *The Story of the Borgias*, London, G. Routledge and Sons, 1932, pp. 12–245; Michael Mallett, *The Borgias. The Rise and Fall of a Renaissance Dynasty*, London, Paladin, 1971, esp. pp. 79–227.
54. For a useful overview of the role of papal physicians in sixteenth-century Rome, see Richard Palmer, 'Medicine at the Papal Court in the Sixteenth Century', in Vivian Nutton, ed., *Medicine at the Courts of Europe, 1500–1837*, London, Routledge, 1990, pp. 49–78.
55. On Gaspar Torrella see José María López-Piñero et al., *Diccionario Histórico de la Ciencia Moderna en España*, 2 vols, Barcelona, Península, 1983, vol. 2, pp. 356–58; Jon Arrizabalaga, 'Práctica y teoría en la medicina universitaria de finales del siglo XV: el tratamiento del mal francés en la corte papal de Alejandro VI Borgia', *Arbor*, 153 (604–5), 1996, pp. 127–160: particularly pp. 131–3, 157; and the bibliography there referred to.
56. On Pere Pintor see López-Piñero et al., *Diccionario Histórico*, vol. 2, pp. 178–9; Arrizabalaga, 'Práctica y teoría', pp. 127–60: particularly pp. 130–31, 155–7; and the bibliography there referred to.
57. On the French Disease at the papal court of Alexander VI see Hesnaut

[pseudonym of Louis Thuasne], *Le Mal Français a l'Époque de l'Expédition de Charles VIII en Italie, d'après les Documents Originaux*. París, Marpon et Flammarion, 1886, pp. 49–50; Lorenzo Gualino, 'L'infezione celtica', *Storia Medica dei Romani Pontefici*, Turin, Minerva Medica, 1934, pp. 257–331.

58. Pere Pintor, *Agregator Sentenciarum Doctorum Omnium de Preservatione Curationeque Pestilentie*, Rome, 1499, (henceforth, *Agregator*). For Guy de Chauliac's opinion in this respect ('Scientiae enim per additamenta fiunt') see his *Chirurgia Magna*, Lyons, 1585, p. 1.
59. P. Pintor, *De Morbo Foedo et Occulto his Temporibus Affligente*, Rome, 1500 (henceforth *De Morbo Foedo*), sigs a3r, a3v–4r, a7v, d7v.
60. Gaspar Torrella, *Tractatus cum Consiliis Contra Pudendagram seu Morbum Gallicum*, Rome, 1497 (henceforth *Tractatus*), sig. a4v.
61. For a detailed account of the early names of the French Disease, see Jean Astruc, *De Morbis Venereis Libri Novem*, Venice, 1748, vol. 1, pp. 4–6. Some of these are more fully documented in Ernest Wickersheimer, 'Sur la syphilis aux XVe et XVIe siècles', *Humanisme et Renaissance*, 4, 1937, pp. 157–207, particularly pp. 159–75.
62. On Pico see Eugenio Garin, *Giovanni Pico della Mirandola. Vita e Dottrina*, Florence, Le Monnier, 1937, pp. 169–93; Shumaker, *The Occult Sciences*, pp. 16–27.
63. G. Torrella, *Dialogus de Dolore cum Tractatu de Ulceribus in Pudendagra Evenire Solitis*, Rome, 1500 (henceforth *Dialogus*), sig. a5v.
64. Giovanni Pico della Mirandola *Disputationes Adversus Astrologiam Divinatricem*, ed. by Eugenio Garin, 2 vols, Florence, Vallecchi, 1946–52, vol. 1, pp. 60–63.
65. He believed that God's anger was a continuing cause of the disease: Pintor, *De Morbo Foedo*, sig. b6r. For more information Pintor directs the reader to his *Agregator*, sig. b3v.
66. Pintor, *De Morbo Foedo*, sigs av, a1v, a7v–bv.
67. Pintor, *De Morbo Foedo*, sigs dr–dv.
68. Torrella, *Tractatus*, sigs a4v–b1r, c4v–d1r, e1r, e2r; *Dialogus*, sigs a6v.
69. Pintor, *De Morbo Foedo*, sigs er–e3v.
70. Pintor, *De Morbo Foedo*, sigs e3v–e4r, fv–f1r.
71. Pintor, *De Morbo Foedo*, sigs f1v–f3v.
72. Torrella, *Tractatus*, sigs. c3v, d2r, d4r–v, e1v–e2r, e2v, f3r; *Dialogus*, sigs e2r–v.
73. Pintor, *De Morbo Foedo*, sig. e5v.
74. Pintor, *De Morbo Foedo*, sig. er.
75. On Bertomeu Martí, see Pelegrín Luis Llorens-Raga, *Episcopologio de la Diócesis de Segorbe-Castellón*, 2 vols, Madrid, CSIC, 1973, vol. 1, pp. 237–42; Johann Burchard, *Diarium sive Rerum Urbanarum Commentarii (1483–1506)*, ed. Louis Thuasne, 3 vols, Paris, E. Leroux, 1883–85; vol. 2, p. 521; C. Eubel, *Hierarchia Catholica Medii et Recentioris Aevi*, 3 vols, 2nd edn, Munich, L. Regensbergianae, 1913–23 (facs. repr.: Padua, Il Messagero di S. Antonio, 1960), vol. 2, pp. 23, 55.
76. Pintor, *De Morbo Foedo*, sigs ev–e1r.
77. Pintor, *De Morbo Foedo*, sigs e1r–v.
78. Torrella, *Dialogus*, e6r.
79. P. Trapolino, *De Morbo Gallico Tractatus*, in Luigini, *De Morbo Gallico*, vol. 2, p. 47.

80. On 11 April, the Ferrarese anonymous diary announced that the corpse of someone accused of murder and robbery who had been hanged in Ferrara was transferred 'to physicians in order to be dissected (*per fare nothomia*) with the purpose of seeing where the French pox came from, since he suffered from this disease'. See *DFA*, pp. 199–200.
81. Dall'Aquila, *Interpretatio*, ff. 186r–v.
82. See *Morbi Gallici Curandi Ratio*, Basel, 1536: the collected tracts of P. Mattioli, J. Almenar, N. Massa, N. Pol, Benedictus de Victoriis and A. Bolognini.
83. Nicolò Massa, in *Morbi Gallici Curandi Ratio*.
84. Gabriele Falloppio, *Opera Omnia*, Frankfurt, 1600, p. 682; Giovanni Pascale, *De Morbo Quodam Composito*, in Luigini, *De Morbo Gallico*, p. 192.
85. See Leonhard Schmaus, *De Morbo Gallico Tractatus*, in Luigini, *De Morbo Gallico*, vol. 1, p. 331; Antonio Scanaroli, *Disputatio Utilis de Morbo Gallico et Opinionis Nicolai Leoniceni Confirmatio contra Adversarium eandem Opinionem Oppugnantem*, Bologna, 1498 (reproduced in facsimile in Sudhoff, *The Earliest Printed Literature*, pp. 315–45): p. 320 (sig. a3v).
86. See Trapolino in Luigini, *De Morbo Gallico*, vol. 2, p. 44.
87. Trapolino in Luigini, *De Morbo Gallico*, vol. 2, p. 44.
88. On the 'whole substance' theory, see Linda Deer-Richardson, 'The Generation of Disease: Occult Causes and Diseases of the Total Substance', in Wear, French and Lonie, eds, *The Medical Renaissance*, pp. 175–94, 326–30.
89. Falloppio, *Opera Omnia*, p. 682.
90. G. Vella and Trapolino use *fomes*. See Luigini, *De Morbo Gallico*, vol. 1, p. 179, and vol. 2, p. 44.

CHAPTER TWELVE

Anatomical Rationality

Roger French

Introduction: difficulties and opportunities in writing a history of anatomy

Writing a history of anatomy is rather like writing one of infectious disease. In the latter case the historian can be tempted to see the pathogen as the ultimate reality and accordingly work out how people in the past responded to its manifestations.[1] In anatomy the human body can be seen as a similar unchanging reality against which we might measure the efforts of people in the past to describe it.

In practice such a procedure does not work very easily. In the case of disease, we can for example trace 'tuberculosis' back to 'consumption' with little trouble. But 'scrophula' and 'struma', although linked by the historical use of language to the idea in our mind of the disease, were things very different from the modern disease. Different in name, signs, symptoms and causes, these historical diseases were constructions of the people who saw them and described them.[2]

Can we write a history of anatomy in which the body is an unchanging constant, against which we can measure the success of anatomists in describing it? This chapter argues that we cannot, and that anatomy, like disease, is a construction, here that of anatomists. In this case, there can be no simple narrative history of anatomy as an attempt to describe the human body. But there are some things we can usefully say about the history of 'anatomy' conceived in broad terms. First, it is a characteristic feature of Western medicine.[3] Other large civilizations did not have medicine with this character.[4] The medicine of the chosen father of Western medicine, Hippocrates, was not based on anatomy. But from the high Middle Ages Western medicine employed on an increasing scale systematic dissection of the body for teaching and discovery, whether forensic or medical.[5] By the time Europeans began to move into large distant parts of the earth, Western medicine was firmly anatomical.

Second, anatomical knowledge gained in this way came to be extremely detailed. Since surgery was comparatively limited in its practical scope it could have no use for intimate knowledge of internal parts. At first sight the same seems true for medicine, for the physician's routine armoury of interventionist techniques in the practice of internal medicine – promoting the flow of blood and other humours, of sweat, urine, feces, vomit and so on – seems coarse in relation to the detailed knowledge of the internal parts that the anatomists were building up.

This chapter examines this notion – that is, that anatomical knowledge had more detail than was medically useful. If this were so then it could be argued that the anatomists were building their subject for their own purposes. In testing this thesis we shall look at two different styles of anatomy, the complexional and the structural–functional, and at two main scholars who used these styles, Gentile da Foligno (who taught in Perugia and died during the Black Death) and Gabriele de Zerbi (whose textbook was written in Padua and who was killed in 1504), one at either end of the period covered in this volume.[6]

Since our medicine has a strong anatomical component, we naturally see medieval and Renaissance medicine as undergoing development as it became more anatomical. At one level this idea is unexceptionable, for medicine was ultimately able to use the accumulated anatomical knowledge in a much more direct way than before. But the causes of change were contemporary and did not come from the future. There is no objective historical way of assessing if it was more effective in terms of cure because it was anatomical. Nor can we say that the wide distribution of this kind of medicine was due to its being anatomical.

Anatomy of complexion

When doctors of the Western high Middle Ages tried to reconstruct the medicine of the ancients and of the Arabs, Galen became important. There were three main reasons for this. First, Hippocrates had long been admired in the West as the father of medicine, and Galen called himself a Hippocratist, and gave a structure to Hippocrates's medical wisdom that allowed it to be built up into a system. This was useful in the teaching in the new corporate *studia* of the West. Second, part of Galen's rationalization of Hippocratic medicine was based on Aristotle's logic and natural philosophy, which were fundamental to the arts course of the new *studia* and very convenient for the teaching of medicine. Third, Galen addressed himself on some occasions to beginners, which gave the new medical teachers some suggestions about what should come first in an agreed and structured curriculum.[7]

One of Galen's important introductory books was *De Sectis*, in which he discussed the medical sects of his day, in second-century Rome. As is well known, *De Sectis* outlined the rival approaches of the rationalists, who believed that the structure and function of the body could be known and that the doctor could rationally work out how to intervene;

the empiricists, who thought the body was ultimately unknowable and that experience was a surer guide to practice than reason; and the methodists, who held that disease was a simple change within the body and that medicine could be learned quickly.

The doctors of the new *studia* sided with the rationalists. This was consistent with Aristotelian logic and natural philosophy and with the image they chose to develop of being learned and rational. This professional image meant that the old empiricists of Rome became the new empirics outside the universities. The move towards rationalism was already apparent in the commentary on *De Sectis* by John of Alexandria. This commentary is important for the story of this chapter because John identifies dissection as characteristic of the rationalists. Direct knowledge of the body seemed to be necessary if one were to argue properly about how it works, goes wrong and can be put right.

John says anatomy is the skilful cutting of the body and the revealing of what is hidden. This was influential in the West, along with the other lessons of *De Sectis* about beginners and teachers and the attractions of rationalism. It meant, first, that anatomy was not merely knowledge of structure, but also the process of dissection by which it was gained. Second, John's elaboration of 'what is hidden' gave a multiple choice for anatomists who saw the body in different ways. In what amounts to a physical *accessus*[8] to the body, John gives a list of six things to be noted as the body is dissected. The anatomist should look at each organ in turn and note its number, substance, position, size, shape and connections. Apart from the simple first category (in which for example the anatomist would note there was one liver and two kidneys) the rest are largely morphological – position, size, shape and connections. An anatomist following this simple prescription was writing a morphological anatomy. Mondino's anatomy of *c.*1316 perhaps comes closest to a morphological anatomy, but as an organizing principle for texts, John of Alexandria's six observables was very widespread in the anatomical literature.

The remaining category in John's list is *substancia*. This could be interpreted simply, in terms of texture for example, so that an organ was known to be hard or soft, or porous or dense, and so on. But it could also be interpreted as 'complexion', the balance of elementary qualities that characterized each organ. This was a view developed extensively by Gentile da Foligno in commenting on the *Canon* of Avicenna, a task he had essentially completed when he died in the Black Death.

Let us see why such a view was important and what attitude to the body it revealed, before looking in more detail at Gentile's 'complexional anatomy'. The doctrine of the four elements – earth, air, fire and water – and the pairs of qualities they shared was fundamental to the Aristotelian world-view and was shared by all who had completed a university arts course. Natural philosophy was the basis of the theory of medicine and the qualities – hot, cold, dry and wet – were basic to all areas of medicine.[9] Most of the drugs administered by the doctor and the food he prescribed in the patient's regimen had actions determined by the qualities – they had their own complexion. The airs, waters and places of the patient's environment had their effect on him qualitatively. The qualities were the very basis of the macrocosm, where the patient lived, and the microcosm, his body. Disease was most often a disturbance in the balance of qualities and most treatment was a restoration of that balance, the natural complexion. Elements, qualities and complexions are among the things that Avicenna says the doctor *must* believe. They are medical axioms in being without proof, explains Gentile: the doctor has a duty to believe in them.[10] When Gentile looked at the body anatomically he saw locations of complexions.[11]

This is almost certainly because his lifetime intellectual task was to make the *Canon* more intelligible to the Latins by expounding it and raising disputed questions to solve apparent problems. Avicenna was the great systematizer and a consistent rational thread runs through his presentation of the anatomy or 'disposition' of a part, its diseases and treatments. Although vast, the *Canon* was a valuable textbook precisely because it was so highly structured. Galen's works in contrast were 'particular': some on diseases, some on symptoms, others on philosophy, the compounding of simples, or regimen. Following Avicenna, complexion was a major rational thread for Gentile: not only was complexion fundamental in the ways mentioned above but the very function of the organs was determined by their complexion. Thus in discussing the action of nerves and muscles, a central question at a time when 'anatomy' of a part included its function, Gentile's argument is complexional. Nerves, he says, are naturally cold organs, being derived from the cold brain. Muscle, on the hand, is naturally hot, being related to blood. How does the nerve avoid being warmed by the muscle, and so lose its nature? Moreover, the spirit that acts in the nerve is also warm: this is 'incoming' rather than 'innate' heat. Gentile raises the question of whether, perhaps, the nerve was originally made extra cold, so that these warming influences in fact produced the right complexion. In general he had a doctrine of 'resistances' in which local complexions opposed each other, and it was in the resolution of such oppositions that a correct complexion was achieved and the proper function of the organ fulfilled.

A large area where Gentile thought he could refine the theoretical apparatus of medicine was that concerned with the *quantification* of qualities, so that mathematics could lend precision to the doctor's understanding of the action of medicines and the very working of the organs.[12] So strong is Gentile's complexion-rationality that where Avicenna treats anatomy on its own and not as part of a complexion-dominated system, Gentile omitted to comment on it.

That is, the meaning Gentile attaches to the term *anatomia* is distant from the physical 'skilful cutting' intended by John of Alexandria. He often says that Avicenna 'demonstrates through anatomy', but the demonstration is an argument and neither Avicenna nor Gentile has visual demonstration in mind. When Avicenna says that the brain was created cold and wet, Gentile's accompanying disputed question is 'Can anything more be learned of a part through anatomy than complexion and number?'[13] Part of his argument is that anatomy is rather limited and cannot reach the fundamentals of medicine, those things the *medicus* receives from the *physicus* without question, including the axiomatic action of the qualities. Anatomical demonstration for Gentile is simply the pointing out of something that can be rationally derived from fundamentals.

Uses of anatomy

Of what medical use was Gentile's complexional anatomy? How does it help us test the hypothesis with which we began, that anatomical knowledge was more detailed than was medically necessary? The answer seems to come in two parts. First, any amount of detailed anatomical knowledge could be used by the anatomist as a specialist. To the extent that the anatomist was a specialist, a man with his own art and independent of medicine, his knowledge was useful professionally, even politically. To this extent too, he was using his knowledge for his own, rather than for medical purposes. Second, we can see that there were many ways in which detailed anatomical knowledge could be used directly in medicine, if we look carefully at contemporary medical techniques.

Let us look at the second part of the answer first. It might seem to us that knowledge of the structure of the eye or the ventricles of the brain could hardly be of value to medieval doctors. We think this, perhaps, because we cannot see that the medieval doctor could effectively treat such parts. But to think this is to again use modern criteria to judge the past. The medieval doctor thought he could treat these parts and had confident knowledge of how to do it. His success was measured by the expectations of everyone involved. In that sense his anatomical knowledge had therapeutic importance.

Secondly, even where his anatomical knowledge did not direct his therapy, it could be used in argument. The rational doctor's image depended on his learning and the power and extent of his reasoning. In a discussion of causes of disease, for example, a doctor might want to distinguish a 'primitive' (external) cause from a predisposing or conjoint cause. These are (deliberately) technical terms within the learned apparatus, and the doctor could employ them in connection with the most detailed anatomy of the most inaccessible parts. Most would have agreed that a doctor with a knowledge of the causes of things, whether they were treatable or not, was a better doctor than one who did not.

For Gentile, 'anatomy' was also what Avicenna had written. He often says that Avicenna 'demonstrates through anatomy' where in fact Avicenna is making an argument from the axioms of complexion. Gentile too uses such arguments, and can use very detailed anatomical knowledge in doing so. As a commentator on a textual anatomy he had two separate duties: to expound Avicenna's text and to solve difficulties raised by it. The exposition follows complex rules which, however, once understood are easy to follow. The exposition was a matter of identifying and locating places in the text where Avicenna's argument took important turns. Introductory expositions at the beginning of chapters or fens recall what has gone before and reach forward some distance in the text to show how the argument will continue; each subsequent subdivision of the text is a stage closer to where the expositor is in the text and after the final one the exposition can proceed in parallel with the text.[14] Thus in the exposition as in the text the anatomy (mostly in book 3) is presented as a precondition of the discussion on action, disease, signs and treatment.[15]

However, the bulk of Gentile's commentary consists of disputed questions, *dubia*. Above all else, this was the area where Gentile used detailed knowledge that was anatomical in his sense. These questions arise when the text of the *Canon* appears to contradict what is found in other authors. They are also a contrivance for Gentile to work up special topics and a mechanism to allow him to report what is in the technical literature in his subject, medicine from theory to practice. This was a duty of a commentator, and it helps us to locate Gentile intellectually as we compare his absorption with Avicenna with his contemporaries' grappling with the 'new Galen'. Disputation was a classroom technique, exercising the students' logic and extending their knowledge of the authors. Disputation was also part of graduation and in both cases characterized the academic business of medicine. The commentator or teacher who could solve problems in the literature with the full force of academic logic was greatly admired.[16] This was a rewarding areas for the use, in argument, of even the minutest piece of anatomical information.

Let us take an example. Gentile had a special interest in the eye. As a youth he had become interested in the images of things not there which appeared in some illnesses. This led him to the *scientia* of the eye: its structure, how it worked, the faculty of receiving images, the theory of perspective and the diseases the eye was heir to. Its anatomy was well known and detailed, and the names of most of its parts had been settled: cornea, conjunctiva, retina, iris, pupil, vitreous humour, sclerotic (what we call the lens they called the crystalline humour). Conflicting theories of vision (extromission and intromission) supplied opportunity for disputation. Gentile essentially leaves Avicenna's treatment behind in a vastly inflated commentary that (he says) is in the nature of a separate tract. He protests that he is writing at the request of colleagues and he finishes with a prayer, which was his practice only at important places. He asks God to preserve his own sight so that he could go on preserving that of others: Gentile was a *medicus oculista*.

Gentile claims that the whole *scientia* of the eye had been almost neglected. He accordingly follows the systematic mode of presentation adopted by Avicenna and works through the categories of structure, action, diseases, signs and treatment. It might be thought that the eye in particular was out of the range of intervention by the medieval medical man. The couching operation for cataract had a long history by Gentile's time and we need not doubt that specialists who learned by example performed the operation at a time when Gentile was writing about it. Gentile calls such people *operantes*,[17] characterized by action rather than learning. It is clear he had not performed the operation himself and despite all his anatomical learning it was indeed out of range of his intervention.

Gentile does on other occasions enlarge on some treatments for different conditions described by Avicenna. One treatment of removing a growth over the cornea involved the use of an instrument to grind the excess flesh away with an abrasive ointment containing ground glass. This is not the least of such techniques and we are bound to ask how far such methods, undoubtedly in the literature, were actually attempted by the *oculistae* of Gentile's time. Were they reconstructed from the words of the Arabs?

However, the issue here is the use of detailed anatomical knowledge in medicine: Gentile's use of it is to settle the question of where the *imaginationes (apparitiones)* come from. Since they do not represent external reality, they originated in the eye. Since the crystalline was the organ of vision, these disturbances could not occur behind it. It was true, Gentile said, that the humours and membranes behind the crystalline could be affected by vapours from the brain, but these had the power only to weaken sight, not to generate apparitions. The disturbance therefore must lie in the humour and membranes in front of the crystalline. Gentile can use all his detailed anatomy of the eye in the discovery of causes, prompted by theory.

Detailed anatomical knowledge of the eye could be matched by elaborate theory of vision to solve medical problems. Gentile accepted that the crystalline, the seat of vision, was at the apex of a pyramid that described the passage of the visible species of things through the medium of the air and the transparent humours and membranes of the front of the eye. These species, and light, travelled in straight lines and were dealt with by the laws of perspective. The species accounted for vision independently of light, which acted only upon the medium carrying the species (some animals were held to activate the medium by light emitted from their own eyes and so could see in total darkness). It followed that some imperfection or disturbance in front of the crystalline might interfere, in what we would call a geometrical way, with the arrival of visible species and so cause apparitions. But the 'law of perspective' operated only in front of the crystalline, for behind it was the 'law of the spirit' which carried the ever less material species through the retinas of each eye, and up the hollow optic nerves to the point where they crossed: here the two sets of images met and the faculty of judgement was employed upon them.[18]

The vapour that reached the rear of the eye in *apparitiones* and other diseases came directly from the brain, and often indirectly first from the stomach. The notion that the brain would often suffer in some sympathetic way with the stomach was an old one in Greek medicine, for the stomach was the receptacle of food and poor food or poor digestion was the cause of evil vapours, which were at the root of many diseases. While Hippocrates famously said that the body was one conspiring whole, and that, therefore, vapours could move within it, yet detailed anatomical knowledge could lend refinement to the doctrine. Galen taught that the sixth pair of cranial nerves reached the mouth of the stomach to provide sensation there. For physicians of Gentile's time, the same pair of nerves also provided a route for rising vapours, and anatomical knowledge added weight and conviction to a doctor's argument about mechanisms of causation of disease.[19]

In another example, we may wonder of what medical use was a detailed knowledge of the shape of the cranial sutures to the medieval doctor. The answer is that to him the sutures were porous: they admitted medicines designed to act on the contents of the skull and they emitted vapours. In certain conditions of the brain and eye evacuation of the matter of disease was obtained by employing a cautery on the scalp, ensuring that the hot iron penetrated right through to the bone, at a suture. As Gentile said, the location of this is known *ex scientia anatomie*.[20] The coronal suture was cauterized in ophthalmia, and a twist of silk thread in the wound ensured the continuation of the evacuation.

To summarize complexional anatomy and the rationality that went with it, we can say that it was a matter of natural forces and actions, the qualitative nature of the parts, organic resistances, innate and incoming heat and related matters. It all arose from a basically Aristotelian world-view in which the actions of the qualities were local and necessary. It was developed by Gentile in a logical manner, where the logic was 'physical' in being taken to describe the natural actions of substances, rather than being merely an intellectual process. It was medically logical in accepting from natural philosophy certain unquestionable axioms, largely about qualities. When Gentile said that anatomy was the alphabet of medicine and should be learned first, he was thinking of the fundamental complexions of the parts.[21]

Gentile followed the common practice of the time and did not comment on Avicenna's separate treatment of anatomy.[22] It is here that Avicenna presents another kind of anatomy, where the fundamentals are not complexions, but the bones that give structure to the body, the muscles that move it, the nerves that guide the motion and the blood vessels that bring the nutriment, warmth, spirits and humours to the moving parts. It is not clear why this kind of anatomy was avoided in the early statutes of the universities. Gentile says it was a mistake to avoid anatomy in this way, but it is not at all clear that he meant an anatomy of morphology and motion. Perhaps it was avoided because the rationality of complexion was so fundamental to medical theory and practice, and had been so since the great impact made on Western medicine by the translation of Haly Abbas's *Pantegni*. Perhaps it was because morphological anatomy was taught separately: in conjunction with the dissection of pigs in the Salernitan 'demonstrations' and in the public anatomies of the university physicians.

Rationality of structure and function

For those concerned with assimilating the newly available Galenic texts, another kind of anatomical rationality became available, one that resembled the omitted anatomy of the *Canon*. It will be recalled that most of the 'hidden things' made knowable by anatomy in John of Alexandria's accessus to the body were morphological categories, size, shape, position and location. These were suitable for the physician who wanted to locate pain and know which organ was affected and whose knowledge included ways of evacuating most organs, however internal.

But John's accessus said nothing about function. From the authors, of course, medical men in the period between the Black Death and French Disease knew in general of the actions of the digestive organs in preparing blood from food, the production of the other humours, the action of the brain and its nerves, the operations of the faculties and spirits. The first tract of the medical textbook of the Middle Ages set out these things in skeleton form.[23] But a much more elaborate discussion was presented in Galen's most philosophical book on anatomy, *On the Use of the Parts*, commonly known in Latin as *De Utilitate Particularium* (or *De Usu Partium*). This had been translated from the Greek by Nicholas of Reggio a few years after Mondino finished his *Anatomia*.

De Utilitate Particularium was a large text and seems to have been seen as difficult. For convenience the Arabs had made a paraphrase of it, as they made paraphrases of a number of Greek medical texts later used in the West.[24] This paraphrase, which was also truncated, reached the West as *De Juvamente Membrorum* and was available much earlier than the full translation from the Greek. It remained popular and its ultimate source does not seem to have been recognized before the Hellenist scholarship of the sixteenth century.

Of the two texts only the *De Utilitate Particularium* carried the full message of Galen's kind of anatomy. Complexional anatomy depended on the necessary actions of the fundamental elementary qualities, derived from Aristotelian philosophy – we can recall that these were unassailable axioms. The rationality that went with it was ideally syllogistic, and Gentile often points out how he derives his major and minor premise: sometimes from authority, sometimes by observation, sometimes from general consent (e.g. 'the major is known') and the conclusion is designed to 'determine' a disputed question. In contrast, Galen's account of the body owes a great deal to the creative demiurge of Plato. For Galen the body has been put together *rationally* and in a sense voluntarily rather than necessarily, the demiurge making wise choices. It was possible to find in Galen's text a hierarchy of 'use' of the parts: it begins with the necessary complexional 'action' of the similar (homogenous) parts and extends up through the 'use' of the organs,[25] both serving and principal, ending with the combined purposive action of preserving the body. The rationality that goes with it is more elaborate than the syllogism. It is partly the wisdom of the demiurge, for example in choosing the best compromise available when two purposes are in view: the teeth have to be hard, but not, like the hardest substances, brittle. The rationality is also partly Aristotelian. Aristotle had argued that the identity of a thing is what it is *for*. This is its final cause, and although Aristotle is being teleological, the purpose he sees is not the rational or conscious one we may see in Plato's and Galen's demiurge.

The supremacy of the final cause meant that true knowledge of a thing was knowledge of its purpose. It mattered less what it was made from, what made it, or what shape it was; or at least, these were on their own incomplete knowledge. The final cause also made possible the best kind of demonstration. Demonstrated knowledge was certain in taking finality into account. The medievals used the term *demonstratio propter quid* for demonstrated knowledge and worried about how it stood in relation to knowledge derived from sensory observation. In anatomy it is distant from the simple syllogisms framed by Gentile.

Thus in a philosophical anatomy the morphological categories of the *accessus* of John of Alexandria are important only in that they help to explain what the purpose or function of a part is. Function in this sense is central to the other important part of Galenic anatomy, experiment. Galen had been a self-publicist of considerable ability, and the experiments in which he demonstrated his control of the nerves of respiration and voice of a living pig inspired emulation by anatomists of the Renaissance. As a device to convince, this was demonstration with a power to match that which was *propter quid*.

Professional literature

In looking at Gentilian and Galenic anatomy, we are of course not comparing like with like. A commentary on a medical textbook that contains some anatomy, full of disputed questions and designed to generate the best therapy, naturally produces a view of the body different from that of an explicitly philosophical text centring on nature's providence. The two approaches continued side by side until long after the period covered by his volume. Indeed, it is not possible to make like-for-like comparisons within 'anatomy' because no two major works were written for the same purpose or in the same format. Mondino's was short and practical, designed to help with the dissection of the body. Commentators on the *Canon*, like Dino del Garbo and Gentile, wanted anatomy to help direct practice. Another genre of anatomical writing was the textbook, serving anatomy as a specialty. We shall meet that of Gabriel de Zerbi in a moment. Berengario da Carpi's commentary on Mondino's anatomy was a major work and a specialist text (unlike Gentile's on the *Canon*). *Dubia* were appropriate for it, in a way they were not for Zerbi's textbook.

But whatever the purposes and formats of the earlier works on anatomy, the detailed anatomical knowledge they contained was taken up by the later writers, notably Zerbi and Berengario. Anatomical detail multiplied with the growth of the accumulating literature, and with the size of separate treatments: Berengario's commentary and Zerbi's textbook are huge. The problem was that the commentator had the duty of informing the reader of the opinions of the authors. These included the moderns, and for example, Gentile reports extensively on the opinions of Mondino, Taddeo Alderotti, Dino del Garbo, William of Lombardy, Gilbertus Anglicus, Bartholomeus da Varignana and others. Such a procedure cannot be sustained indefinitely. It is difficult to see how another commentary could be made on the *Canon* that took into account even the major points made by Gentile. Gentile himself noted how medical terms tended to multiply, but he was locked into a system which by its nature required the listing of different terms from the different Arabic and Latin authors, not only to identify synonyms and the physical reality to which they referred, but to make the technical literature accessible. Sometimes Gentile was surprised at the variety of names, for example, of *squinantia*, and notes the *magna multiplicitas illorum nominum*. But within the system, there was nothing to be done about it, *sed de hoc non est curandum*.[26]

Professional knowledge and foreign fields

How did Zerbi, at the beginning of the sixteenth century, handle the mass of accumulated anatomical detail? Did he use it in the ways we have identified? He was represented above as the author of a textbook (i.e. not a commentary nor an anatomy-to-therapy exposition). He was, while writing his textbook, a specialist, an anatomist. He had his followers, the *Zerbistae*.[27] In a similar way the followers of Jacobus de Partibus, an anatomist who commented on the *Canon*, were called 'Partists'. These names imply a considerable amount of medical 'faith' given to the master on the part of group. Their professional knowledge was to that extent autonomous.

We need to pause here to recapture some of the circumstances of medieval medical teaching. The *studium* was a corporation. It was in the first instances a decision of the masters to co-operate in a group rather than compete: having the group sanctioned by the authorities meant that it became a legal person. There were theoretical discussions about the right of voluntary associations as well as practical moves to construct them. Teaching masters essentially formed a guild, whose activity was teaching and whose stock-in-trade was knowledge. As in the other guilds the masters themselves decided what the method of business would be – how teaching was to be done – and what was to be taught. The authorities that recognized the group did not attempt to control the nature or content of the teaching unless it conflicted directly with their own interests (the Church would not for example have allowed the teaching of heresy).

Within the *studium* the medical faculty also had some features of an incorporation. Like the *studium*, it had statutes that defined who the great authorities in the subject were, and the faculty had its own professional stock-in-trade knowledge. The physicians' professional identity rested on these things and there were pressures to preserve rather than change them. The university doctors' claim for a monopoly of internal medicine rested on general agreement that university medicine was better than other kinds. This rested in turn on the mode of teaching and the weight of the authorities. Once the doctors had agreed on these there was little pressure from outside for change.

The medieval conventions about incorporation were matched at an intellectual level by use of Aristotle's doctrine on the relationship of the various branches of knowledge. Medicine's closest neighbour was natural philosophy; and while it was generally admitted that medicine was subordinated to philosophy, it was also commonly accepted that where the philosopher finished the physician began. In the northern universities medicine was a higher faculty than philosophy, but again it was widely accepted that the principles of natural philosophy had to be taken in to medicine as axioms that were, in medicine, indemonstrable.[28] The innumerable philosopher–physician disputes (for example on the place of origin of the blood vessels and nerves) were less medieval attempts to find the physical truth than demarcation disputes where the stock-in-trade knowledge of the two fields overlapped.

The teaching guilds also had an internal ethic. Zerbi says that the medical teacher, *docens*, should teach without fee and by example. This recalls the Hippocratic Oath, which was becoming more noticeable in Zerbi's time.[29] The teacher and his group were a sort of family, with ties of respect. One often comes across the use of the word 'faith' in these circumstances: the pupil has a duty of faith to his teacher and must believe him. Medical men as a whole and anatomists in particular should have faith in Galen, the teacher of all physicians. It was for these reasons that so many bitterly condemned Vesalius when he broke faith with Galen.[30] Zerbi was one of the few authors of the late fifteenth century to devote his time to a system of medical ethics. Here he paid a lot of attention to the behaviour of the medical student. He dwelt on the faith, honour and belief that the student must give to his teachers.[31] This was more than a set of rules to ensure efficient teaching, and it extended to the whole learned tradition of medicine, from Galen himself, to whom all faith should be given.[32]

In other words there is a strong sense in which anatomical knowledge was the professional stock-in-trade of the anatomist. This is what made him an anatomist, and as a stock-in-trade was to a degree protected from other professionals. Anatomy was not a subdivision of medicine, not a species of a genus, but a separate art. Zerbi clearly had a medical 'hat' as well as a philosophical one, and what he said depended to a large extent on which one he was wearing.

The key word is 'art', *ars*. An art could be productive – a manufacture – as well as cognitive. The bigger disciplines constructed histories for themselves (the so called *translatio studii*) to emphasize the different origins, aims, methods and dignities of their particular arts. In education the seven liberal arts were supreme before the coming of the 'three philosophies' in the new *studia generalia*. A man who professed the liberal arts was accordingly an *artista* and 'artist' became the general term for the teacher in the arts faculty. It is well known that the term 'humanist' was coined in the same way for the man who taught 'more human letters', the *litterae humaniores* of the older universities. The noun *artista* is feminine in form probably because *ars* is feminine, and as a result other words ending in *-ista* and formed in the same way are feminine in form but masculine in gender. When Gentile called Mondino a *famosus anathomista* it looks uncomfortable on the page, as if there were a confusion of gender. Likewise Gentile uses the term 'oculist' for a medical specialism, the practitioner being a *medicus oculista*. His contemporaries saw what he meant: a university-trained medical man practising his own art.

We shall see that Zerbi speaks of anatomical knowledge as that which is proper to anatomists, as if they were some incorporation holding autonomous professional knowledge; which is how the medical men talked of philosophers. Something similar can be said about medical men and theologians. Occasionally and on special occasions men like Gentile and Niccolo Falcucci addressed the God of the Christians directly. But in general all reference to divine providence, all expressions of piety, are made by quoting Arabic medical authorities. Where Zerbi talks of God as Creator, he takes it from a Jewish source, Maimonides.[33] The Church fathers, recent masters, the *Sentences* are all the stock-in-trade knowledge of the theologians, and the physicians had no desire to trespass or poach. When the Hellenist Leoniceno began to attack Pliny and Avicenna, shortly before Zerbi's anatomical textbook appeared, one of the combatants was the lawyer Collenuccio, who expressed considerable reservation about using his 'sickle in a foreign field', that is, where professional faith and knowledge were being attacked from outside.

We can see, then, that one of the circumstances of the construction of anatomical knowledge was the professional arrangement of anatomists. How far did this constructed knowledge relate to the physical body? In what ways was it medically useful? The problem is analogous to that of the philosopher–physician disputes, like those about the origin of the nerves or veins. If we dismiss these disputations on the grounds that the disputants should have looked at the body, we misunderstand the nature of the disputation. In now wearing an anatomist's hat, and now a philosopher's, a man could change his allegiances, authorities and modes of generating knowledge; but did he abandon physical truth in the process? Did not the physical body offer some restraint to this process?

I think we have to recall the analogy with disease. All the attributes of a disease slip through our fingers when we try to trace it back historically, and we are unable to use the notion of the pathogen. In a like way we cannot use our notion of the body to see its attributes in the past. When the Chinese looked at the body they saw colour, and more technically, channels for the passage of the *chi*. On an occasion when the body of a criminal was dissected, what was recorded of the event was mathematical, the dimensions, capacities and weights of the parts. Clearly the enquirers had a different way of looking at the body, for such a list of observables was not used in the West. Western medieval anatomists of course held that they were recording the physical structure of the body, but this was knowledge that was not to be generated by examination of the body itself. This knowledge pre-existed, and was to be recovered by scholarship. Opening the body provided sensory images to complement textual knowledge and to strengthen the memory. The medieval anatomist did not expect to make discoveries in the body; what he as an individual saw was a particular of observation, not a universal, the truth of which was conformable to reason. He was not an author and had no authority. For him the body was a set of signs that pointed to anatomical knowledge located elsewhere.

When we look in more detail at what Zerbi wrote we can see how it related to the topics we have met. His anatomy reflects the image the learned and rational doctor wanted to project. It indicates where the sources of anatomical knowledge lay, and how the body pointed to them. It demonstrates how anatomical knowledge was a stock-in-trade, for which an anatomical faith was proper; and how the anatomist built up his stock-in-trade for other than medical reasons. We can look at these five topics in turn.

Image

Zerbi chose to spend a year of his life writing out a vast textbook. What were his purposes? Although in writing the book he was in a sound sense an *anatomista*, he had not always specialized. He taught philosophy and medicine in Bologna until 1484[34] when he moved to Rome. He moved to Padua in 1494 as an *ordinarius* teacher, one of those who gave the principal lectures in medicine. The anatomy text appeared in 1502. Zerbi was above all a university medical man,[35] a member of a rational and learned profession and he lived and died in practice.

It is arguable that what he wrote was determined by this. Let us first look at his book of advice to young doctors, the *De Cautelis Medicorum*, written a few years before his anatomy textbook. It is a handbook teaching what to do and how to behave as a practising doctor. It does not indicate how to let blood or take the pulse but how to act in relationship to other doctors, the patient, the bystanders, the apothecaries and the fee. It is a booklet of 'ethics', but almost every rule it lays down had the effect of bolstering the image of the university doctor among the class of people who could afford his fees. The university-trained doctors now thought of themselves as a group and realized that bad behaviour on the part of one of them would tarnish the collective image. Zerbi advises against putting things in writing, lest they be used against the doctor if things go wrong. The appearance of piety and charity can be achieved by treating the poor without asking a fee. Perhaps his severest warning is not to publicly disagree with another: experts who disagree cannot be experts.[36]

The image of the university doctor was maintained by his faculty in a number of other ways. The ceremonies attending graduation proclaimed his learning and reason to all observers. The statutes that claimed the right to a monopoly of the practice of internal medicine emphasized the dignity of the licensed doctor by encouraging the denigration and prosecution of the unlicensed. The public dissection was a statement that this is what learned and rational physicians did: their medicine was based on anatomy and their rationality was anatomical. The dissection was literally a piece of theatre, housed in a special construction that allowed a large number of people to see what was happening.[37] The Paduan statutes of 1468, in operation when Zerbi arrived, use strong language in emphasizing both the public dissection and the suppression of unlicensed practice.[38]

Thus it may be that Zerbi had in mind that a large book of anatomical learning and rationality, the latter now of the Galenic structure–function kind, would not only fill a gap in the literature, but also burnish the image of the university physician, especially of Padua. Likewise when, twenty years later, Berengario da Carpi wrote his commentary on Mondino, part of his purpose was to rehabilitate his own predecessor at Bologna, where both he and Mondino had been *practici*.[39] At the very least what Zerbi wrote had to be consistent with the reputation of the university doctor as rational and learned; and he chose anatomy and Galen.[40]

At the same time Zerbi was bound to defend the *effectiveness* of his learned medicine in order to sustain the claim about the benefit to the public that accrues from learned physicians having a monopoly of practice. In consequence his *modus doctrine* emphasizes the *certainty* of knowledge gained by the use of sight and touch in learning anatomy. In describing how the hands rather than imagination or ratiocination are important Zerbi is invoking the authority of Galen. He is also invoking that of Aristotle, for what is seen are 'the singulars that are better known to us, because close to the senses'. Knowing the animal books as well,[41] Zerbi makes the connection between this methodological statement of Aristotle's and his famous justification of animal dissection.[42] In order to support the claim that the kind of medicine he was promoting was the most effective, Zerbi has to show the utility of anatomy to surgery. He does not do so with much enthusiasm. There may be a number of reasons for this. First, his primary aim was to write a work which depended on learning for its impact, and it is essentially, as he said himself, a gathering together of especially Galen's anatomy into one perfect doctrine. But like everyone else he was aware that there was a considerable gap in status between true theoretical knowledge and a practical art. Surgery was above all a practical art and Zerbi had to be careful not to debase the image that he was cultivating of a learned medicine. While it is true in Italy that surgeons could be educated along with the physicians, there is little doubt that in practice their standing was lower. When the faculty examined and licensed unqualified practitioners, the licence was surgical.[43] During the Paduan anatomies, only those reading surgery needed to go forward to the cadaver and see how the dissection was done.[44] Berengario da Carpi recalled that successful physicians despised and had long since forgotten how to perform surgery. They characteristically took along a Jewish surgeon to difficult cases to do the work and share the fee.[45]

In practice Zerbi does not discuss surgery extensively. Included in his *accessus* is the remark that surgeons, as well a philosophers and physicians, should be well exercised in the dissection of animals[46] that resemble man, as well as in the human body, of both sexes. He goes on to recommend the employment of the senses in the manual operations of dissection, but there is nothing that relates to the surgeon *qua* surgeon. Indeed among his sources, apart from those that relate to the philosopher–physician disputes, those he is most critical of are the surgeons. He saw Mondino the *practicus* of Bologna as writing a surgical anatomy, and indeed Mondino's practical instructions for the 'manual operations' of dissection are more numerous than Zerbi's.[47] Zerbi disagreed with Mondino in more than half his references to him; and the surgeon Guy de Chauliac was effectively dismissed by Zerbi as being 'barbaric'.[48]

Possibly he had met Guy's text in the vernacular, or thought his Latin coarse; his dismissal is that he is only mentioned perhaps four or five times in the entire work. He has high praise for a contemporary lithotomist,[49] records an ingenious operation to drain fistulae of the eye through the nose,[50] has remarks on perforations in the chest for drainage[51] and borrows a description from Avicenna of cautery with *ferrum ignitum*,[52] but there is no systematic argument from anatomical knowledge to surgical efficiency. There are some pieces of advice on operating on the head and a little borrowing of modern surgical names of parts of the body,[53] but it is clear that Zerbi has opted for the strategy of learning, rather than effectiveness.

Dissection as a guide to anatomical knowledge

The bulk of Zerbi's anatomical textbook is divided into sections headed *Textus* and *Additiones*. The 'text' is designed to be read in conjunction with the dissection of the body, and the 'additions' in moments in between. It was then, designed as a guide to practice, perhaps at the public anatomy which said so much about university medicine. The additions consequently contain matter that does not require a sight of the body, perhaps textual material, like the difference between old and new translations, perhaps broader discussions about the nature of anatomy and, significantly, often diseases. In a fairly direct way the physical body, handled in the *textus* according to a rote of observables, was a pointer to anatomical knowledge located elsewhere.

Within this arrangement Zerbi uses a number of devices to handle the great bulk of the technical literature. The first of these devices is that he divides up his description of the body according to the observables suggested by John, the Alexandrian commentator on Galen's *De Sectis*. Since John's day the list had become somewhat extended, and now Zerbi, in dealing with each part in turn, has nine separate headings, Substance, Complexion, Quantity, Figure, Number, Site, Connection, Function and Disease that the part is liable to. These categories structure the text (and provide the only relief in the dense text of the double column format). It is very notable that one of the newer categories is 'function', for Zerbi can now use the Galenic structure–function rationality of Galen. A principal feature of Zerbi's anatomy is that the dissection points to Galen and *De Utilitate Particularium*. Zerbi's mastery of this difficult text is apparent, and the result was to make anatomy a very different business from the complexional anatomy of Gentile. Perhaps it had taken the intervening century and a half for the Galenic text to be assimilated in the European medical tradition. Its dominance is shown by the fact that in another half century's time it was the main point of departure for the anatomical 'revolution' of the mid-sixteenth century.

The medieval anatomists also dissected, and vivisected, animals. Zerbi reports having an ape with a thin and dry body, which prevented Zerbi from 'anatomizing him before he had died'; after death, Zerbi found all the organs healthy, despite the animal's appearance in life.[54] The only peculiarity was a coarse humour in the pericardium, which Zerbi also found when he cut open a cock. He also describes how a heart cut from a living animal continues warm and pulsating for a time: no author's name is directly attached to the remark and it may be Zerbi's own.[55] The same can be said of a vivisectional division of a tongue of an animal, which reveals a mass of arteries and veins.[56] Zerbi seems to have had a special interest in the tongue as the organ by which the uniquely human faculty of speech is performed. He also knew of Galen's vivisections, and no doubt appreciated their force as demonstrations. Zerbi knew of the experiments in which Galen had exposed the heart and brain of a living animal, and demonstrated that it was the brain that controlled the motion and life of the animal, not the heart, which could be handled roughly while the animal 'cried, walked and expired'.[57] Such vivisectional experiments and Galen's arguments were central to the old problem of whether the heart or brain was the dominant organ, but they were contained in a text, Galen's *De Placitis Hippocratis et Platonis* that was not available to Zerbi, who had to depend on Maimonides's report of it.

Zerbi's language suggests that animal dissection and vivisection were routine.[58] He gives more detailed instructions for the dissection of an eye of an animal than for most parts of man 'if you wish to anatomize the eye of a dead animal'.[59] No author's names are attached to this and it reads much as though Zerbi has done the dissection.[60] Nor does Zerbi cite authorities when discussing the eyelids of birds, fish and quadrupeds, although there was material in Aristotle, Avicenna and Albertus Magnus, and Zerbi, like Pliny, made it a point of honour to name his authorities.[61]

If we can take absence of authorities as an indication that Zerbi is making some argument of his own, then he seems to have a special interest in the sense organs and brain of man. We have seen his remarks on the tongue and eyes. There is a change of tone in his writing when his description reaches the head, the third of the traditional three venters of the body. After describing the vivisection of the tongue, Zerbi goes on to its movements, anxious to show it anatomically rather than by the 'dialectics' of the [pseudo-]Galenic *De Motibus Liquidis*.[62] The problem was how people could stick out their tongues, since all muscles contract, all voluntary motion was muscular and the tongue's motion was voluntary. The number of authorities cited drops as Zerbi continues, to complete this very large section on the throat and its contents. Dealing with the tongue as a sense organ and organ of speech, discussing talking animals and telling a parrot story, Zerbi passes to the reasons why the head, as the centre of the senses, is held high: is it, with Aristotle, to temper the heat of the heart? Or with Galen, to place the senses to best advantage? This was a view elaborated by Avicenna, and a standard topic of the *Canon* commentators.[63]

The size of Zerbi's text, partly due to his extensive reporting of these authorities, has deterred historians from examining it closely. Its format – double columns of densely contracted type on a large page – well known in the schools, which were its market, has had the same effect. That the biggest anatomy text before Vesalius has been the most ignored cannot help us form a picture of medieval and Renaissance anatomy.

Zerbi declares what he believed anatomy to be by means of another device of the schools, the *accessus*. This was another formal rote of questions, developed in Alexandrian Aristotle scholarship and applied to medicine as it became a formal doctrine. The *accessus* questions were designed to help the teacher take his class through a text unknown to it. The questions related to the purpose of the author, the content and organization of the work and its relation to knowledge as a whole. As applied to the discipline of anatomy, Zerbi's *accessus* asked about the purposes of the discipline of anatomy, the use and excellence of anatomy, its name, how anatomy is taught, its relationship to other knowledge and how his book is divided up.[64]

Now, in the first of these, Zerbi describes the purpose of anatomy in terms unexceptionable to us as being to provide a knowledge of the body by dissection as far as it helps the medical man do his business, but Zerbi at once qualifies it on the authority of Galen's *De Usu Partium*, the doctrine of which, Zerbi declares, he will always follow as far as he can: Zerbi, as anatomist, had abundant *faith* in Galen. But Galen's text is thoroughly philosophical, addressed as much to the natural philosopher as to the medical man and certainly not limited to that anatomical knowledge that a doctor can use in achieving and preserving health. Zerbi consequently asserts that he will include *all* parts of the body, irrespective, that is, of both the capacity of medicine to reach them and of their ignobility. This is a good example of the anatomist building up anatomical knowledge for his own reasons, not merely medical ones.

Zerbi takes the matter a great deal further in the second point of the *accessus*, the utility of anatomy. Although by anatomy the medical man may know the use of the parts (achieving health is not mentioned) yet anatomy, says Zerbi, is more important to the philosopher, who is trying to gain a knowledge of the whole of nature. Again the explicit model is Galen's text on the use of the parts, and Zerbi is following the text where Galen speaks of the wonders of nature's construction of the body being incomparably greater than the mysteries of the religion of Samothrace and Eleusis. Galen's language indeed is generously 'natural–theological' as he invites his reader to see the hand of a creator in the created bodies of animals and man. For Zerbi of course this is a Christian message and he takes it up enthusiastically, knowing that it will be consistent with the views of his audience and that by adding Galen's name to it he will be adding authority to the philosophical and religious aspects of the anatomy and hence to the medicine that he was promoting.

Zerbi makes a related point in the sixth point of his *accessus*, the *ordo doctrine*. Here he makes it clear that as a branch of knowledge, a *scientia*, anatomy is 'subalternated' to natural philosophy. Like it, it is theoretical knowledge and does *not* immediately teach the kind or method of action. Zerbi bases his argument on the fact that knowledge of the 'naturals,[65] which include the parts of the body, was agreed to be theoretical in this sense. Clearly here anatomy was not to be admired for its direct medical and surgical practical utility. The question of whether medicine was a practical art or a theoretical *scientia* had been discussed by Zerbi's Arabic sources and was used by his predecessors when negotiating a remunerative trade into the universities, and it is easy to see why he too wanted to defend his kind of medicine as not only learned but possessed of real learning, *scientia*.

Apart from these scholastic devices that Zerbi uses to handle the literature, give structure to his work and promote his kind of anatomy and medicine, he has at the beginning of the work a proem in which he additionally pursues these objectives and gives his reasons for writing. Beginning with Aristotle's justification of the knowledge of animals for philosophical purposes and with the story of Heraclitus at the stove, inviting in his hesitant friends by saying there was something divine in everything, Zerbi is clearly announcing the philosophical worth and the divinity of anatomical knowledge. He moves directly to the harmony and beauty of the human body as a noble object of study; more than noble, it is in part celestial, for God has given us a soul. For Zerbi the Christian vehicle of immortality is also the rational soul of the ancients, and he can derive authority for his views from what the ancients had said about the intellective processes, the internal and external senses and even what Galen had said about the insane thirst for knowledge of the greatest philosophers. All this lends dignity to Zerbi's picture of anatomy and gives him an expressed reason for writing. By writing, he said, not only will he make medical men more learned – more like his own ideal – but by becoming learned they put themselves in a position where later on they can charge high fees. This is not a slip, or even an incongruity on Zerbi's part. As we shall see later, money was status and status was important for the kind of medicine and doctor that Zerbi was promoting.

Anatomical faith

His expressed reasons for writing are largely concerned with his admiration for Galen as an anatomist. The author of *De Usu Partium* was the pontifex of anatomy. There was no error in his works and he did not contradict himself. Zerbi judged other authors partly on how faithfully they interpreted Galen, and Haly Abbas scored high on that account.

A traditional problem of course was that Galen often disagreed with what Aristotle had said. While Aristotle was the *summus vir in omni scientia*, Galen was the 'most diligent observer of all things'. In other words, Zerbi says they were not engaged in the same enterprise: Aristotle's was reasoned knowledge, Galen's more sensory observation. Zerbi's effort is directed towards lessening the force of any perceived impact between differing authorities. His technique is not the resolution of the disputed points, which is what a commentator would do (and which Berengario came to do in his commentary on Mondino) but of minimizing the problem. His general principle was that anatomy had a history, and had been young in Aristotle's day.[66] So Aristotle could not be blamed for his contemporaries' ignorance, nor could he be expected to have developed anatomy single-handedly. Another principle of Zerbi's is that all of Galen's disagreements with Aristotle are best seen as additions, not contradictions. The seeds of anatomy were laid in antiquity, says Zerbi, to be cultivated by Galen. Zerbi felt some urgency to publish because the anatomists of his own time (he does not name them) had not observed these principles and had mangled the job of reconciling Aristotle and Galen.

There is another way too in which Zerbi sidestepped the problem of Galen and Aristotle. He often makes it clear in the bulk of the text that in writing the book and teaching anatomy he has, as it were, put on an anatomist's hat. It is his duty as a medical man to follow Galen;[67] he will here follow the *schola medicorum* and deny some details of what Aristotle had to say on the origin of the nerves or the veins.[68] As a medical man Zerbi says he will adhere to the doctrines of Galen in anatomy 'as to an anatomical and sensual doctrine more comformable to experience'.[69] He does not mention (as the reader feels he might well in some other book) that Aristotle, as the master of reasoned knowledge, might be considered nearer the truth.[70]

He first deals with the relationship between anatomy and natural philosophy. He argues that elements, matter and form, the very bases of school natural philosophy, although the body is composed of them, are not part of anatomy, which is only concerned with things formed out of them.[71] The heart of the matter is that the first principles of natural philosophy cannot be seen and are therefore not proper parts of a sensory exercise like anatomy. This is in complete contrast with Gentile da Foligno, for whom the first principles of natural philosophy, because they were incontrovertibly accepted from philosophy, were the firmest foundation for complexional anatomy. By the end of our period, anatomists like Berengario, Massa and Zerbi were avoiding a tight link with philosophy and emphasizing sensory observation. Prompted by the old question of whether the vena cava arises from the liver or heart, Zerbi says that according to Galen, the physicians and anatomical appearance, it is from the liver, for 'medical thought is always according to sense'.[72] Judgements made *not* according to sense are consequently not part of anatomy – which was in this way limited – and room was left for Zerbi to accept some of what Aristotle had to say on the centrality of the heart. This technique was used by Hali Ridwan in his commentary on the *Tegni* (whom Zerbi follows), an important source for later commentators who wanted to define the different but compatible roles of the philosopher and physician.[73]

Apart from the invisible principles of natural philosophy, another category of invisibles that did not fall within anatomy for Zerbi were those of function, where function had no medical significance. An example is the faculties of the brain, which Zerbi says are recognized by the medical men only in so far as they relate to health and disease. Their classification was therefore simpler than that of the natural philosophers and for example, they regarded the *sensus communis* and the *fantasia* as a single faculty. The philosophers are 'most exact' and separate them, said Zerbi.[74]

As observed above, it was not Zerbi's technique to resolve or 'determine' philosopher–physician disputes, as a commentator like Gentile or Pietro d'Abano had done, but to state the opposing opinions and fly a flag of medical convenience by agreeing with Galen. 'Galen' was only wrong where the work in question had been wrongly attributed to him, like *De Juvamento Anhelitus*, 'with which in the present work we disagree', said Zerbi. In this case 'in the present work it is wiser to agree with the learned physicians' than the pseudo-Galen or Aristotle, he concluded.[75] Where the work was truly Galenic, then Zerbi's purposes were best served by following him; but his lack of conviction is clear. On the question of the function of the liver, Zerbi chooses the Galenic view of sanguification over Aristotle's view that the liver tempered the body, notwithstanding Galen's Platonic leanings here: 'The Platonic Galen, whom we follow in this anatomy'.[76] Likewise, dealing with the function of the testes, he is wearing a medical hat for the occasion: 'According to the doctrine of the medical men and of Galen, whose doctrine we are following closely in the present work'.[77] Sometimes it is almost as if it is group loyalty that decides what Zerbi believes; 'Since we are medical men we think with Galen that the brain is the organ of these powers, against Aristotle ... '.[78] At other times Zerbi seems to distance himself from both sides and simply report the opinions of 'Galen and the medical men' and 'Aristotle and the peripatetics' without choosing between them, for example on the medical view that the brain receives spirits from the heart and the philosophical opinion that it receives its powers from the heart.[79]

Despite making anatomy an affair of the senses rather than reason, in practice he often has rational rather than sensory ways of arriving at anatomical descriptions. Indeed, Zerbi uses *rationabiliter* constantly. This draws on a tradition closer to Gentile's kind of anatomy in its dependence on logic and complexion. Thus Zerbi says the complexion of the spleen is found first by touch, that is, by comparing its complexion to that of the hand, and secondly by a syllogistic method, by rationally comparing its complexion to that of other organs, on the basis of function.[80] Function was of course part of anatomy, for as all philosophers knew, real knowledge of a thing included knowledge of what it was for. Reason was the link between form and function; Zerbi attacks those who thought it 'irrational' that the heart should have veins of its own, when it was full of blood: he says it was very rational, because the heart's function was to prepare blood for other organs, not for itself, and so had to draw its own blood, through its own veins, from elsewhere.[81] Sometimes the rationality is that of nature or the creator, and the structure of organs is said to have been made 'rationally' in view of their function, so that for example, vessels carrying watery liquids are made slender; there are 'rational' purposes for one kidney being higher than the other, of the right being more masculine than the left; of thin nerves traversing only short distances.[82] Zerbi's *nihil irrationabiliter* is Galen's 'nature does nothing in vain' and the model is of course *De Usu Partium*.[83]

Zerbi certainly has the Christian God in mind when he speaks of *Creator noster*. Very often too he speaks of organs having been 'created' rather than 'made', which implies God rather than nature. But often enough it is nature rather than God, which is a Greek philosophical position rather than a sixteenth-century Christian one. (Even when it is God rather than nature, the authority he draws upon is Arabic.)[84] Zerbi accordingly finds himself in difficulties when dealing with the passage where Galen, dealing with the appropriate length to which the eyelashes grow, mocks the idea that the 'God of Moses' is omnipotent and that the eyelashes know his purposes and worship him.[85] Here then is the Prince of Anatomists[86] displaying his paganness by attacking Christianity or Judaism, and a Christian Galenist would be hard pressed to resolve the question. So would a Jewish Galenist, and indeed Maimonides had taken issue with Galen on the point of God's omnipotence. Zerbi attempts a reconciliation of Galen and Maimonides.[87]

Zerbi's sources

Zerbi's is overwhelmingly Galenic anatomy. Galen is the pontifex and prince of anatomists, without error or contradiction, and has to be imitated. The story behind Zerbi's anatomy book is the imposition of *De Usu Partium* on fragments of anatomical knowledge derived from other sources. It is the explicit model. Zerbi cites it so often that no part of his text is free of its shadow. Zerbi is nearly as free with the early, corrupt and truncated form of the work, known as *De Juvamentis Membrorum*, but, although recognising that they are closely related, he does see that the former could supplant the latter. Galen is cited on average about ten times on every page, or approximately 2 000 time in the entire work. Most of these are references to the two anatomical texts just mentioned, and a much smaller number to Galen's book on pathological anatomy, *De Locis Affectis*, known in the Middle Ages as *De Interioribus*; to the *Natural Faculties*; to *De Voce* (which seems to reflect Zerbi's special interest in the tongue) and to the (pseudo-)Galenic *Introductorium seu Medicus*. He may have known of Galen's *Anatomical Procedures* through Maimonides's use of it.[88] Part of Zerbi's express plan was to pull together some of Galen's specialist anatomical works and he refers in the appropriate places to the texts on the anatomy of the uterus and of the eyes. He also makes use of the (spurious) *De Motibus Liquidis*, the books on semen and complexions, the *Tegni, De Methodo Medendi* (known as *De Ingenio Sanitatis*), *De Morbo et Accidenti* and Galen's commentaries on the Hippocratic *Aphorisms* and *Acute Diseases*.

He refers to other Galenic works, but he has not seen them. Galen was supposed to have written a pair of texts on the anatomy of the living and of the dead, but it was thought they had not survived. The important *De Placitis Hippocratis et Platonis* was available only – as we have seen – to Zerbi through reports of it by Maimonides. Zerbi seems not have read, or found useful, Galen's books on the motion of the muscles and on the causes of respiration. He did make use of a text known to him as *De Utilitate Anhelitus*, but he was not sure whether Galen had written it.

The picture of Zerbi's anatomy being very Galenic is reinforced by his use of Avicenna. This is his second most popular author, being cited just over half as many times as Galen. Most of the human anatomy of the *Canon* was derived from Galen and Zerbi found little discordance between the two authors. Another popular author for Zerbi (fourth in terms of frequency of citation, rather less than half the frequency of Avicenna) is the Arab, Haly Abbas, whom Zerbi found agreeable mainly on the basis of his being a faithful interpreter of Galen.

Complementary to this Galenic picture is the Aristotelian. Zerbi resorts to Aristotle less often than to Avicenna (about a third as often as to Galen). But Aristotle's anatomy was animal, that of the books on the 'history', the 'causes' and the generation of animals. These three works were regarded as one by the Arabs, and Avicenna wrote a paraphrase of them; many of Zerbi's citations of Avicenna are not to the *Canon* but to this. Zerbi also makes extensive use of the paraphrase of the same Aristotelian books by Albertus Magnus. The Aristotelian animal books were not part of school natural philosophy, which apart from the *parva naturalia* and Aristotle's book on the soul was limited to the non-living part of the natural world. But then neither was Zerbi's anatomy part of school medicine, which insisted on a literal reading of Mondino at the anatomy. Clearly the development of anatomy at Padua was something additional to the statutes.

Commentators and the generation of the embryo

In book three of the *Canon*, Avicenna, dealing with the generative organs, has a chapter on the generation of the embryo. It is part of his structure–function–malfunction sequence and is not primarily anatomical. It was, however, picked up and developed as a topic in anatomy by the university anatomists of our period. They presented it as an anatomy of the pregnant uterus. Anatomical knowledge of this kind highlights the thesis we are examining. Neither surgeons nor physicians could have any professional and practical interest in the development of the foetus, which was out of range of surgery and which could not report on the part of the body where it felt pains. As a body enclosed in another, the physicians did not have access to it for administration of medicines or for securing evacuation. The interest of the physicians in the topic was necessarily not directly medical in a practical sense. More than any kind of anatomical knowledge, this had to relate to the other reasons the physicians had for accumulating knowledge. The topic of human reproduction was of natural interest to humans; and the doctors 'medicalized' it, making it an appropriate subject for medicine, and thereby become authorities on it.

Their method of dealing with the topic, too, indicates that this was to be part of learned and rational anatomy, the kind of anatomy appropriate for university medicine and for Faculty monopoly of internal medicine. Dino del Garbo,[89] dealing with the question in the high scholastic manner, is before our period, but his son Tommaso belongs to the time after the Black Death, and having taught in Perugia, Bologna and Florence, died in 1370. He, his father, and Jacoppo da Forli, all have an elaborate formal analysis of Avicenna's text, and all break it for *lemmata* at the same points. Dino and Jacoppo use two scholastic devices in tandem, the commentary and question. The question format also provided an abundant source of materials for those who needed arguments for and against a thesis in a disputation, and almost certainly the format was adopted with this in mind. In this case the question itself was after all a traditional one, relying on the different accounts of the generation of the embryo found in Galen and Aristotle. (According to Aristotle the superior heat of the male alone was responsible for generation, supplying form while the female supplied only matter; for Galen, both sexes contributed semen, from a mixture of which the embryo developed.) So all in all these formats would be powerful in a university setting where the apparatus of textual analysis, the authorial learning of the commentary and the dialectical determinations of *dubia* would be demonstrations of the rationality and learning of the university doctor. The disputation was not only an educational device but also part of the ceremony at graduation, where the new master demonstrated his skill in the characteristic action of a master.

Zerbi's treatment of the topic also helps us form a picture of why physicians should write on generation. His discussion forms a final item in his anatomy textbook of 1502. It follows book III, but is not called book IV and was probably intended to be in some degree a separate exercise. But like the rest of the anatomy, it follows John of Alexandria's observables, and Zerbi says that the generation of the embryo and the anatomy of the pregnant uterus are the same topic.

Zerbi also says that what characterizes his *sermo* is that it is put together from the best sources.[90] He is not claiming, that is, that this exposition of those sources is better than anyone else's – which is the implicit claim of Gentile's *dubia*. In practice Zerbi is saying that he has collected together fragments of the writings of authors whose opinions can best be used to represent the learned and rational doctor of his own time. He is colonizing an area of study for professional reasons.

These professional reasons include promoting the image of the rational and learned doctor. In Zerbi's Padua the public anatomy was an arresting spectacle and carried a plain message about the anatomical basis of the medicine of university physicians. But although it demonstrated powerfully that learned and rational physicians knew about the body, it had a negative side. To most people cutting up a dead body into the smallest significant bits was perhaps as disgusting a practice as it appears to us. At all events such public dissections could not be allowed to generate the notion that the learned doctor was callous. Zerbi has to say often that a feeling humanity itself prohibits vivisection of humans.[91] It is notable that this moral sentiment, like scholastic expressions of piety, is derived from old medical sources (Galen and Haly Abbas): it is professional piety.[92]

The image of the learned and rational doctor that Zerbi wished to get across to his reader was constructed partly from sources in the technical literature. Undoubtedly they performed anatomies in Padua, but what they signified, their message about the nature of university medicine, was often taken piecemeal from the old authors. It is again professional piety when Zerbi indicates how excessively cruel it would be to vivisect a pregnant woman,[93] and more cruel still to do it systematically in order to view the stages of the development of the foetus.[94] It is a topic he has taken from his sources, and on which he repeats himself. Passages in Zerbi's text which seem to suggest direct experience of dissection may also have been selected from the authors to construct an image of experiential learning. When he says that cruelty to humans obliges the anatomist to use apes and pigs 'and other animals like a woman', he may have had practical experience in mind, for dissection of pigs had been part of medical training since Salernitan times, and we know that Zerbi possessed an ape. But his *via experimenti*, a 'way of experiment', is derived from Avicenna, and even there it is secondhand, for Avicenna talks of experimenters who have investigated pregnant goats, apes and pigs. Perhaps it is a reflection of a real anatomy when Zerbi discusses the fragility of the embryonic membrane called *biles* by Avicenna and *alancoidea* by Galen: it is readily broken at a light touch, he says.[95] It is certainly a contemporary story when Zerbi says that sometimes at birth the innermost embryonic membrane remains unbroken and still surrounds the infant, giving it the appearance of being dressed in a monkish habit: often the parents take this to be a sign, and dedicate the child to a monastery.[96] We might also suppose that a doctor of Zerbi's time had experience of aborted foetuses. Discussing the 'quantity' of the growing foetus under one of John of Alexandria's headings, Zerbi observes that its growth can be readily seen in aborted foetuses.[97] An aborted male foetus of 40 days, he explains, is so small that it may fall to the ground with the discharge of humours and be unnoticed. But if it placed in cool clear water and separated from the humours, it will be seen to be about the size of a large ant. Its parts are to be clearly seen and the eye and penis are very large in comparison to the other parts. No authorities are given for this account (although some details are confirmed from Avicenna) and it looks like fifteenth-century medical experience. But it is not. The whole story comes from Aristotle[98] and Zerbi probably acquired it from Avicenna's *De Animalibus*.[99]

Conclusion

We have seen that the detailed anatomical knowledge built up by the anatomists did have some use. It was used in a fairly direct medical way because the doctor believed he had techniques for evacuating even deep and small structures. It was used by the doctor in constructing disputed questions and refining the medical knowledge of earlier doctors, both of which were of use to the doctor in his professional and educational activities.

But it is also true that the anatomist was a specialist. While anatomical knowledge could be used by the doctor in professional ways, the anatomist could use it with greater profit. To the extent that anatomy was a separate field or specialism, the successful anatomist was one who had anatomical knowledge of a certain kind, and in a certain quantity. Scholastic medical knowledge was divided into compartments, each with its guild-like body of stock-in-trade knowledge, a conventional set of authorities and agreed boundaries. To this extent the knowledge of the anatomist was medically useless, because it was not designed for medical use. When, beyond the *terminus ad quem* of this volume, Vesalius attacked Galen, his object was to be a better morphological anatomist than Galen, not to make medicine more effective.

Notes

1. See the Introduction of Jon Arrizabalaga, John Henderson and Roger French, *The Great Pox, The French Disease in Renaissance Europe*, New Haven and London, Yale University Press, 1997.
2. For an account of scrophula, see Roger French, 'Surgery and scrophula' in C. Lawrence, ed., *Medical Theory, Surgical Practice*, London, Routledge, 1992, pp. 85–100.

3. In the most general terms it was characteristic of Western, Christian society that physical mutilation of the body was a physical, terrestrial and hence a temporary thing. In other cultures the punishment that lay behind the lopping the hands or noses of thieves and other criminals was the fear of mutilation in the afterlife, but in a world that believed in the general and miraculous resurrection of bodies that had died and decayed there was no such fear. Likewise where one's fear in this life was the fate of one's soul in the next, the condition of the body was of little concern.
4. See for example Shigehisa Kuriyama, 'Visual Knowledge in Classical Chinese Medicine', in Don Bates, ed., *Knowledge and the Scholarly Medical Traditions*, Cambridge, Cambridge University Press, 1995, pp. 205–34. Dissection was not impossible in classical Chinese medicine, but was limited to the bodies of executed criminals and was never frequent or regular. See Shizu Sakai, 'Concepts of Anatomy in Traditional Chinese and Japanese Medicine', in Teizo Ogawa, *History of Traditional Medicine. Proceedings of the 1st and 2nd International Symposia on the Comparative History of Medicine – East and West*, Osaka, Taniguchi Foundation, 1986, pp. 287–302.
5. The Church had little antagonism towards medicine, but rather more towards doctors. Christ had a traditional role as a healer, but doctors were seen as engaged in a lucrative business. Nor did the Church condemn surgery, and its dislike of clerics shedding blood had more to do with clerics being enticed into a lucrative trade. Nor did the Church condemn dissection of the body, although there was papal repugnance at the practice of boiling the flesh off the bones of dead crusaders so that the bones could be brought home for burial. The reports of the Council of Reims and the Lateran are given in J. D. Mansi, *Sacrorum Conciliorum nova et amplissima collectio*, vol. 21, Venice, 1776, cols 459 and 528. See also R. Somerville, 'Pope Innocent II and the Study of Roman Law', *Revue des Etudes Islamique*, 44 (1976), pp. 105–14.
6. Zerbi was sawn in half between two planks by the Turks. See L. R. Lind, *Prevesalian Anatomy. Biography, Translations, Documents*, Philadelphia, The American Philosophy Association, 1975, p. 141. Zerbi's book is *Liber Anathomie Corporis Humani et singulorum membrorum illius*, Venice, 1502.
7. When medicine in the West began to be incorporated and a textbook was assembled for teaching, a central text was the *Tegni* of Galen. This was a major component of the new textbook, which came to be known as the *Articella*, which almost always began with the *Isagoge* of Johannitius, regarded as an introduction to the *Tegni*. Anatomists in the period covered by this chapter often justifed their anatomy because of what Galen said about the importance of anatomy in the *Tegni*. Thus the *Anatomia Ricardi Salernitani* of the twelfth century begins *Galieno testant in Tegni quiscumque interiorum membrorum corporis humani dispositionem scire desiderat*. Closely related is the *Anatomia Magistri Nicolai*, the incipit of which is *Galienus testatur in tegni quod quicumque interiorum membrorum connitur esse desiderat eum in anatomia esse oportet diligentem*. Gloucester Cathedral MS. 18. London, British Library, Sloane 1610 also has the text.
8. See Roger French, 'A Note on the Anatomical Accessus of the Middle Ages', *Medical History*, 23 (1979), pp. 461–8.

9. These doctrines remained central to medicine down to the seventeenth century. Zerbi takes due note of them early in his textbook. Zerbi (1502) f. 5v.
10. *Avicenne medicorum Principis Canonum Liber una cum lucidissima Gentilis Fulg. Expositione, qui merito est Speculator appellatus*. Venice (heirs of Octavian Scot) 1520, ff. 10r–v. (Hereafter *Canon*.)
11. Gentile does have some anatomical and morphological rationality, for instance that of nerves and muscles when discussing the *tortura faciei*. He can refute a notion that spasm pulls organs up and paralysis down by a detailed knowledge of the muscles of the face. This knowledge is not of direct medical use, like most detailed anatomical knowledge, but he can *use it in argument*. See *Tertius Can. Avic. cum amplissima Gentilis fulg. Expositione. Demum commentaria nuper additur videlicet Jacobi de Partibus super fen vi et xiii. Item Jo. Matthei de Gradi super fen xxii quia Gentilis in eis deficit*, Venice, 1522, ff. 131v. Gentile's commentary on the third book of the *Canon* is continued in *Secunda pars Gentilis super tertio Avic cum supplementis Jacobi de Partibus Parisiensis ac Joannis Matthei de Gradi Mediolanensis ubi Gentilis vel breviter vel tacite pertransivit*, Venice, 1522.
12. *Canon* I, 14v. On quantification of qualities see the work of Michael McVaugh, for example 'The Nature and Limits of Medical Certitude at Early Fourteenth-century Montepellier', *Renaissance Medical Learning. Evolution of a Tradition*, eds Michael R. McVaugh and Nancy G. Siraisi (*Osiris*, 6, 2nd series) 1990, pp. 62–84.
13. *Canon* III, fen 1, tract 1.
14. On structure of exposition see Roger French, 'Berengario da Carpi and the use of commentary in anatomical teaching' in A. Wear, R. French and I. Lonie, eds, *The Medical Renaissance of the Sixteenth Century*, Cambridge, Cambridge University Press, 1989, pp. 42–74.
15. Discussing Avicenna's sequence of exposition Gentile says because the doctor wishes to control the diseases that are in the parts, anatomy is necessary, as in the second fen of Canon I, doctrine 3, chapter 1. (*Canon* III, 315v.)
16. It is said that when Dino del Garbo began to teach from Pietro d'Abano's *Conciliator* without revealing his source, his audience greatly increased. See Per-Gunnar Ottosson, *Scholastic Medicine and Philosophy. A Study of Commentaries on Galen's Tegni (c.1300–1450)*, Uppsala, 1982, p. 23.
17. *Canon* III, f. 184v.
18. *Canon* III, f. 225v.
19. *Canon* III, f. 165r.
20. *Canon* III, f. 167r.
21. Zerbi, (1502), 3v also saw Gentile in this light.
22. That is, on *Canon* I, fen 1, doctrine 5, summae 1–5. The anatomy was still omitted from the statutes of Bologna in 1406. See C. Malagola, *Statuti delle Universita e dei Collegi dello Studio Bolognese*, Bologna, 1888, p. 275. If post-mortems for legal purposes were indeed the first anatomies of the thirteenth century, then it seems that the doctors had persuaded the lawyers of the anatomical rationality of medicine. This would seem to be related to the natural-philosophical rationality that was used to justify medicine as a learned university discipline.
23. The medical textbook was the 'Articella', sometimes known as the *Ars*

Medicine and the *Ars Commentata*. Its first component was generally the *Isagoge* of Johannitius.

24. The first versions of Greek works like the Hippocratic *Prognostica* and *Regimen Acutorum* in the *Articella* were Arabic paraphrases. The practice was not uncommon in relation to philosophical and medical texts: the first version of Aristotle's *Meteorologica* to be taught in thirteenth-century Oxford was a translation of an Arabic paraphrase (see for example London, British Library, Royal 12 G II); for the paraphrase of Galen's *Du Usu Partium*, see Roger French, 'De Juvamentis Membrorum and the Reception of Galenic Physiological Anatomy', *Isis*, 70 (1979), pp. 96–109.
25. Galen's distinction between 'action' and 'use' can best be found in his *De Usu Partium*. See the edition by C. G. Kühn, *Medicorum Graecorum Opera quae exstant. Volumen III continens Claudii Galeni T. III*, Leipzig, 1822.
26. *Canon* III f. 267v.
27. In the same way the followers of Jacobus de Partibus (Jacques Desparts, d. 1458)) were *Partistae*. See Jacopo Berengario da Carpi, *Carpi Commentaria plus multis Additionibus super Anatomia Mundini*, Bologna 1521, f. 301r. 'Galenist' was a term used by Zerbi when defending Galen against the Aristotelians: *Albertus Aristotelicus quam id magis quam Galienista*, Zerbi (1502) 113rb. At 121vb Pietro d'Abano is said by Zerbi to be a peripatetic rather than a *Galienista*.
28. Gentile says that the indemonstrable axioms taken into medicine from philosophy are the nature of the elements, their qualities and the actions of the qualities. He bases his logic directly on the qualities, which is the underpinning of his complexional medicine. See *Canon* I, 1, f. 9v.
29. The added attention given to the Hippocratic ethical work perhaps prompted Zerbi to write his own *Opus perutile De Cautelis Medicorum*, Padua, 1495. I have used the edition included in 'Pantheleon', *Pillularium omnibus medicis quam necessariam*, n.p., 1528. The Hippocratic Oath was sometimes included in late editions of the Articella.
30. Zerbi (1502) f. 12v expresses the duty a medical man had to follow Galen. For defence of Galen as the great teacher see, e.g., Bartolommeo Eustachio, *Opuscula Anatomica*, Venice, 1563 (introductory material and the sixth 'antigramma').
31. Zerbi (1528, f. lxxi^{v}) says that the duty of the medical *docens* is to reach the art without reward and through action. If the teacher really taught without asking a fee then he perhaps expected more faith from his pupils.
32. Zerbi (1502), ff. 3v, 102r says there is no error in Galen's practical books. But it is clear that his faith in Galen is of a professional nature. At f. 26v he observes that Galen 'platonizes' when he places part of the soul in the liver: Galen 'whom we follow in this anatomy'. He depends on Galen only when writing anatomy (41r). The obedience that he feels is owed to the master, Aristotle (131vb), does not interfere with medical faith: it is not proper to believe that Galen or Avicenna (his admitted interpreter) contradict themelves (ff. 43r, 63r.) We teach, says Zerbi, that Galen must be believed (102v). 'Since we are medical men' we follow Galen (f. 116r).
33. Zerbi (1502) f. 133v. The context was the problem of how it comes about that the eyelashes are just the right length. Galen's great admiration for the Platonic, creative demiurge is great, and he mocks the God of Moses. For a Greek, omnipotence was deeply unphilosophical.

34. See V. Putti, *Berengario da Carpi saggio biografico e bibliografico seguito dalla traduzione del 'De Fracture calvae sive cranei'*, Classici Italiani della Medicina, no. 3, Bologna, 1937, p. 18; Lind (1975), p. 141.
35. As an *ordinarius* of medicine he was an important man in the studium. He is mentioned in its statutes as being freed of the necessity of voting: *Statuta almae Universitatis D. Artistarum et Medicorum Patavini Gymnasii*, Venice, 1589, f. 61v.
36. Zerbi was particularly bitter that his world of practice included some learned physicians who did, in fact, disagree in public. Since they were learned, he could not reject the kind of medicine they professed, and the law offered him no protection from their competition. His words seem to betray some resentment at being patronized by these learned doctors when they publicly contradicted him. These were the 'collegiating' doctors, almost certainly from the Paduan or Venetian College. Whereas the Paduan student *universitas* was responsible for the education of the students, the graduation of the student depended on a separate professional body, or college, of doctors. The college doctors, especially an inner circle, were influential. As practitioners they did not necessarily have the same view of medicine as the teachers in the *universitas*, and may have looked down their noses at them. If Zerbi had some new ideas about the nature and role of anatomy (and his half a million words suggests he might have had) they might well have had other ideas.
37. An 'anatomy' was a public dissection and a stark business: a newly executed criminal was stripped, washed, shaved and put on the table in front of a crowd of individuals whose business took them there. The corpse was incised with a great cross-shaped cut from ribs to pubis and from flank to flank: the flaps of the membranes were folded back, briefly discussed and the guts dealt with quickly before they began to putrefy. The theory of the thing demanded that the body be reduced to its smallest undifferentiable parts, which were at the end of the performance gathered up and given a decent Christian burial.
38. The anatomies were also part of the student's training and part of what Zerbi was doing in teaching anatomy was equipping the young doctor for a world in which he might be called on to perform a post-mortem examination, or at least to make pathological judgements on the members of an opened corpse. For example the French Disease had become a new plague some six or seven years before Zerbi finished his anatomy book and it was not uncomon for its victims to be cut open after death to try to find what part was affected. (Sometimes the doctors claimed to have found a white mucilage associated with the bones and nerves.) To be able to do this might seem like a good reason to go to anatomies as a student, but in fact in an anatomy text like Zerbi's there is no great interest in pathological appearance. Much more to the point is that dissections of the dead in civil life, outside the university, was another display of the nature of university medicine. The very expectation that post-mortem examination would reveal the cause of death is testimony to the pervasiveness of the anatomical rationality of university medicine.
39. To Berengario's eyes Mondino represented a tradition of practical, even surgical anatomy, which centred on discovering the truth about structure by the use of the senses, by judging the authors and commentators according to the same criterion, by excluding the philosophers, by settling

disputed opinions in a full scholastic way, by a humanistic historical evaluation of texts and by the use of diagrams to provide demonstration when words failed, in short, to do a number of things that were foreign to Zerbi's aims and methods.

40. Zerbi may well have been promoting the Paduan form of learned medicine. He is generally negative in his remarks on Mondino, perhaps because he regarded him as a commentator, perhaps because so much anatomical literature had been recovered since his time. Perhaps in view of this Zerbi wanted his own textbook to be adopted as statutory. Certainly he wanted Paduan anatomy to be superior to that of the statutory Bolognese author, Mondino. Whether this was because Mondino's was old-fashioned anatomy or because it was Bolognese is not clear.
41. We should also note that in addition to the medical material in the *Canon*, Avicenna had much to say on the bodies of animals in his *De Animalibus*, derived from Aristotle's three works on animals, the *Historia Animalium*, the *De Partibus Animalium* and the *De Generatione Animalium*.
42. See D. M. Balme, *Aristotle's De Partibus Animalium I and De Generatione Animalium I*, Oxford, Clarendon, 1972, p. 644b.
43. See in general Katherine Park, 'Medicine and Society in Medieval Europe, 500–1500', in Andrew Wear, ed., *Medicine and Society. Historical Essays*, Cambridge, Cambridge University Press, 1992, pp. 59–90.
44. *Statuta* (1589) f. 42v.
45. Berengario (1521) f. 58r.
46. Probably anatomists in the fifteenth and early sixteenth century often had to make do without a human body. Animals provided an alternative source for demonstration. Galen had offered advice on what kind of animals to use. They had dissected pigs in Salerno and such a practice may have been in use even outside medical circles. Alberto Pio and Berengario da Carpi, under the tutelage of Aldo Manuzio, 'had to dissect a pig' (Berengario's dedication to his *Isagoge Breves: A Short Introduction to Anatomy*, trans. L. R. Lind, Chicago, University of Chicago Press, 1959.) Zerbi discussed pigs, although his words do not betray any personal involvement with dissection (ff. 79r, 83r (the size of the mouth); f. 112v (pig's fat, from Aristotle). It is equally unlikely that he dissected the elephant he refes to: f. 82v: almost certainly his account is from Galen or Aristotle.
47. In proportion to the size of the two works.
48. Zerbi (1502) ff. 15v, 47v: *barbarus Cauliacus*; f. 20v: *cauliacus sermone barbaro*.
49. Zerbi (1502) f. 49v.
50. Zerbi (1502) f. 132r.
51. Zerbi (1502) f. 59v.
52. Zerbi (1502) f. 83v.
53. Zerbi (1502) ff. 89v. 99v, 106v, 109r; 123 (i.e. 137) rb, scliroticha as a surgical term for the outermost membrane of the eye; Zerbi derives it from the dura mater.
54. Zerbi (1502) f. 61r: *impeditus eram anathomizare priusquam moreretur* .... He later reports he found two 'heads' or 'cusps' in the heart, f. 70r.
55. Zerbi (1502) f. 62v; he continues, however, with the remark from Galen that the greater heat of the left ventricle may be felt by a finger inserted into such a heart. Perhaps the whole story is Galen's.

56. Zerbi (1502) f. 95r.
57. Zerbi (1502) f. 121v.
58. For example on ff. 8v, 22r, 58r, 120v and 122r he gives practical instructions for dissection. 18v: dividing the omentum in a living animal; 48r: he has experimental inflation of hollow organs to show their shape; 61r: dissection of the dessicated ape; 61v: elephants; 63r, 69vb: separated heart continues to beat; 70r ape anatomies; 76r *Immo procedat dissector excoriando collum ...* ; 74r inflation of lungs with bellows; 97r: big interest in the tongue; 95r: vivisection of tongue; 94v: anatomists misled by apes; 121v: vivisections and the heart/brain dispute. Also 116v and 116r: parts that cannot be seen without actual anatomical observation.
59. Zerbi (1502) f. 126 (e.e. 140)r: *Si vero mortuo animali accipiens oculum anathomizare*, says Zerbi, choose one that is rugged, and watch for the flow of a humour as soon as the cornea is cut.
60. Zerbi (1502) f. 126r.
61. Zerbi (1502) f. 120v.
62. Zerbi (1502) f. 96r; it is not clear that Zerbi thought this text was genuine.
63. Zerbi (1502) ff. 97v, 98r.
64. *Intentio doctrine, utilitas anatomie, titulus, modus doctrine, ordo doctrine, divisio operis.*
65. A 'subalternate' field of knowledge took its fundamental axions from another field, and while relying on the axioms in an unquestioned way, extended its own arguments beyond those of the other field. The 'naturals' were seven: elements, mixtures, compositions, the parts of the body, its powers, its functions and its spirit. They are thus defined at the opening of the *Isagoge*, the first work in the medieval textbook of medicine, the *Articella*. See for example the *Articella* of Venice, 1483, f. 3r.
66. For example Zerbi (1502) ff. 3v, 59v.
67. For example 67r: *Galienus autem quem imitandum duximus.* 68v: ... *doctrinam Galieni quem imitamur ...* .
68. Zerbi (1502) f. 17v: Aristotle is far from the medical men and truth; 22v: it is *maturius* to follow the medical men in this work.
69. Zerbi (1502) f. 65r: Anatomy is needed *sensualiter* to understand heart valves; 69v: the perceptibly beating heart is important to medical men; 128r, 129r: often the *rete mirabile* is not apparent to the sight while anatomizing.
70. See also Zerbi (1502) ff. 70v, 73v.
71. Zerbi (1502) f. 5v: *Neque est anathomici negocii partes humani corporis primas considerare materiam videlicit primam et ultimam formam, sed propinquiores integrantes partes et membra: ut etiam elementa inquantum huius excludamus ab hac consideratione ...* .
72. Zerbi (1502) f. 30v: *Consideratio enim medicinalis semper est secundum sensum.*
73. See Roger French, 'Gentile da Foligno and the via medicorum', in J. D. North and J. J. Roche, *The Light of Nature*, Dordrecht, Nijhoff, 1985.
74. Zerbi (1502) f. 116v; he takes it from Haly Abbas. 117v: the order of perception in the brain is a business outside the boundaries of anatomy; 117r: in relation to mental powers the doctors distinguish only what is relevant to the art of curing and preserving health.
75. Zerbi (1502) f. 22v.

76. Zerbi (1502) 26v: *concoquendique gratia adest, Galienus quoque platonicus existens quem sequeremur in hac anathomia.*
77. Zerbi (1502) f. 41r: *Verum secundum doctrinam medicorum et Galieni: cuius doctrine maxime imninitimur [sic] in hoc opere.* Compare f. 59v: *Medici autem et Galieni praesertim quos imitamur in presenti* ... (on the diaphragm, unknown to Aristotle) and f. 62v: *Nos vero Galienum volumus in hoc imitari* ... (on whether there are nerves in the heart).
78. Zerbi (1502) f. 116r: *Nos tamen ut medici opinamur cum Galieno 2 tegni cerebrum harum virtutum esse organum: contra Aristotelem ibidem: licet a Galieno quem imitamur non satis distincte habeamus quis ventriculorum cerebri sit harum virtutum sedes*: ' ... even though we do not have a distinct enough idea from Galen of which of the ventricles of the brain is the seat of these powers ... '.
79. Zerbi (1502) f. 77r. Another example is 77v.
80. Zerbi (1502) f. 22v.
81. Zerbi (1502) f. 30v.
82. Zerbi (1502) ff. 30v, 32r, 36r, 40r, 44v, 69v.
83. Zerbi (1502) f. 71v.
84. His source is Avicenna: Zerbi (1502) ff. 48r–v.
85. Zerbi (1502) ff. 133r–v. Zerbi's discussion about the creator comes from Maimonides, not Western theology.
86. Zerbi (1502) ff. 92v, 100v, 121r.
87. Zerbi (1502) f. 133r.
88. Zerbi (1502) f. 70r.
89. Dino del Garbo, who commented on parts of the *Canon* and who died in 1327 must not be confused with Dino Dini, who flourished just after the plague, was the third in a line of veterinary surgeons, on whose business he published a treatise in 1359.
90. He seems to have put it together rather hastily, for there are a number of repetitions.
91. Zerbi (1502) f. 1r: *Et licet hec scrutari in vivis saltem in specie humana ipsa humanitas prohibeat.*
92. It would of course, says Zerbi, be doubly cruel to vivisect a pregnant woman, because it would claim two lives. Merely to discuss and deny the possibility of human vivisection was to keep the topic, derived from the story about Herophilus and Erasistratus, alive.
93. Zerbi (1502) f. 1r.
94. ... *nam crudele et inhumane fuisset multas mulieres pregnantes aperuisse ferro ut id videretur corrumpendo germen et necando matrem*: Zerbi (1502) ff. 9vb–10ra.
95. Zerbi (1502) f. 8r.
96. Zerbi (1502) f. 9r.
97. Zerbi (1502) f. 13r: *quod in aborsibus facilius est videre.*
98. *Historia Animalium*, 583b.
99. In only one particular does Zerbi's account differ from that of Aristotle, for he says the ant-like foetus responds to a prod from a sharp point with a motion of contraction and expansion, 'which shows that it is animated'. Zerbi (1502) f. 14v.

Index